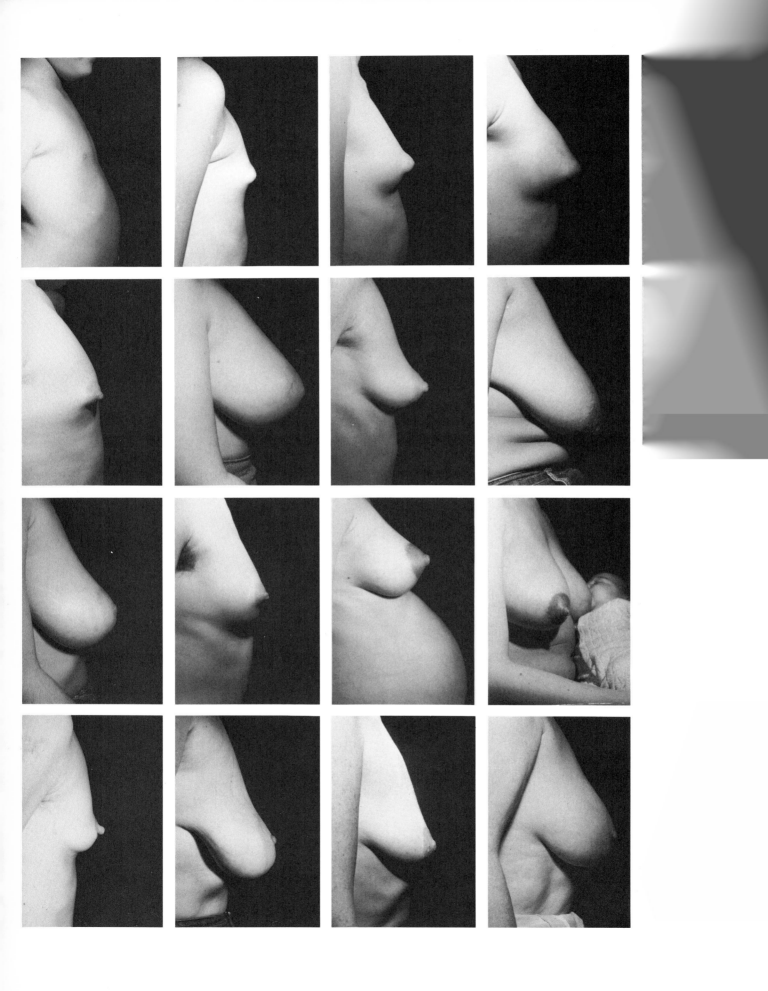

BREASTS

Women Speak About Their Breasts and Their Lives

Daphna Ayalah and Isaac J. Weinstock

SUMMIT BOOKS   NEW YORK

The authors gratefully acknowledge permission to reprint the following:

Excerpts abridged from pages 79, 146, 83–84, 79–80 in *Male and Female* by Margaret Mead. Copyright 1949 by Margaret Mead. By permission of William Morrow & Company.

Marshall McLuhan for material from his introduction to *Subliminal Seduction* by Wilson Brian Key. Copyright McLuhan Associates Limited, 1972.

Excerpt abridged from page 161 in *Going Too Far* by Robin Morgan. Copyright 1977 by Robin Morgan. By Permission of Random House, Inc.

Excerpts abridged from the article "I'll Cry Tomorrow but I'll Strip Tonight," by Victoria Hodgetts. Reprinted by permission of *The Village Voice*. Copyright © The Village Voice, Inc. 1976.

"Dear Abby" © 1978 by the Chicago-Tribune–New York News Syndicate, Inc.

Excerpts from the article "My Life in a 36DD Bra, or, The All-American Obsession," by Eve Babitz. Copyright Ms. Magazine, Corp., 1976. Reprinted with permission.

"VP aide nude in Hamptons" and "Baring it" reprinted by permission of the *New York Post*. © 1977, New York Post Corporation.

"Topless Bathing Sunk," courtesy the Associated Press.

"Mother's Milk Ideal for Growing Brain," reproduced from *The Times*, London, by permission.

"Mother Sues Over Ban on Her Breastfeeding," © 1978 by the New York Times Company. Reprinted by permission.

Sufi Inayat Khan quote reprinted with permission from *Education: From Birth to Maturity* by Sufi Inayat Khan. © 1962 International Headquarters of the Sufi Movement, Geneva, Switzerland. (Published by Sufi Publishing Company.)

How to Talk Dirty and Influence People by Lenny Bruce, through the courtesy of the Estate of Lenny Bruce, Kitty Bruce, administratrix.

"Whose Liability." Copyright Ms. Magazine Corp., 1977. Reprinted with permission.

Excerpts from pages 12, 13, *Our Bodies, Ourselves*, by the Boston Women's Health Book Collective (Simon & Schuster, Inc., rev. ed., 1976).

Copyright © 1978 by "Majority Report," all rights reserved.

To our parents, Lea and Eddy Kaplansky, Elsa and Manny Weinstock

Copyright © 1979 by Daphna Ayalah and Isaac J. Weinstock
All rights reserved
including the right of reproduction
in whole or in part in any form
Published by Summit Books
A Simon & Schuster Division of Gulf & Western Corporation
Simon & Schuster Building
1230 Avenue of the Americas
New York, New York 10020

Designed by Elizabeth Woll
Manufactured in the United States of America

1   2   3   4   5   6   7   8   9   10

Library of Congress Cataloging in Publication Data

Ayalah, Daphna.
    Breasts : women speak about their breasts and their lives.

    1. Women—Psychology.   2. Breast.   3. Body image.
4. Women—Attitudes.   5. Self-perception—Case studies.
I. Weinstock, Isaac J., joint author.   II.   Title.
HQ1206.A9   301.41'2   79-4533

ISBN   0-671-40021-5
       0-671-40095-9 Pbk.

Acknowledgments

We wish to thank Arthur Cohen, Elaine Lustig Cohen, Dorothy Crouch, Betty Dodson, Betty Harris, Gary Kennedy and the Nova Scotia College of Art, Ziva Kwitney, Lucy Lippard and Charles Neighbors for their support and enthusiasm in the early stages of the book; the late Margaret Mead for finding time in her busy schedule to meet with and encourage us; Bob Forrest, Stuart Kleiner, Marguerite Livingston, Regina Rollin, Robin Schuman, Steven Weinstock, Ron Wyenn and Sue Wyenn for their creative input and feedback; and our beloved friends and family for being there when we needed them.

We are also grateful to Lynn Nesbit, our agent, for lending her professional stature to the project; Jim Silberman, our publisher, for sharing our vision; and especially Christine Steinmetz, our devoted editor, for her extraordinary effort in helping us realize that vision.

Most of all, we are indebted to the hundreds of women who courageously contributed to this book in words and pictures. Thank you!

Contents

tomy at age thirty-nine. "The *worst* thing that can happen to a woman is to lose a breast!"

Note: The names of the women interviewed for this book have been changed to protect their anonymity.

"I Have Breasts, Therefore I Am!"

The tale of how this book came to be—the process by which it evolved—is its perfect introduction. The idea actually came to us one day while we were shopping and taking care of errands. The evening before, a friend who worked in advertising had said in passing, "The revolutionaries of the world would reach a far greater audience if they wrote their manifestos on women's breasts. The first law of advertising is *Tits Sell!*" All through the next day, this "Law" of the world of commerce lingered in our minds.

It was not really a revelation to us. We had long been conscious of the way that images of women's bodies pervade our visual environment. They are everywhere— at newsstands, at checkout counters of grocery stores, in drugstores, in countless ads in every magazine, and even on television. In effect, it is the female body that is being sold—the product is secondary. As artists involved in visual media, we also knew about the incredible power of cultural imagery to shape the individual's ideals, behavior, and perception of reality.

But on that day as we went about our daily routine, we were very aware that it is particularly the image of women's breasts, either partially or completely exposed, that is *everywhere.* The entire environment is "titillated" by images of breasts.

We are confronted everywhere with pictures of partially dressed seductive women . . . The solution for the peculiar difficulties of a puritan society does not lie in a series of pin-up girls whose breasts, tailored for love, are explicitly not meant for the loving nourishment of their children.

—Margaret Mead

We also realized that these images served up to the public in the media are *unreal*—they are airbrushed, photo-retouched fantasies, the idealized illusions of photo technology. And we wondered what the effect of such an exclusive diet of unreal images was on people, particularly women. We assumed that it was probably harmful, but how and to what extent we could not imagine.

Later that day at a newsstand, we were struck by the irony that although women's breasts are displayed everywhere in the media, images of *real* breasts, as they actually are in all stages of a woman's life, are almost never seen. Since there is such a strong cultural taboo about women exposing their breasts in the everyday environment, we rarely see "the real thing," and the breasts we do see in the media are of women of a very restricted age range. So, it became clear to us that the unreal media images of young, "new-bile" breasts have become *the breast* in our cultural consciousness.

Advertising is an environmental striptease for a world of abundance. But environments as such have a way of being inaccessible to inspection. Environments by reason of their total character are mostly subliminal to ordinary experience.

—Marshall McLuhan

●

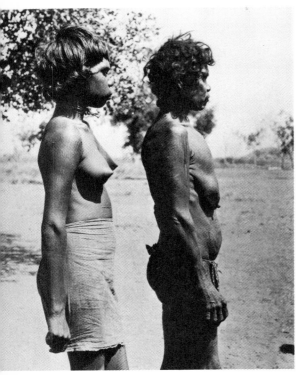

Aborigine women

Walls separate us from each other at most of the important moments of our lives . . . clothes separate us from our own bodies as well as from the bodies of others. The more society . . . muffles the human body in clothes . . . camouflages pregnancy . . . and hides breastfeeding, the more individual and bizarre will be the child's attempts to understand, to piece together a very imperfect knowledge of the life-cycle of the two sexes and an understanding of the particular state of maturity of his or her own body.

[The child needs] assurance that there is a continuous series of steps between [her] small body and that of an adult . . . [and] needs to be one of a series of girls, up through the nubile girl with budding breasts to the mature young woman, and finally to the just pregnant, the fully pregnant, and the post-parturient and suckling mother. . . . In those primitive societies in which the body is hardly covered at all and most of the major bodily changes are present to the child's eye . . . the full pageant of human development from early childhood to full maturity is visible.

—Margaret Mead

The book was born that day in the spring of International Women's Year. Buoyed up by the new spirit of the women's movement and wishing to create art that would have social as well as aesthetic relevance, we were inspired to collaborate on a project that would incorporate both elements.

We wanted to produce a photographic catalog of the breasts of women of *all* ages, without makeup or special lighting effects, unretouched, and without bias toward the preconceived cultural ideal of "beautiful breasts." Our intention was simply to compile a book with pictures of hundreds of women's breasts in all their variety of shape and size and age, arranged in chronological order, from puberty to old age. The photographs would thus create a life cycle through which one could witness, perhaps for the first time in our ultraclothed culture, the growth and change of breasts throughout women's lives.

In addition to serving as an antidote — rare visual imagery — to the standard media images, we hoped that such a collection of pictures would help nurture in women an acceptance of their own breasts and an appreciation of the uniqueness and dignity of their individual bodies.

Women are a colonized people . . . Our bodies have been taken from us, mined for their natural resources (sex and children), and deliberately mystified . . . We must begin, as women, to reclaim our land, and the most concrete place to begin is with our own flesh.

—Robin Morgan

Consciousness raising — the collective efforts of women revealing themselves to one another and thereby replacing stereotypes and myths with reality — is one of the foundations upon which the women's movement was built. As our vision of the catalog crystallized we became intrigued by the idea of celebrating the women's movement, specifically the process of consciousness raising, through the metaphors of "breast baring" and "making a clean breast of it."

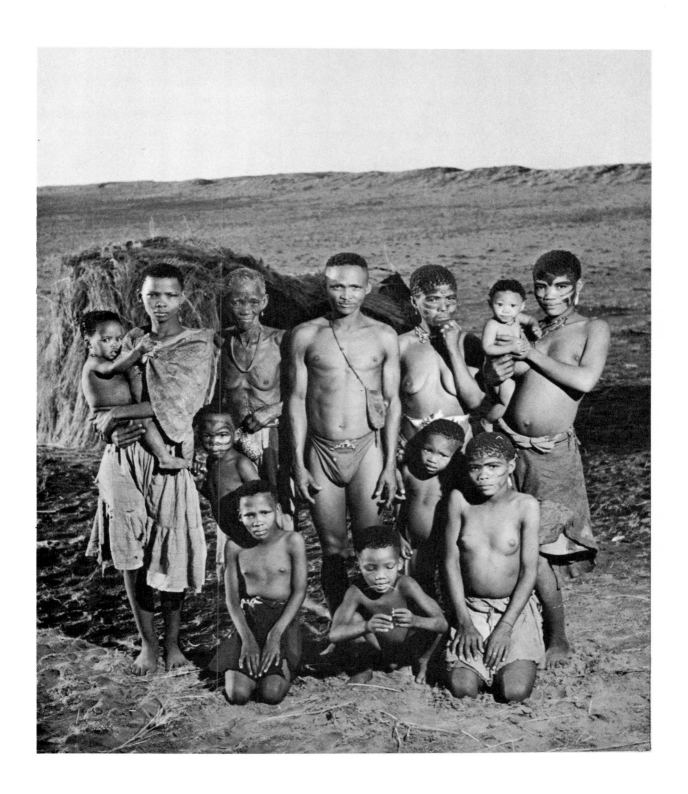

In the first flush of our enthusiasm, the task of photographing women's breasts seemed simple enough. As a woman, Daphna would contact potential subjects and do the actual photography. We didn't think we would have trouble finding subjects. After all, there were friends, and friends of friends. There was the local college and even women's groups where women who would be supportive of the project could be found.

To our amazement, many women said flatly, "No!" Some were even horrified! Others gave some very "reasonable" rationalizations. One woman in her mid-fifties explained, "At my age, I feel that I no longer have to do things that make me uncomfortable." We hadn't anticipated such reactions—not from all these "liberated" women.

We soon realized that gathering the photographs would be harder than we expected . . . a troublesome thought. Yet at the same time, women's resistance and even refusal to be photographed was a direct acknowledgment and expression of the need for such a catalog. So we dug in psychologically and prepared ourselves for the difficult job ahead.

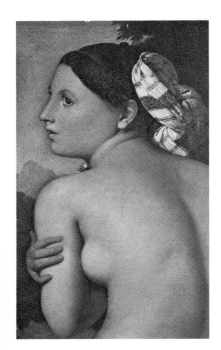

Often those women who agreed to be photographed had great difficulty actually going through with it—"It wasn't as easy as I thought it would be. . . ." Intellectually, they saw nothing wrong with the project, but deep-rooted self-consciousness and embarrassment about their breasts were something over which their intellect had no control. The simple act of exposing one's breasts in front of another woman for a moment or two, though it was for a "good cause," often provoked tremendous anxiety.

In fact, many *apologized* for not having "nice breasts"! In an effort to be helpful, they said things like, "My neighbor has beautiful breasts—real beauties! Why don't you photograph hers instead?" No matter how many times they were told about the purpose of the pictures—that we didn't need "beautiful" breasts but just their "average" breasts—most women remained self-conscious throughout.

There were some who sat hunched with their arms crossed over their breasts, only disentangling themselves when the camera was focused and Daphna's eyes were well-hidden behind it, ready to shoot. One woman kept her bra on until the very last second. Then, as soon as the camera clicked, she yanked the bra back on and *ran* to "make some coffee." There were many similar reactions, all of them very poignant and saddening. Some women described their feelings in these ways:

• *When you were photographing me I thought about the ickies that I have—the little pimples and stretch marks. I hoped they wouldn't show up and waste your film.*

• *The only person who ever sees my breasts is my husband, so it feels weird to have a perfect stranger see them . . . even though it's for a book.*

• *I felt a little self-conscious about sitting there without anything on top. If anyone had walked in, I would have run for the hills!*

• *I usually am more embarrassed exposing my breasts to a woman than a man. I wonder if she's comparing her's to mine and whether she thinks I have terrible-looking breasts. With men I don't feel that way. So I couldn't help but think that you would be judging me.*

• *When you first asked me if you could photograph my breasts, I felt that you might not want to when you met me because I don't have big breasts. Then I thought, "Jesus Christ, I'm just telling myself the same thing that gets shoved down my throat by men all the time! If I think that way, what can I expect from men?" Just to see that in myself, to realize that was a part of my reaction, amazed me.*

• *While you were photographing me I tried to control myself because I was* shaking! (Laughs.) *I'm more self-conscious about my breasts than any other part of my body, so zeroing in on them like this was devastating! It's the thing I feel most vulnerable about. To have my breasts photographed, when they are so different from anything you might see in* Playboy . . . (sighs) . . . *is a very uncomfortable situation.*

• *My breasts have always been long and pendulous. They're just not as nice as the breasts of those more perfect creatures with the pink titties which are so lovely to certain kinds of men. I wouldn't mind at all looking like a* Playboy *bunny. Who wouldn't? I wish I hadn't jumped rope so much as a teenager! (Laughs.) Even at my age [forty-five] I still have an inferiority complex about my breasts.*

The tremendous anxiety and self-consciousness that women exhibited while being photographed, another factor we hadn't anticipated, confirmed our notion that women were negatively affected by the ever-present media images of "ideal" breasts.

Of course, the women's reactions varied, and some thought as little of taking off their shirts and exposing their breasts as they would of removing overcoats or gloves. Some women were intrigued by the idea that their breasts were being photographed and would ultimately be published for the world to see. "I like the idea that these stretched-out breasts that would certainly be rejected by any magazine or beauty contest are actually going to appear in print!"

For a few, being photographed was a consciously political act, a reaction to the taboo against exposing their breasts that they believed was oppressive to women. For some others, it was an opportunity to outrage and shock the Establishment, like the prank of "mooning" (dropping your pants and displaying your ass in public), only in this case it was breasts being exposed.

And there were even a few more exhibitionist reactions. "When you said you wanted to photograph my breasts, I fantasized that you would take 'dirty' pictures of me! I don't know why, but I got really excited by the idea of exposing myself the way they do in the magazines. To be honest, when you didn't want me to pose, but to just *sit* there, well, I was disappointed."

Photographer Janet Beller was visiting friends, and after a pleasant hour of snapping their garden and dog, she was ready to go. "Just give me a parting shot," said Janet. "My friend got this twinkle in her eye, and before her boyfriend could even turn around . . . flash!" Janet is not sure what it means but she says it was the fifth time it happened to her in the last year.

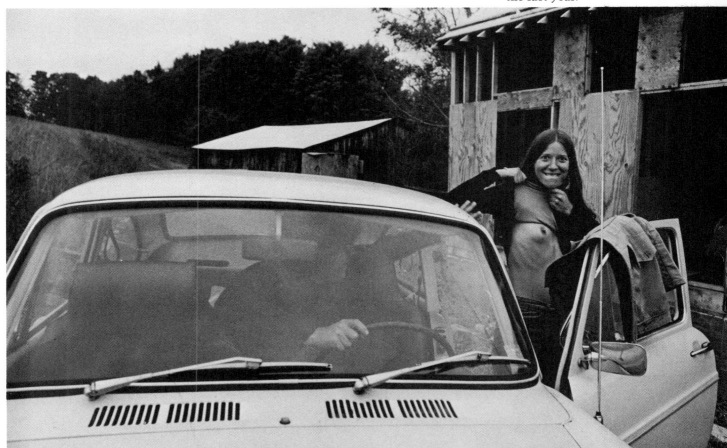

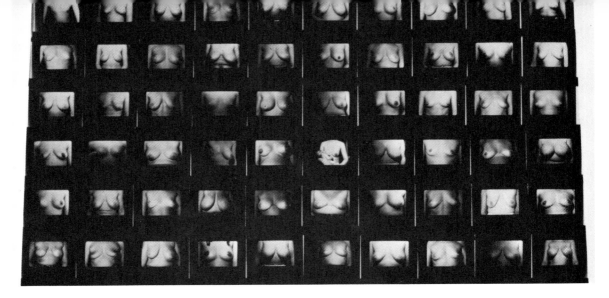

As our collection of pictures grew, they were shown as encouragement to women who were reluctant to be photographed. In this case a picture was often worth a thousand words. Indeed, women found the photographs to be very reassuring because of their concern about anonymity. Even though women were told again and again that the photographs were completely anonymous, actually seeing that faces were not included frequently elicited a sigh of relief!

The reactions women had upon seeing how other women's breasts actually looked were very interesting. Initially, they were often a bit squeamish — the women's breasts were not "pretty." As one woman said, "There is such a contradiction in society between the images of breasts projected at us and the reality of what they look like, that I always feel surprised — a flickering sensation — on seeing anybody's breasts in real life, or even looking at my own in comparison to the media images. There's been a tremendous proliferation of girlie magazines, and in some of the cheaper ones where they can't afford to airbrush and make the breasts look absolutely perfect, in spite of myself I find that the breasts look grotesque. I can't quite get used to the fact that women really *don't have* ideal breasts!"

Often women expressed curiosity or disbelief at how women with such unattractive, "unsexy" breasts had the courage to reveal them for the camera. But as a result of looking at the photographs, they were usually reassured or even inspired by the evidence that other women's breasts were no more "beautiful" than their own. Underneath it all, this was a big concern, so seeing the pictures was often the deciding factor in a woman's personal dilemma about whether or not to be photographed. Usually she would reluctantly agree: "Okay. If *they* can, I guess I can."

After being photographed, relaxed now that the ordeal was behind them, many women wanted to look at the pictures again so they could study them. "Look at *that* one," they'd say, intrigued by a particular photograph. "How *small* she is . . . tsk, tsk!" or "God, she's *huge!* Did she have silicone or something?" Surprisingly, some women had never seen a nursing mother's breasts before and they commented on the "abnormal" nipple color or size.

On seeing the photograph of someone who had a mastectomy, one woman confessed, "I was once asked by a woman I know if I wanted to see her mastectomy, and I just couldn't. It was painful because she really *needed* to show it to me, if you know what I mean. But I was too frightened. Now that I've seen it, it's not as bad as I imagined."

Another, captivated by the withered breasts of an eighty-year-old woman said, "I have never really taken a good look at an elderly woman's breasts or body, and I certainly never had the opportunity to see anything like *this.*"

A very common reaction to the photographs involved guessing the ages of the women whose breasts they were shown. "How old is this one?" women would ask, seeing a photograph of pendulous breasts. "She looks like she's in her fifties." They were *amazed* that the woman was actually in her early twenties and often commiserated, "Poor dear." Then they might study the photograph of a particularly upright pair of breasts and hesitatingly ask, "In her twenties, isn't she?" When told that the woman with "twenty-year-old" breasts was actually fifty-one, they were incredulous: "It's unbelievable!"

The one observation that most women made during their brief exposure to the photographs was about the variety of breasts. "I always thought breasts looked pretty much the same. How amazingly different they all are. They seem to have different characters—like individual faces." "How different they are from what you see in the magazines." One woman remarked, "They all look like moonscapes!" They also wondered out loud about how the women *felt* about their large, small, unusually shaped, or whatever, breasts—"How does she feel about being lopsided like that?"

We were very excited by the women's reactions to the photographs. Each woman got a sneak preview of the catalog-in-progress and the responses it provoked were very encouraging.

●

We felt that in order to demonstrate the astounding variety of breasts and thus have its full impact, the catalog should have hundreds of pictures. And having largely solved the problem of persuading women to have their breasts photographed by showing them pictures already taken, we were confident that we could accomplish the task.

Our plan required scheduling several photographic sessions a day and spending as little time as possible with each woman. But something unexpected happened. During the sessions the women, almost without exception, began impulsively to talk about themselves, at first making offhanded remarks—a self-conscious commentary on their breasts:

• *My breasts are one of my best features, but if I could wave my wand and change them, maybe I would make them just a little bigger.*

• *One of my breasts is larger than the other and it's obvious and disturbing to me. I wish the bigger one was smaller. In fact, I've often wished both my breasts were smaller.*

• *Men have told me that I'm not well-endowed on top and that the hair around my nipples is "disgusting." But I happen to think my breasts are beautiful!*

• *I'm one of those women who won't share a dressing room when the big department stores have their sales. I think my breasts are* disgusting!

• *A man once said that I had the second nicest pair he'd ever come in contact with. He didn't tell me who the first was! It really made me feel good.*

• *My breasts are sort of average . . .* hah! *That's a cop-out. I don't really think they're great to look at. I wish they were firmer and not pendulous because that's a no-no in our culture.*

• *My breasts are smaller than my ass in relation to my body. I don't think my body is well-proportioned. To be perfect, either my breasts should be larger or my ass smaller. So I think about my breasts in terms of my* ass!

More often than not, these remarks were the trigger for a flood of associations—memories from the past and anecdotes from the present. Obviously provoked by the opportunity to talk about something they usually didn't speak of, many women initiated lengthy and intimate conversations . . . or were they rather acts of unburdening?

This was interesting, but it took up precious time—scheduling had to be cut back. Our first reaction to these "interruptions" was, we admit, *annoyance*. We hoped that they would turn out to be the exception rather than the rule. Yet, to our growing dismay, the women persisted. Whether it was intimacies or just plain breast-lore, the women talked!

We resisted acknowledging it at first, but as we discussed these revelations we finally had to admit that they were indeed fascinating:

• *I always sit around my apartment without my shirt on in the summer because I don't have air conditioning. Just the other day the phone rang and before I ran to answer it, I grabbed my shirt to put it on, without even thinking about it. I just couldn't believe it!*

• *I used to work for a bus company and we had to wear clingy polyester uniforms. One day I went to work without a bra and I was the talk of the whole office. My boss called me in at noontime and said, "When you go home for lunch I want you to put on a bra or a full slip. Your nipples are showing and that's not the way to dress for business." I was furious!*

• *I once had a roommate who had three nipples! The third one was off center and looked like a mole, but if you looked closely it was in fact a nipple. She said it didn't have sensitivity, but she knew it was a nipple because it had a tiny aureole and a doctor had told her when she was very young that it was a "supernumerary nipple." It used to really bother her. We went to the beach once and she had makeup over it because it wasn't concealed by the bathing suit. After all, it was a nipple!*

• *Once at a bus stop a man wanted me to show him my breasts. He said he had a gun, but of course it turned out to be the old finger-in-the-pocket trick. Well, I wouldn't do it. I would have shown him my breasts if I thought he was going to shoot, but it was in the middle of the afternoon and thousands of people were around. So then he clawed my breasts and left. It was just awful! I started screaming at him, but everyone looked at me like I was crazy because they didn't see it happen. I felt like an idiot!*

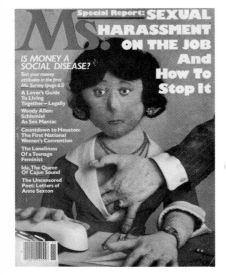

• *I worked in an employment agency and, honest to God, some companies call up and ask for "someone with big knockers." It really happens even now! Often women with bigger breasts get preference in secretarial jobs—receptionists, for instance. I know for a fact that female bank tellers are sometimes hired because of their "vital statistics." The presence of a well-endowed woman supposedly eases the flow of financial transactions. You'll be inclined to worry less about the payments you're making on that bank loan or mortgage.*

If you're small-breasted and your competition for a job is a woman who's got "big tits," many men will hire her even though she may have the brain of a peanut. I know I've missed out on jobs because my breasts are "too small"!

• *With my large breasts I've never had trouble getting a job. The trouble begins once I have the job. Always . . . Always! Flirting, leering, comments, and even jokes, you name it! I worked with one man for three years and every time he saw me his eyes fell directly on my breasts and never once rose throughout the conversation. I'm certain that if someone asked him to describe my face, he couldn't have done it!*

• *On my wedding night, when my husband saw my breasts for the first time, he exclaimed, "They're incredible!" as if my breasts were completely detachable. He didn't say I'm incredible. I often wished that I could cut my boobs off painlessly and hand them to him on a silver platter with a sarcastic remark like, "If they do so much for you, here they are!"*

As I've gotten older, I realize that to many men all that matters is boobs, but I don't think it's entirely their fault. I think it's because our breasts are covered up and people usually crave the things that are hidden from them.

• My breasts never used to be an erogenous zone. In the last few years, though, whenever my boyfriend sucks or licks my breasts, I get a very strange sensation. It's hard to explain, but there is a word in German, Weltschmerz, which translated literally means "world sadness." That sort of describes what I experience. Enormous feelings of wistful, lost sadness and sexual longing flow over me, but I don't know why. Any intense stimulation of my nipples immediately triggers that sensation — it's like pushing a button. It can only be described as wanting to laugh, cry, scream, shout, eat, and be fucked all at the same time.

• As a seventy-five-year-old woman, I've had a lot of experience in life. I've come to the conclusion that women get breast cancer because men handle their breasts too much!

• When I read books or am engrossed in thought, I often find myself holding my breasts or stroking them. I think this is comparable to a man stroking his beard while he thinks. It relaxes me and helps me concentrate, but I only do it when I'm alone.

• I can't stand the word "tits!" It drives me crazy, and I think it's because my breasts are so small and pointy, like tits on a dog. When I think of "breasts," I see them as full and nicely shaped, and since mine are little and pointy they are just "tits," because "tits" is a short and kind of pointy word.

• My friends and I have gotten into using a new expression — "Get your tits together." For example, if we plan on going to the movies but are still all sitting around, we'll say, "Well, let's get our tits together." It sounded strange to me the first time I heard it, but among women I thought it was neat, so I picked it up.

• When my dog had a litter I had an unusual experience. The puppies crawled all over me and one of them started to nurse on my breast. It was incredible! I don't know what happened but it put me on another level — it made me experience the strong feeling of what it might be like to nurse a child.

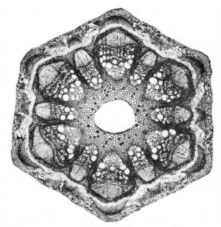

Microscopic cross section of a twig

• Mystically, I feel that breasts give off a special energy. I always think of the breast as a cosmic spiritual symbol because it is the shape of the circle, the mandala, the Great Round, which symbolizes the Feminine. The breast is not only one circle, but it is a circle within a circle within a circle . . . and that's very significant.

Concentric circles are often used as a symbol of infinity or time, like the solar system, the rings inside a tree, or an embryo inside the womb inside the woman. So to me, breasts symbolize innate power, the essence of a woman and her ability to give out. She holds the mysteries of the universe within her breasts.

• Sometimes I've had the experience of hearing a voice inside my head and it only happens when I have my hands on my breasts. It feels almost sacrilegious to speak about it now, but I think God lives in my breasts.

• There's something I've always wondered about and I've never discussed it with anyone because I was afraid they'd think I was crazy. As a child I was forced into a mother role of being responsible for my brothers and sisters. I just wonder if I didn't possibly develop my large breasts out of that role. Maybe there's some connection.

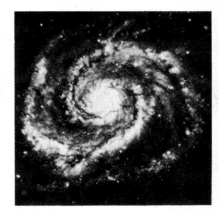

Whirlpool galaxy

What did this spontaneous unburdening, this act of "getting it off my chest" mean? It seemed as if the physical act of baring one's breasts for the photograph, the intimacy of that gesture in a culture where it is taboo, actually provoked a corresponding reflex in women to bare their intimate feelings about their breasts . . . and inevitably about themselves.

Then it dawned on us that our initial inspiration—to celebrate the women's movement through the visual metaphor of "breast baring"—was no longer just a metaphor, and that we could no longer ignore the significance of what the women were saying. So we decided to revise the concept of the photographic catalog to incorporate the feelings and experiences that the women were revealing. The revised catalog would still consist of the photographic life-cycle we were compiling, but it would also include a variety of interesting statements by the women about their breasts. We drafted a few questions to guide the conversations informally and began to record each session on tape.

When we listened to the tapes for the first time, we realized that what the women said was as important as the photographs of their breasts and that quoted material from their personal testimonies could be enormously beneficial to the women who would see and read the book.

We were determined to gather as much of this material as we could and, ironically, what began as an "obstacle" to our plan became the major focus of our efforts for several years. In this organic way, the seed of our initial idea continued to change and evolve throughout the process of compiling the book.

As more and more women spoke of their experiences, our list of questions grew until, quite unintentionally, we had developed a questionnaire and the informal conversations had turned into actual interviews.

Often during the interviews women suggested areas they were curious about and questions about breasts they wanted other women to answer. Many of these issues and questions never would have occurred to us:

• *I'd like to find out about women's experiences when their breasts first began to develop, because when I went through it I couldn't really talk about it. I was just too self-conscious and shy.*

• *I'd like to know whether or not most women are generally stimulated sexually through their breasts, and whether they seek sexual satisfaction by touching their own breasts.*

• *I think you should interview somebody who can, honest-to-God, without faking it, have an orgasm just by having her breasts touched or kissed or whatever! I wonder, is there more sexual feeling in breasts if they are larger?*

• *Well, I always wondered what it's like to have large breasts. I have a friend who has them and I'd like to ask her how it feels, but it's not the kind of conversation women can usually get into.*

• *I wonder about people who have little breasts—how they felt growing up when everybody was supposed to look like Raquel Welch or Marilyn Monroe.*

• *I would be interested to know how a Playboy bunny feels about her breasts. I went to the opening of a Playboy Club and I was amazed at how the girls' breasts were pushed up in such an incredibly artificial way—they were practically spilling over! It must be uncomfortable, but I wonder if it also has some unhealthy emotional effect.*

• *I'd like to know what it's like to be a topless dancer and how women who've done it feel about it.*

• *I'm curious about women who have had implants or surgery on their breasts.*

• *I'm thinking of having a baby and I'd be curious to hear what changes other women's breasts went through during pregnancy and how they felt about the changes. I'd also like to know what it feels like to nurse a baby and how you get your breasts back together again afterward.*

• *Faced with the choice of using their breasts to nurse a child or not, I'd like to know if other women's breasts were as tied up with their vanity as mine were.*

• *The one thing that terrifies me is breast cancer and that is probably why I don't get checkups. I wonder if most women feel as threatened by it as I do.*

• *I'm curious about women who have had a breast removed — how they tried to overcome it and, if they're married, how their husbands and children are taking it. How does a woman relate to herself sexually and how does a man relate to a woman in sex after a mastectomy? I would love to learn more about that.*

• *I wonder if there are many women like myself who would like to go topless at beaches.*

• *I have a friend who never exposes herself if she's changing in front of me. I'm sure she doesn't even let her husband feel her breasts! I'm really curious what gives women such hang ups about their breasts. Is it normal?*

• *I'm particularly curious if other women feel as insecure and embarrassed about themselves because of their breasts as I do. Why can't we grow old gracefully without feeling self-revulsion and trying to look like eighteen-year-olds? Why do we all want our breasts to remain at shoulder level? Why are we all so nuts about them?*

• *I'd like to know what happens to women's breasts when you reach menopause.*

• *How do older women feel about their breasts? I wonder if they can stand looking at their breasts in the mirror when they're saggy and wrinkled.*

Sometimes an unusual experience described in the course of an interview would shed light on a new aspect of women's experiences with their breasts, so we incorporated pertinent questions in future interviews. Thus, directly and indirectly, the women created the questionnaire *themselves!* It was almost as if they were interviewing each other, asking and answering their own questions, and as though we were simply the medium through which this dialogue took place.

Although we were gratified that in setting up the agenda of their concerns the women were deepening the spirit of the book, we began to feel overwhelmed by the immense territory they wanted documented. The modest photo book we'd envisioned was evolving into a breast *encyclopedia* — The Whole Breast Catalog! Since we are artists, not writers or researchers, we almost balked at the magnitude of the task before us. How could we find all the women who'd had the experiences that other women wanted to know about?

What saved us was the women themselves. Time and time again they suggested women they knew who "had to be" interviewed — a neighbor who was breast-feeding her baby, an acquaintance who had been a topless dancer or a model for *Playboy*, a friend who had a mastectomy and might be willing to share her experience, an outspoken grandmother . . .

In so many ways, it seemed that the book's evolution was a natural outgrowth of each woman's enthusiasm for the subject. Many offered to make preliminary telephone calls to friends and acquaintances to tell them about the book — about being interviewed and photographed.

On a few occasions women who heard about the book through the grapevine contacted us on their own initiative, some with very specific experiences they wanted to share and others just out of interest or curiosity. As one said, "When I heard about your project I was immediately fascinated by it. I'm interested in all kinds of women's issues, and as a dance therapist I'm also very involved with the body and how we relate to it. So naturally I wanted to be a part of what you were doing."

Women continually nurtured and sustained the book, their collective efforts making the impossible possible.

To our amazement and good fortune, surprisingly few of the women who were approached refused to be interviewed. In fact, some women felt "honored" that they'd been asked to participate, or that somehow it had even been "fated." One woman said, "I'm just the person to talk to. After what I've been through I could write a book. I can tell you *all* you need to know about breasts!"

But there were also women who were not as enthusiastic — who felt the entire idea was ludicrous or boring, inconsequential to them personally or irrelevant compared to other women's issues. There were even a few who thought that the subject wasn't radical enough — that breasts were passé and that most women had long ago left behind in consciousness raising whatever hang-ups they had about their breasts. And then there was the eighty-five-year-old woman, plagued by a nagging thought following her interview, who declared, "This isn't for women's liberation, is it? I'm *against* women's liberation, you know!"

Some women initially felt negative toward the project because their upbringing had taught them that the subject of breasts was "taboo," "risqué," or "dirty." In most cases, this point of view was quickly overcome with explanation. The most extreme reaction came from one woman who actually hung up the telephone upon hearing the word "breasts," before she was told what the book was all about!

Another woman confessed during her interview, "The only obscene phone call I ever got was from a guy who was into a whole breast number. So, when you asked me about being interviewed for a book on breasts, I couldn't figure out whether it was serious or not, and I didn't want to get involved in some sort of sleazy and perverted thing. But then, after giving it some thought, I realized that I was being paranoid and ridiculous, so I decided to relax and trust you."

When asked for an interview, a woman who had modeled for a bra manufacturer twenty-five years ago reacted in a very ambivalent and apprehensive way although reassured that the interview would be anonymous. After several days of consideration, she finally decided that she wanted to "go through with it," but at the last minute her husband got wind of it and actually *forbade* her!

Many of the women interviewed would have explained her husband's reaction in terms of the proprietary feeling a man may have toward his wife's body. As one woman put it, "Many women have been hurt by men *because* of their breasts — men who have just owned them and taken them away from a woman's body. They suck them and touch them and don't want them to be shown to anyone else. There are too many women I know whose breasts belong to their men and not to themselves!"

Though husbands were sometimes nervous and belittled the book — "What the hell do you have to say about your tits?" — most men did not interfere. One remarked after his wife emerged from a two-hour interview behind closed doors, "I know women like to talk a lot but *really* . . . !"

Another man, more positively predisposed, said, "Well, what did you talk about? Give me one question." His wife responded, "I can't — you wouldn't believe it anyway. Just wait for the book to come out." Then he asked, "Do you think I'll be able to pick your breasts out?" And she replied, "You should be able to — you look at them a lot more than I do!"

On one unusual occasion a woman's husband was present during her interview. Upon hearing her admit that she was unhappy with her breasts, he remarked, "I love my wife and respect her, but it dismays me that she has this idea that her breasts are ugly. I love her breasts because they're *hers* and it saddens me that despite this very positive reinforcement from me she still feels so badly. It makes me feel as though society has *poisoned* her."

There was a typical response from some women who reluctantly agreed to be interviewed because the value of the book for *other* women appealed to them, but who felt that personally they had nothing of interest to contribute — "My breasts are just *there*. I really don't give them much thought. I'll probably give you a very boring interview."

But time and time again, the questions asked during the interview revealed buried memories and feelings, and these women would often find themselves talking for hours:

• *I had no idea how this interview would go, or what I was going to say, because I had never consciously thought about my breasts. But the more questions I was asked, the more I began to think about all these things for the first time. I must say it was very positive and enlightening to really* think *in a systematic way about something so deeply personal.*

• *At first, my attitude about the interview was, "Gee, I don't know if I'm going to have anything to say." Once I agreed to do it, the prospect of answering personal questions made me self-conscious. But I'm glad I did it. I never had any kind of intelligent discussion about developing breasts and growing up with my mother, so it was really good to go back and review that crucial part of my life. It's made me think of things that I haven't thought about for years.*

Talking about their breasts was easy enough for most of the women, but for some the interview evoked strong emotional responses. They experienced moments of nervousness or outright embarrassment and even pain:

• *Frankly, I was reluctant to answer some of the questions and at times I was really embarrassed, especially when you asked what I like having done to my breasts sexually. But I have been as honest with you as I can be. There were moments when I was very uncomfortable and I apologize for that because I was really trying my best.*

• *On the whole the interview felt okay — the only part that freaked me out a little was the question on breast cancer. I hate having to think about it.*

• *I've told you things that I wouldn't tell anybody! Things that wouldn't ever come up in a conversation. I'm sure it would have been much harder if there were other women here. On the other hand, in a group I might have been reminded of things that I'd forgotten or chose to forget. But for me it's easier talking about this one to one.*

• *I was so nervous that I was even chain-smoking for the first twenty minutes! I thought I wanted to talk about my breasts, but when you got here I wasn't sure I really* did. *I still feel guilty about having had the breast operation, so I was afraid of your rejection in a way — that you would pass judgment on me and think that it was a* horrible *thing to do. And I was worried you'd think I'm nuts for having so much anxiety about it. You know, it's the feeling that I'm the* only one *who's gone through a horrible experience with my breasts!*

And a great many women felt that the interview had been a consciousness-raising experience:

• *While I was talking, I heard myself saying so many negative things about my breasts that I sort of resolved to try not to hate them anymore.* (Laughs.) *And you know, somehow I do feel less negative about them just from hearing myself say all that out loud. I said a lot of things I'd never even heard myself* think! *So the interview has been therapeutic for me . . . even cathartic.*

• *I felt good about the interview. Watching my reactions to some of the questions has really raised my consciousness. It's made me think about a lot of things besides* my breasts, *so I actually discovered some things about myself that I didn't know before.*

The realization that the actual process of being interviewed had been "therapeutic" and "consciousness-raising" for many women inspired and encouraged us throughout the extremely arduous and time-consuming task of transcribing, studying, and editing the tapes. It was another confirmation of what we now *knew*—women wanted the book to happen, wanted to be a part of it, and wanted to overcome the taboos and begin a dialogue. "I really like the fact that together with other women I am helping all women learn about themselves. I feel good about myself when I talk about all this. *Really!* How often do we get a chance to talk about our breasts?"

●

While putting the book together, we examined en masse all the material we had gathered. The cumulative insight gained from so many women discussing their lifelong experiences with their breasts in detail made us aware of a recurring pattern of cause and effect within each woman's story. A woman's current feelings about her breasts were often linked to or a result of particular attitudes and experiences—both positive and negative—she encountered in her life from earliest childhood, through puberty and adolescence, on into adulthood.

As each woman traced her life through the focus of her breasts, without realizing it she usually uncovered the hidden patterns of causality leading to her present feelings. Occasionally the women themselves recognized and commented upon the way that their breasts have influenced their lives:

• *I recently told a friend that I thought smaller breasts would look very elegant. He said to me that he didn't think I'd be who I am if I had small breasts, and when I thought about that, I agreed.*

• *After my divorce I went to a therapist and, to my surprise, the first thing he said to me was, "For starters, how do you feel about being small-breasted?" I couldn't believe it!*

• *I was not breast-fed and I wonder if my entire relationship to sex would have turned out differently if I had been.*

• *I went topless until I was ten or eleven, and one day long before I began to develop, putting on a shirt became a rule. I really resented that. It was just another example of the privilege boys had. Whenever being a girl was called to my attention, I hated it! At thirteen, when I finally reached what was my mature breast development—I'm flat-chested!—I was very satisfied that it wasn't worse. I've often thought I controlled the way my breasts developed by my attitude.*

• *I was ashamed of my breasts so I went around bent over since puberty—that's how I faced the world. I carried that around with me for years!*

• *I had some very ugly, traumatic sexual experiences with my breasts as a teenager—pinned to the back seat of a car, et cetera—and so my breasts have never been a turn-on. Maybe it's a rationalization, but I always thought it was because of those negative experiences.*

• *I've had trauma my whole life since the development of my breasts. When I was younger I felt that everybody prejudged my whole character because they were big. They'd say, "Oh, you're going to have ten children and spend your life taking care of them and changing diapers. You'll never have a career." Breasts can be like a prison!*

• *Breasts were used by my peers as a sign of being more or less of a woman, of being mature. So my being flat meant I was inferior and it was used to ostracize me. I found myself on the fringe, not really knowing how to make friends. I was forced to turn inward. My prime concern became my work and my thoughts.*

• *My heavy breasts made me inhibited and shy and physically restrained. And it carried over into other parts of my life not directly related to my breasts—I put a lot of emphasis on intellectuality, spirituality, philosophy, and other nonphysical interests.*

• Having large breasts helped me think of myself as a sex symbol. Everyone else did! That attitude certainly didn't encourage me to do anything with myself intellectually. I never thought about having a career.

• My breasts have caused me to have an angry, hard attitude toward men. I had something they wanted, the shitheads, but I learned that men weren't really sensitive to me! I felt like, "Okay, you schmucks—you like tits? I've got tits! I know that's all you want!" That tough, cynical attitude is a result of the defensive feelings I had about my breasts which turned into paranoia, and has greatly affected the way I relate to myself and to the world.

• It just occurred to me that all the men I've known well became involved with me because of my breasts.

• Sometimes I feel as though I've been having to adjust to my breasts all my life!

• I've often wondered if my breasts were different, whether my life would have turned out differently.

In one interview after another, as we observed the numerous and varied instances of causality which linked a woman's breasts to her personality or life-style, we were amazed at how basic and profoundly fundamental the experience of having breasts actually was in women's lives. Some women seemed to have a sense of this themselves:

• How women are has a great deal to do with how their breasts are—our breasts are so involved with who we are. My breasts have always been a real point of my identity.

• My breasts are kind of perky—they make me feel impudent, shameless. There is a famous Greek play called Lysistrata *based on a true event in ancient Greek history. The women were fed up with their men going off to war so they organized a sexual boycott. Their slogan was something like, "Make love, not war!"*

There's a funny scene where the women use their sexual charms—their breasts— as weapons to excite the men so that they'll do anything for sex, even make peace. The leader of the protest has her shoulders drawn back so her pointy nipples are thrust out proudly.

That is an image I have of my own breasts, and of myself, too, I guess—impudent and sassy!

• My breasts are the focal point of my existence and for the way I feel—good or bad—about my body. If anything terrible were to happen to me, I feel that it would happen to my breasts.

• When I'm not being receptive and open, my breasts lose their sensitivity and ability to respond in sex. In that way, they help me be more in tune with my sexuality and even more in tune with my world in general.

• My breasts are the region where I am bothered, physically and mentally, in every way! This has been my big inferiority complex for as long as I have lived. I hate my breasts and I hate myself!

• My breasts are a very important part of my self-image. They were something I always fixed on to feel confident about myself. More than any other part of me, my breasts gave me assurance and sensuality—they gave me power!

• While I was breast-feeding I felt closely linked to the billions of women before me who had nursed their babies. I felt as if it was one of the things that truly made me a woman.

• What scared me before the mastectomy was that somehow I thought I would

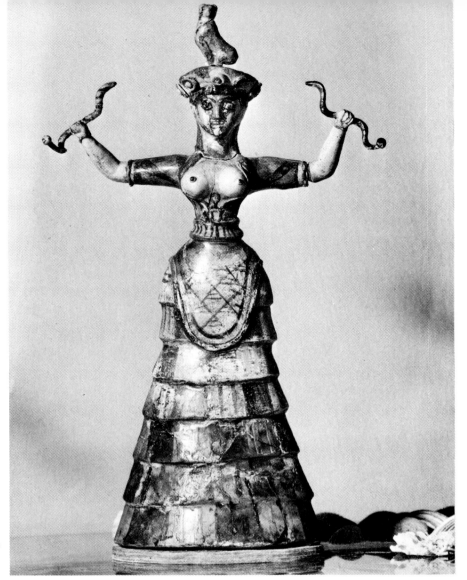

Earth Goddess; ancient Crete, where the uncovering of the breast was a sacred act.

be changed and that my relationships with people would change. That something would be taken away—like the breast—everywhere in my personality!

• Recently, I read about an ancient Minoan culture that worshiped the Mother Goddess and where women were the high priestesses. They lived on the island of Crete around 3000 B.C. Carved in one of their temples was a statement that proclaimed, "I have breasts, therefore I am!" It struck me, so I thought about it for a while and, you know, I think there's something to it.

Now we realized that our book was not only about women's breasts, but also about women's lives today and the timeless experience of being a woman. As one of the women interviewed put it, "In my mind, the subject of anything is the subject of everything. I can't talk about my breasts without talking about being a woman."

●

When we first decided to incorporate women's feelings and experiences into the photographic life cycle, we thought we would intersperse interesting quotes—fragments from the interviews—throughout the book to answer the basic query, "How do the women whose breasts appear in the pictures feel about their breasts?"

Yet, as our understanding evolved, it became evident that this format was no longer appropriate. In addition to answering that one question, we also wanted to provide all the evidence that demonstrated that how a woman feels about her breasts is a result of her unique life experience. So once again we felt compelled to revise the structure of the book. It's final form is now based on the photographic life cycle and a selection of complete personal stories from a limited number of women, rather than a more fragmented documentation of the feelings and experiences of the over two hundred women who were interviewed.

So many women had something of interest to contribute that it wasn't easy to decide which of their stories should be included. We tried to select those which provided the widest possible spectrum of experiences, attitudes, and feelings. In some instances the uniqueness of a woman's particular experience, and in others a woman's ability to express her involvement with her breasts articulately, were the deciding factors in our selection. Some of the stories selected may seem extreme or even exotic. For each woman in the book, however, we did encounter many others who described similar feelings and experiences, the difference being in degree.

Whether a woman has an orgasm through sexual stimulation of her breasts, or if her sexually insensitive breasts make her feel "abnormal"; whether she is obsessed with dressing to reveal her cleavage, or with dressing to cover and even disguise the existence of her breasts; whether she feels that her breasts give her womanly "power," or whether the small size of her breasts causes her actually to question her gender; whether she hates her breasts so much that she undergoes surgery to make them larger or smaller, or whether she has lost a breast because of cancer; whether she has been threatened with arrest for "indecent exposure" while sunbathing bare-breasted, or whether she earns her living as a topless dancer, a model for *Playboy* magazine, or as a call girl whose primary attraction for her clientele is her large breasts; whether her experience of breast-feeding is mystical, whether having her breasts sag is traumatic, whether her menopausal symptoms center entirely on her breasts . . . all women will be able to identify with those whose stories are presented in the book. Even within the most unusual stories there are universal elements about the uniquely female experience of having breasts to which all women can relate.

A series of childhood, puberty, and adolescent breast pictures appear in the beginning of the book and initiate the photographic life cycle which continues throughout. The thirty-eight women's stories that follow, most accompanied by a picture of the woman's breasts, are arranged in loose chronological order in keeping with the life-cycle theme of the book. But the stories may be read in any order, according to the individual interests of the reader. In addition to the frontal or profile pictures accompanying the women's stories, there are several groups of breast photographs unaccompanied by text throughout the book. Their purpose is to illustrate further the astounding variety of breasts.

There are also two sections, "The Models" and "Pregnancy and Breast-feeding," whose format is different. "The Models" begins with three individual stories—Sherry, Jackie, and Gail briefly describe their childhood and adolescent experiences with their breasts—followed by responses to questions about nude modeling for men's magazines. We felt it was important to include this material in order to provide a behind-the-scenes look at this media phenomenon which is so much a part of our cultural fascination with breasts.

The "Pregnancy and Breast-feeding" section is illustrated with a series of pertinent photographs and is compiled from excerpts of many different women's interviews, expressing a variety of experience and opinion about these profound events in a woman's life. Questions from our interview are used throughout the section to guide the reader from one subject to another. The complete questionnaire is included in the Epilogue.

●

Often, inspired by their interviews, women expressed their hopes for the book and its effect upon its audience. These were usually reflections of their own individual needs and aspirations. In conclusion, we want to share with you some of their hopes:

• *I hope the book helps women realize that we are uniquely beautiful no matter what our breasts look like. Women will now be able to see that our breasts all vary and that "so-and-so's" do not look better or worse than yours, just* different!

• *The range of normalcy in the shape of the physical body is enormous and so it is very important to correct misconceptions. I hope this gets rid of the* Playboy *stereotype of the "ideal" breast because it's a vast misrepresentation and it is very intimidating to women.*

• *The thing I especially like about this book is the message of variety. During my field studies among bare-breasted cultures, I used to experience a feeling of elation just seeing all the physical differences of the women's breasts. It was obvious to me then how hard our society tries to conceal and homogenize these differences. So what we're left with is the insanity of large-breasted women wanting to be smaller and small-breasted women wanting to be larger. I hope the book makes women aware of the fact that although the grass always* seems *greener on the other side, it usually isn't!*

• *If men read the book, too, maybe they'll stop wishing their wives had some-thing they don't have.* Enough *already!*

• *I hope that women who are anguished because of their small breasts will be helped by the book. I know some women whose self-images have been shattered and who've wound up on psychiatrists' couches because some doctor told them that the reason they're "flat-chested" is because there's something wrong with their hormones and they're not really women. I want everyone to realize that there is* nothing *wrong with a woman if she's flat-chested!*

• *I hope the book shows women that some of us have gone through* hell *because of our breasts . . . and it's* not *worth it!*

• *As a nurse I ran across a lot of women who didn't want to breast-feed because they were afraid of what it would do to their breasts. I really want the book to break people's stereotypes about the beautiful breast so that more women breast-feed, because that was one of the greatest experiences of my life. And since we now have bottle-feeding, it's easy to forget about the function of breasts. So I hope the book makes women think more about what their breasts are for.*

• *I'd really like to see less emphasis on the sexuality of breasts because it has screwed up women in many ways. Breasts should be more of an everyday thing.*

• *Husband of interviewee: Unfortunately, chances are that the effect of the book will be to bring even* more *attention and hysteria to breasts as a special part of the body.*

Interviewee: *I don't think so because the moment you use the word "breasts," instead of "tits" or "boobs," that's already stating a certain approach, an attitude. People will be clued in that the book is about something other than the sexism that's normally associated with that part of women's bodies.*

• *Men should read this book—every last one of them! I always hated being put down for something over which I had no control, like pendulous breasts. So I'm hoping for more sensitivity on the part of men about how women feel, instead of the usual condescending attitude about "tits." I don't think men really understand the extent that women are insecure about their breasts and how much they have to do with it. The book could make for better understanding between the sexes and that would really help everyone.*

• *Most women are terribly self-conscious about their bodies and haven't been able to share their feelings with anybody. Suppose a woman suffers all her life* thinking, *My breasts are so ugly! I must be abnormal!* But then she reads that many women feel the same as her—she's not alone! *That's got to be the greatest revelation.*

• *I want people to realize how much breasts have become a symbol of a woman's worth in our society, and that, like a big cock, big breasts—or breasts period—are not the be-all and end-all of a woman's existence!*

• *I hope that women who have had mastectomies are reassured that they can still hold the affection of another human being and continue to be sexually active.*

• *In my mind, the most important message of this book is for young girls. I really hope it helps women feel better about their breasts so they can relax and be more open with their daughters, especially when they're going through puberty. That seems to be the most painful period of life; at least it was for me.*

• *Our youth-fixated culture, which focuses on a woman's youth, isolating it as an ideal against which the rest of her life is devalued, causes so much fear of getting old. We really need to help each other fight the negativity and see the beauty in aging, and I see the book as a step in that direction.*

• *There's a tendency in our life-style today to live and work among people exclusively of our own age, so we don't really have a perspective on the whole process of life. It will be really healthy to be reminded of what an eleven- or fourteen-year-old girl goes through during puberty and to learn how an eighty-year-old woman feels about her breasts.*

• *I hope the book neutralizes the whole "dirty" connotation that breasts have, even today, in the minds of too many people. These experiences that have been hidden for so long are precisely the things that need to be shared and delved into if we are going to overcome the shame we've been taught to feel about our bodies.*

• *Beyond being a presentation of all the different possibilities that exist around these two things—breasts—that you have for your whole life, women are talking about how they really feel. And interesting things start to happen when a lot of people talk about something they haven't talked about before. They look up and see that there are other people who share their feelings and it can change their lives!*

Women are giving it some thought—we're rethinking the menu, folks! And maybe we don't want to sip a Shirley Temple anymore. Maybe we're already through the reaction stage of boilermakers. Who knows, maybe some of us want to try a ginseng cocktail . . . or maybe we'd just like a glass of water. And then again, maybe we're just gonna sit it out because we don't want anything . . . and we don't want to be polite, either.

• *I hope this book gives us back our breasts in a way . . . kind of helps us reclaim them.*

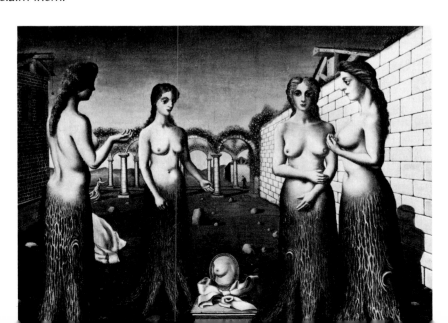

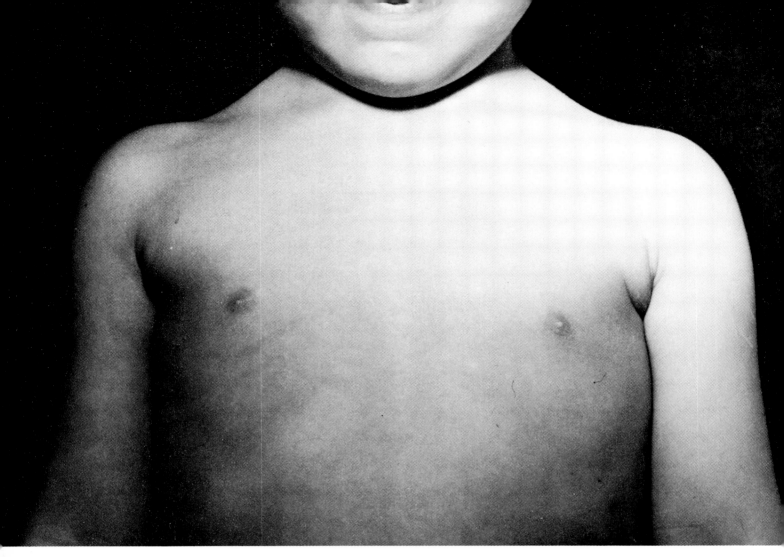

Age 7

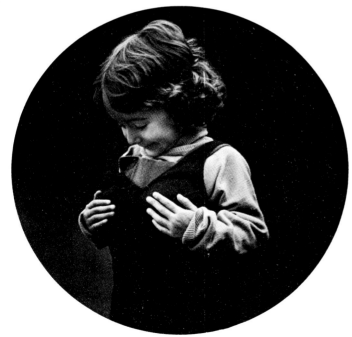

All my daughters looked forward to having breasts when they were younger. When one of them was eleven, she stood in front of the mirror and cried, "Oh, I'll never get breasts!" I said, "Trust me. I know you will get breasts. You have a good history—your mother and your aunts and your grandmothers were all well developed. Don't you worry about it. You'll get breasts."

Since then, whenever one of them lacks confidence or thinks she can't do something, I say, "Don't worry, you'll get breasts," meaning it's inevitable that it will happen and it will be positive for her.

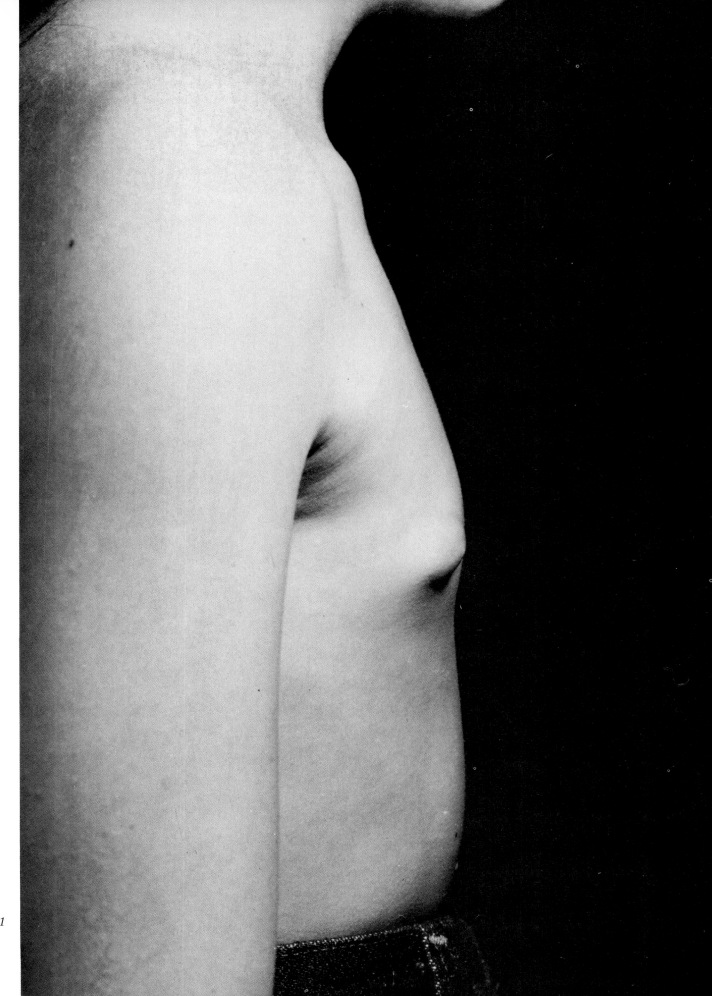

Age 11

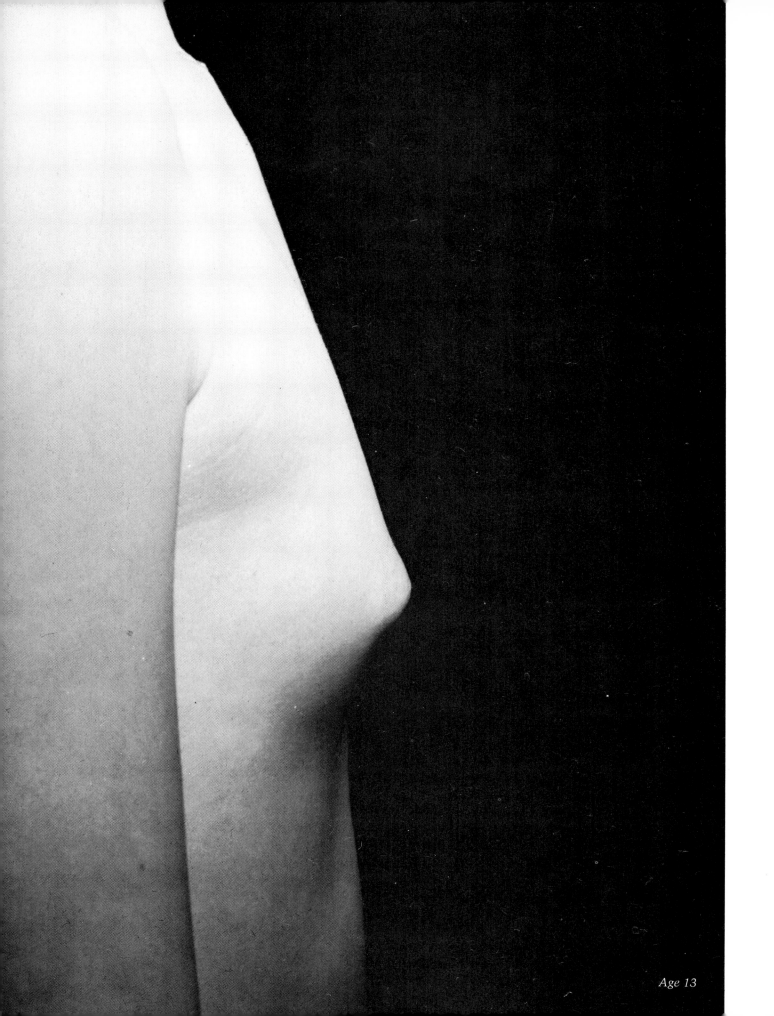

Age 13

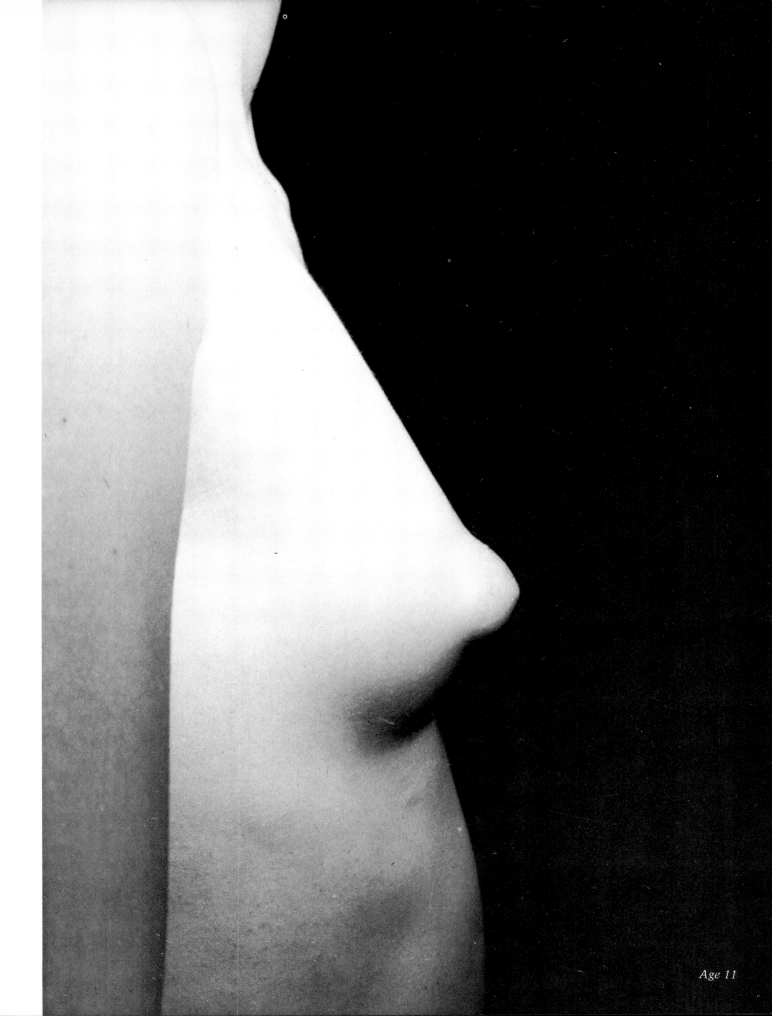

Age 11

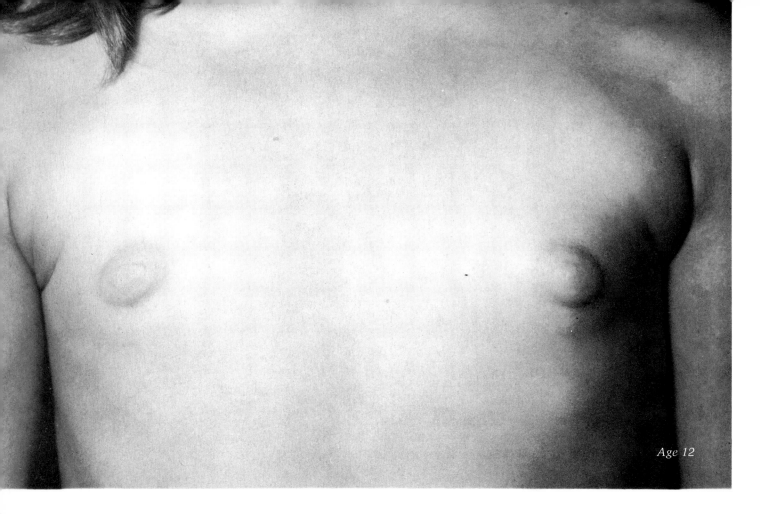

Age 12

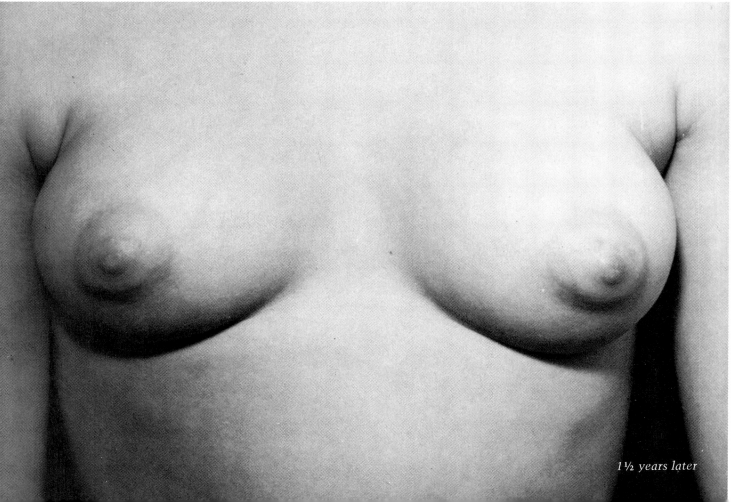

1½ years later

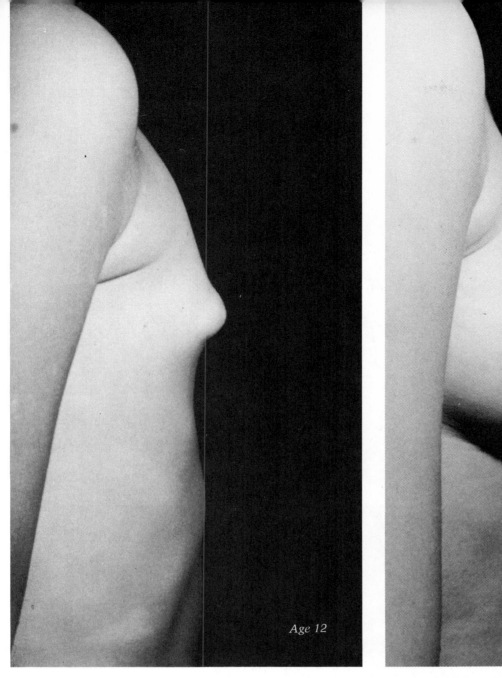

Age 12

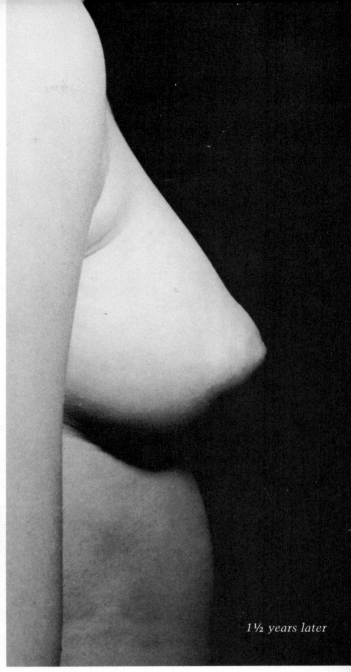

1½ years later

At first they were flat, then all of a sudden the nipples came out like mosquito bites. And three or four days ago I noticed that my breasts were coming out from the sides. When I first started they were just little lumps by the nipples.

●

I can remember my little child's body and what it felt like to be flat-chested. Then I went through an enormous shift when I developed breasts— it was like having two different body transmutations. Now running is a totally different experience from when I was twelve! That's something that men don't experience and it makes us different.

33

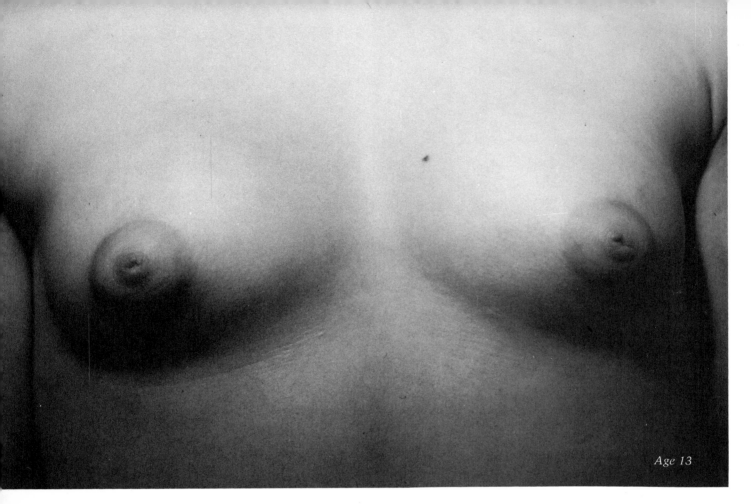

Age 13

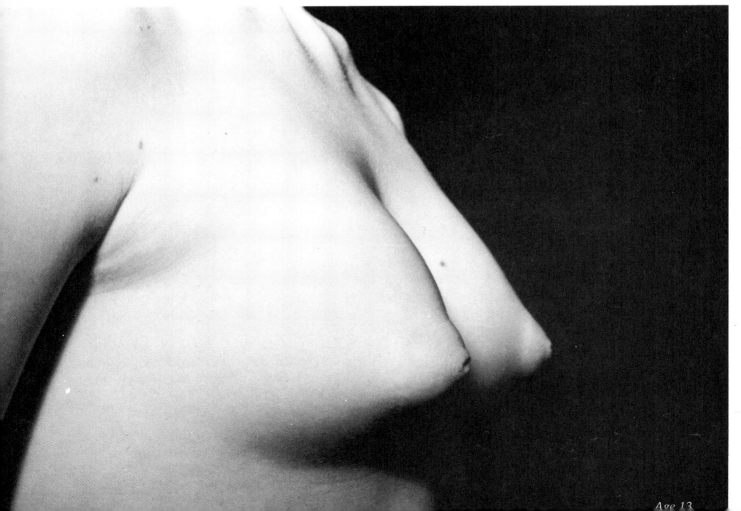

Age 13

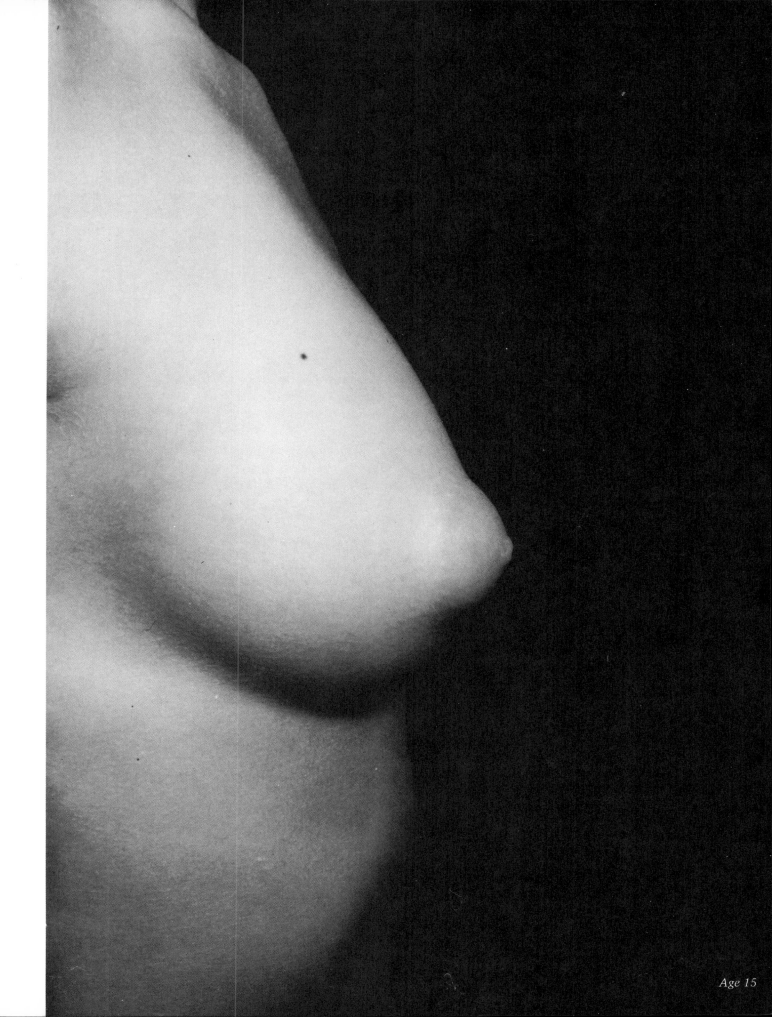

Age 15

Virginia

There is something in acting called the "point of lead." Its three major areas are the heart, gut, and head, and it's used as the psychological basis for the exploration of a character. In the development of my character as a human being, my point of lead has always been my breasts—always! I don't remember when that happened, but I'm consciously aware of it now. It's like people who don't comb their hair in the back. When I get dressed, the only part of me that I really dress and admire and look at is my breasts. The rest I don't pay too much attention to!

I don't think of my breasts as a real large part of my body. But I had a teacher in college who never knew my name but used to describe me by the typical gesture "oomph!" (extends arms out in front of chest, as if to hold a Z cup). I guess that he meant zaftig [voluptuous] so that my impression of my breasts and how they affect other people is quite different. I think of them as strong and firm and beautiful.

A lot of times I characterize myself as a "glit and tit" girl—scrumptious! A couple of months ago a man and his girlfriend and I were going out for drinks. She had on something low-cut and he was flipping out! He didn't like it because a lot of men were looking at her and it was making him uncomfortable. She said to him, "You work with Virginia every day and her breasts are always showing," so he said, "Oh, that's just Virginia." It's like it's gotten to be my trademark. A certain protocol concerning my breasts is suspended among my circle of friends, because they know that's just the way I'm going to be around them. Even when it's freezing outside, my breasts are still the only part of me that is naked!

My mother has huge breasts—huge. I think she likes her breasts a lot. She is a very large woman, yet she has a lot of dignity—she is very stately. I remember as a little girl, when I saw her put on a bra, I would be very excited because I never saw either of my parents really touch their bodies very much. She would hook her bra in the back and then lean over and tuck her breasts in one by one. It was so beautiful I couldn't believe it. She cared for them like they were beings outside of her body. She put each one in and then she would look in the mirror and there they were. When I was really little I thought that she was putting her breasts to bed, and I loved that.

I was really excited about the ritual that surrounded breasts, rather than the breasts themselves. I was excited about bras. In school, girls had to wear white slips under their blouses so that their bras wouldn't show—they were very concealed. There was always such an effort by the school authorities to conceal bras that I couldn't *wait* to have one. And it took me so much nerve to just *ask* for one. I didn't really *need* one, but I felt I did—I was beginning to develop enough so that I thought I warranted the *sacred treasure.*

Bras were "sacred" because they were a mystery. People who wore bras were very mystical to me. It was almost an occult kind of thing because the bras didn't show and they went under everything. Going through puberty, we would guess who had one and who didn't. It was the same as who had breasts and who didn't. I just got such a kick out of it.

When I was twelve, I had a best girlfriend with whom I played a game called "photograph." We would pose like Playboy bunnies on a bed, and *all* the poses had to do with our breasts. We would pretend we were photographers and take each

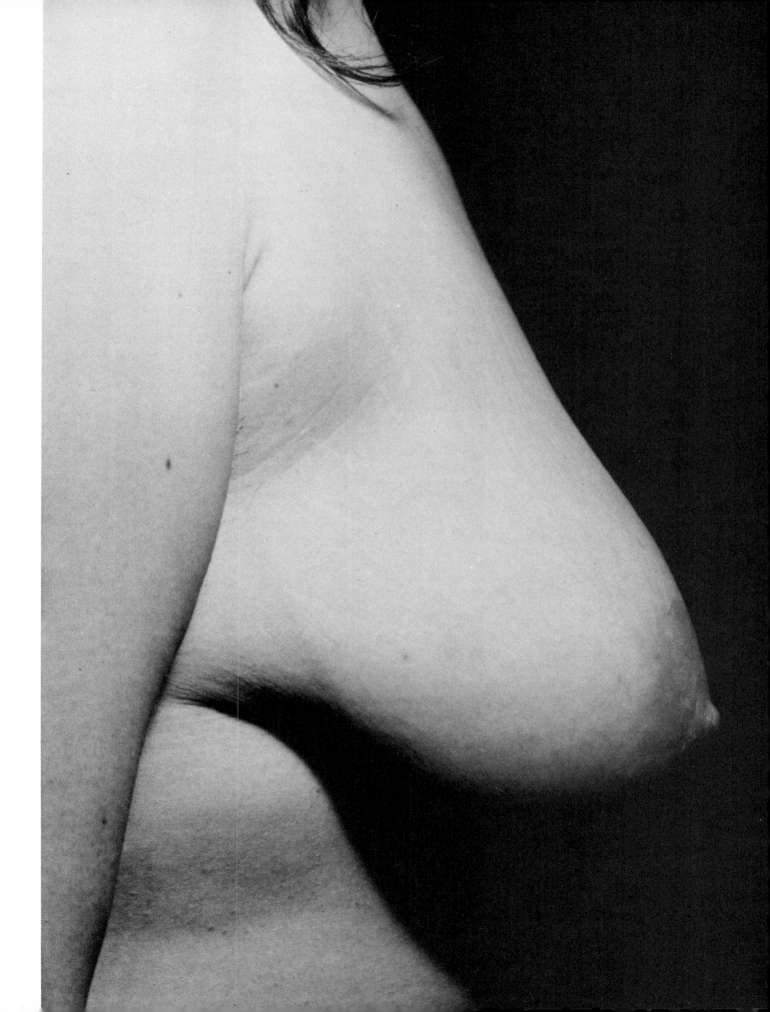

other's picture. The idea was to see how many original and bizarre contortions we could get into. We would also play a card game where, if you lost, the winner got to touch you. That was a big penalty! And it *always* seemed to involve each other's breasts.

My girlfriend had much larger breasts than I did and they were two different sizes, which I thought was so terrific! I was so upset that mine were the *same* size. At twelve I wasn't burdened by certain points of view about what was beautiful. I thought having two different-size breasts was so much better than having two the same. There was more variety, like having two different friends instead of twins. I was so excited for her. She's miserable now, but then it was quite an honor.

I always wanted my breasts to be high on my body, so they have always been a very important factor in my posture and the way I walk. I never wanted them to sag—that was just something that I learned really early, that sagging wasn't as pretty as high breasts. Also I always wanted darker nipples because I'm really fair and a lot of women that I had seen in magazines had white skin and dark nipples, so I thought that was just beautiful.

I always wanted to be five feet two inches, blond, and skinny, and here I was, all brunette, five feet eight inches, and fat. My relationship to my body was different from that of most of the girls I grew up with because I had a very different body than they did. I never had a "figure" in the traditional sense of the word—I had *my* figure. I never coveted a style other than my own because there was no way I could fulfill it.

The archetypal woman of the South where I was raised was small. Her breasts were small, she was small, her intellect was small, her personality was small—all in all she was very manageable, and didn't create too much disturbance wherever she went. As my breasts began to develop and grow large, they became a very determining factor in my largeness as a human being—my not being manageable or "easy."

None of the popular and successful girls in high school had large breasts—cheerleaders didn't, majorettes didn't, even the National Honor Society students didn't—it went that far! So having large breasts was a real big factor in my personality, especially because they weren't manageable by boys. Guys made fun of them and were frightened by them.

I grew up during a time when large breasts were "out." My father and his cronies were of the generation that thought of big breasts as a sign of something attractive and desirable—a kind of status symbol. By the time *I* came around, things had reversed and large breasts became something to hide.

When I started feeling that it wasn't cool to have big breasts, I used to wrap Ace bandages around my chest so my breasts wouldn't stick out too much. I almost *fainted* once because I couldn't breathe!

The only way that I could deal with an environment in which my body provoked a lot of shame because of its size was to love my breasts. So I began to show them. This was at a time when no one showed their body, but I always wore low-cut things with my breasts showing on top. It used to flip my mother out—she couldn't stand it! But it got me the same kind of attention as someone with a good figure. It was my way of getting the positive attention that I needed in adolescence—attention that I would never have gotten otherwise because of my untraditional body.

In high school I had a million fantasies about petting—it was the big step! I went out with the ugliest boy in the school! He couldn't kiss girls very easily because his nose was so big—he played Cyrano de Bergerac in the school play with no makeup. When all the other boys were kissing, he had to feel girls up because kissing was just not a successful part of his interaction. He and I went parking in front of the principal's house after the junior prom. We were just sitting in the car and talking and it was getting more and more awkward. The tension was building and finally he just pushed me over on the seat and touched my breasts. He was sort of brutal and crude, but it was so innocent that I really appreciated it. Neither one of us had ever had an experience like that before and he really didn't know what breasts were for. He was just as awestruck as I was. In a certain way, he helped me be proud of my breasts because he was really enamored of them.

●

Breasts are symbolic for me, but not always in ways that I admire. There is both the seductress and the sorceress in me. The sorceress is much more the spiritual woman whom I admire, but my breasts are also a symbol of the manipulative part of my magic. I don't admire my manipulation and, oh, my God, I'm such a manipulator! I tease men with my breasts and I make them forbidden. My breasts are always exposed like those peep shows where you put in a quarter and the movies run out till you pay another quarter to see more. But I don't condemn décolletage entirely because I really enjoy certain playful aspects of the mating situation, and my breasts are a very playful part of me.

Yet I am always much more excited by *mystery* than the revelation of mystery. Breasts can be very mysterious but sometimes they are *overexposed.* I like to have work to do—when I look at somebody I like to be able to mentally undress them.

I don't ever like to *completely* expose my breasts—I like to imply them. When you walk around naked in front of someone, when there's no anticipation, it makes the body less interesting. I think of my body as my temple and when exposing it becomes an everyday thing, it somehow becomes less sacred.

Revealing my breasts is like giving a present. When I'm being unwrapped they're the prize or the treasure, and not just for sexual reasons, but because breasts are particularly inspiring to me artistically—how they've been painted and conceived and sculpted all through history. To me breasts are the artwork of the human body. Even when I doodle, most of the drawings that come out are breasts.

Are your breasts sexually arousing?

Yes, but not to an extreme degree. Interestingly, the area *between* my breasts—my cleavage—is quite sensitive. When my breasts are partially covered, they are much more sensitive than when they are totally bare.

I've learned things about self-love from touching my breasts that I would have had no other way of learning. I enjoy touching my breasts much more when I am looking at myself in the mirror.

The *anticipation* of having someone near my breasts or touching or sucking them is much more exciting to me than the actual act itself. It's the whole principle of forbidden fruit. I think of the sex act as the conclusion, rather than the event—the conclusion of a creative experience. The process is always much more exciting to me than the product, and my breasts are involved with the process. Sensuality is the source of my sexuality and my breasts are the aesthetic manifestation of that.

I can't think of anything that makes me feel more pure and peaceful than cuddling against a woman's breasts. A lot of times I dance with women to find out how it feels for a man to hug a woman, but still I can't imagine what it's like to

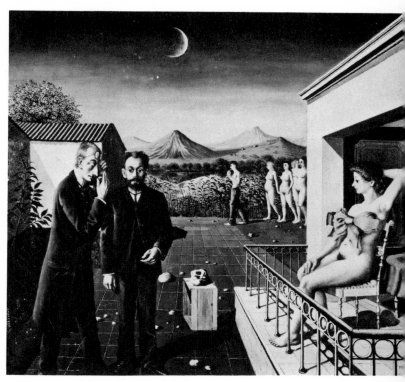

Paul Delvaux, Phases of the Moon, *1939*

have a completely *flat* body and feel breasts pressing against it.

I really am intrigued by breasts. Wherever I am, whomever I'm with, I just want to see *all* of them. They really interest me. My girlfriends always say, "Come on, don't stare, you're embarrassing me," when they are getting dressed or whatever, but I really love to watch.

It's funny—I've seen a lot of men's bodies, yet I never think of the penis as a symbol of variety, but rather as a symbol of the similarity of all men's penises. Breasts are so different, so varied. I don't have a specific image when I say the word "breast." For each woman, breasts are so unique, so much a part of *who* they are. No two pairs of breasts look alike—no two people are the same. To me a penis can be anyone's. (*Laughs.*)

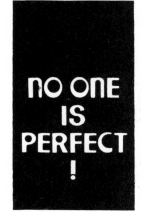
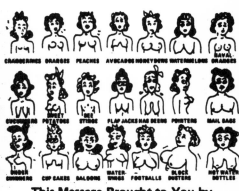

I am convinced that *who* women are has a lot to do with *how* their breasts are. I have a friend whose breasts are firm but low down in the middle of her body, halfway between her neck and her waist. How she moves and even how she feels has so much to do with the placement of her breasts on her body. We call her a "gaucho" girl— a cowgirl. She expresses herself as a woman in a handsome and rugged way which is not necessarily how she feels deep inside her heart. But her body is rugged from the location of her breasts and that has a tremendous influence on her. I think it does on everybody and I think that's why I am so interested in seeing them.

●

I'm *crazy* about bras—I think of them as jewelry. To me they're like the breastplates that they used to have a long time ago. They're really a fun part of my "getting dressed" ritual. When I first started wearing bras my mother would buy me ones that were supportive and big enough and superpractical. I still wear good bras but now they have to fit my costume.

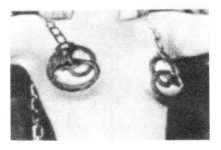

Right now I'm wearing a great red bra which I found on Orchard Street the other day. This little Jewish man with a yarmulke on his head sold it to me. It was so funny! When he went to get it from the window, I got excited and said "It's red, it's red!" Well, he just turned the same color as the bra.

I've worn all kinds of bras. I used to go in stores and they'd say, "We don't make French bras for girls your size, honey." The first time I ever found a French bra that fit I was so excited—it used to make me *hot* to be wearing it. The French bra is cut low and pushes you up—like the women in the movie, *Tom Jones,* and you can see their breasts sticking out of the top of their dresses when they breathe. It was a very exciting day for me when I got my first one.

What's sexy to me has nothing to do with bralessness, but rather with having my chest *exposed.* I can't stand anything on my neck or chest—it makes me feel really uncomfortable. I

wear revealing clothing—low-cut décolletage, anything of that nature. Sometimes I even buy blouses and cut them out.

I pay a price for my freedom—I constantly, *constantly* get hassled in the street by men. A lot of times I don't hear them because I'm too scared to listen. They say things like, "I'd like to get a little piece of that," or "I'd like to get between that pair." It doesn't always make me angry. I know some women who are real hard-core "politicos" who insist that I take offense, and that I should get angry and tell those men to fuck off, but it usually just makes me very sad.

When I was in Italy I really got it a lot. Men in Italy are so enchanted by women's breasts that they don't even relate to a woman's whole body. To them it's like just breasts are walking around! And they really love large women.

I was walking through the train station one night—this is the honest truth—when all of a sudden five Italian men circled me and started holding hands and singing. I didn't understand most of what they were saying, but they'd go, *"Bella, bella, grande, grande."* Then they started to *undress* me! They unbuttoned my blouse and looked inside as though they were unwrapping a package. All five of them exchanged remarks and made noises like "Ohhh! Oooooh! Aaaaah!" Meanwhile, I was *freaking out*—I didn't know what to do. They didn't mean to offend me or hurt me, so when they saw that I was getting really upset, they broke the circle and ran away, and you know what they did? Each one of them came back bringing me a chocolate ice-cream

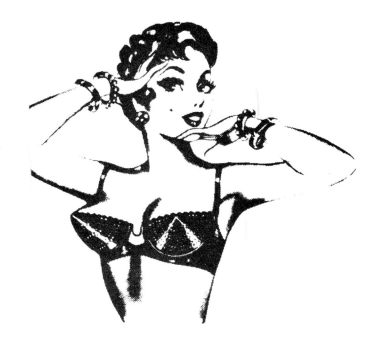

cone, going, "*cioccolata, cioccolata!*" There I was with five chocolate ice-cream cones—it was so weird and wonderful.

●

I saw a picture book one time of African women, and their breasts were the most interesting part of the book. Not only do they burn patterns into their breasts, which is tribal ritual, but also when children are starving in underprivileged cultures, they suck from the breasts of *any* woman, trying to get milk and nourishment. So, many of the women's breasts are literally used up and dried out—the breast is just sucked to a shriveled state at a very early age in a woman's life.

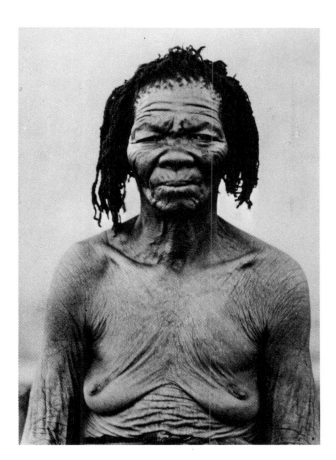

Seeing that had a lot of impact on me because I realized how unweathered our breasts are. Those women's breasts are really like fishermen's faces, with so many lines of experience. Our breasts seem to be artificially preserved and they don't show road maps of certain kinds of journeys, like breast-feeding, that people go through in life.

A lot of times when I am acting or singing, I sort of beat my chest. This is an important gesture for me. It feels good because although my breasts are the most sensitive part of my body (they get sunburned first and so on), they are also a very strong part of my body. I'm proud of that. I know women who are very afraid of their breasts being knocked or accidentally jabbed. It's very painful for them, but not for me. Mine have always been exposed and weathered.

●

In *every* memorable experience I've had my breasts have been involved, because my most memorable experiences have had a lot to do with the "agony and the ecstasy." The ecstasy is pretty self-evident, but when I hurt inside a lot, when I have those agonies, my breasts are very much a part of it.

There are times in my life when I cry my heart out. Then I feel pain underneath my breasts—a real physical pain just drumming and beating so hard inside of me. To just put my hand on my chest when I'm in agony is the greatest comfort in the world to me. There is a poem by a famous poet which I love: "I asked my kindest friend to guard my sleep / I said fold your hands across the drum." When I put my hands to my breasts, it is like folding my hands across that drum inside of me, and it is very soothing.

I often sleep with my hands on my breasts—one hand covering each breast—because in some way it makes me feel that I am closing the energy circuit of my body, creating a circle so energy doesn't escape. Since I was very young it has tucked me into myself for the night—just to sleep and dream and contact the other realms. . . .

Michelle

Age 20 • Raised in Harlem, New York City • Student

The first time I heard the word "tits," it just blew my mind! I never came across it in Harlem. I never knew any people who called breasts "tits." To me they were always "jugs"!

I'm not a sexual being—for me sexuality is something that is very subtle and not very obvious. I mean, no matter how hard I may try, I'll never be the sister who's jettin' down 125th Street in Harlem, lookin' so fine with chest and shape. I just will never be that type of person, and now I wouldn't even try. . . .

I went through a period of denying my breasts. And then I went through a period of intellectually asking myself and trying to understand what breasts represent, and that's when I learned to appreciate them. My breasts have made me deal with the fact that I am a woman, and I haven't always liked it. My breasts and me have gone through some painful times together. . . .

There are a lot of cultural myths perpetuated about black sensuality which are both oppressive and very painful for blacks. One of the things black folks like to say among themselves is, "While white folks was up in the big house gettin' religion, we were down in the cabins fuckin'. And now white folks have to go to Masters and Johnson to learn how to fuck!" (*Laughs.*) I can see the humor in that, and some truth, but blacks have sexual problems of their own, even with their own myths.

I know black girls, and I can speak with some authority about black girls growing up in the ghetto. A black adolescent girl is caught in a bind because if she believes the myths about black sexuality that she hears when she's a kid, she's supposed to be the foxiest, sliest, sexy little momma walkin'! But, if she doesn't develop as fast as everyone else, then she doesn't feel that she's the really sexy person that she's supposed to be, or even that she's really black, and that's frightening!

My breasts growing was the only thing that made me have to deal with the fact that I was developing into an adult, because everything else on me was small. I was very undernourished as a kid. But the fact that my breasts were *there*, no matter how small they were, made me realize that I wasn't a little eight-year-old kid riding on subways anymore. I was developing into a woman and that terrified me! It really did.

I remember feeling two ways—I wanted to de-

velop breasts to be sexy and to feel black, but at the same time I didn't want to. I was frightened. I remember that when the hairs on my vagina started coming in, I got me some Nair and rubbed them all off! Now I know that I was fighting against becoming an adolescent,. because adolescence for me, as a black girl growing up in Harlem, was just too terrifying. Everyone I knew was getting pregnant.

So in a way, because I didn't have the outward manifestations of a "sexy little momma"—I was small-breasted—I was safe. I could still be the person the guys jumped roofs with and just hung out with. In a way, I was glad my breasts were small, and for a time I tried to downplay them even more because I didn't want to be considered a potential "fuckee." I just wanted to be the guys' "little sister" and hear about the other girls they fucked.

I was one of the boys, which was okay with me because I really didn't want to get pregnant. All my girlfriends . . . they'd get pregnant and have to drop out of school, and they were on welfare and they had two or three babies. I didn't want that. So I was in a real bind because I wanted to develop and be sexy and get my peers' approval and be one of them, but at the same time I was terrified of ending up like them.

Another myth in the black community is that *if* you have big breasts, it has nothing to do with your developing. The old wives' tale is, "You can

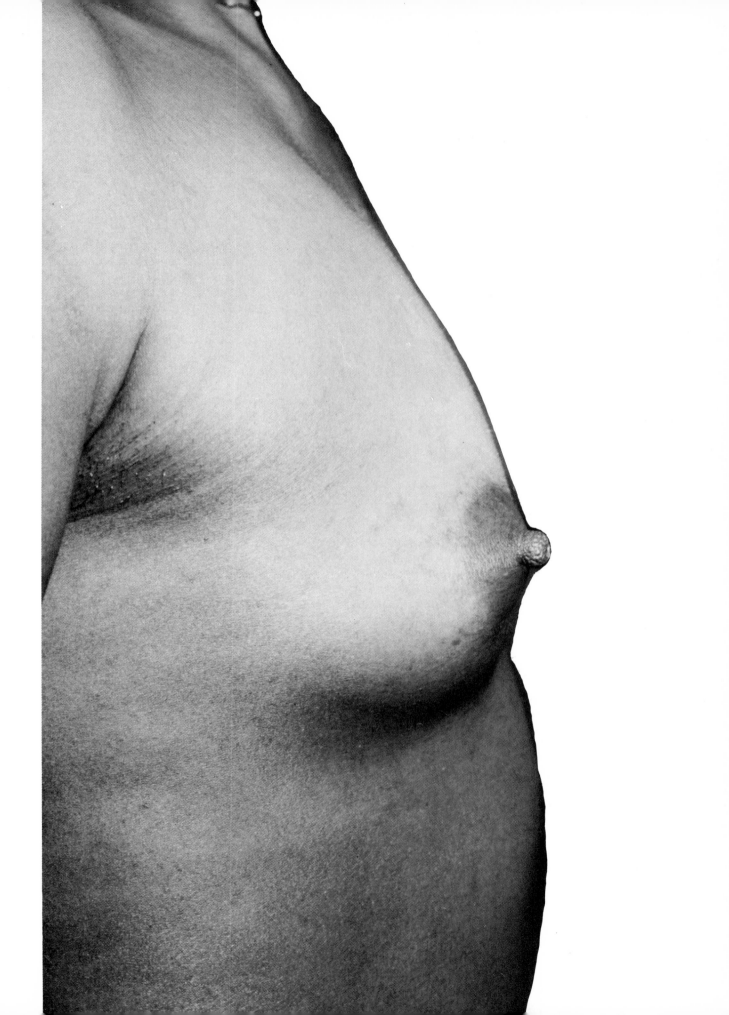

tell who's been fuckin' around." You know, if the girl has got big breasts, even if she's eleven or twelve or thirteen or fourteen, that means she's been fuckin' around with some little boy.

Again I was gettin' two messages from the kids. One was, "Hell, you don't fuck no way!" 'cause they believed the myth, and I didn't have no breasts to prove it different. So I was considered asexual. (*Laughs.*) It was okay, but the other message was that I wasn't worth touching and so I felt lacking, and part of me wanted real bad to be a "little momma."

I had this friend named Yvonne—God, Yvonne was stacked!—and I wanted my breasts to be just like hers. Yvonne was a 36D—Jeesus Ka-rist!—at sixteen no less. All the guys were so turned on to her that when we were together with a group of girls, the guys didn't pay the rest of us no attention. We were just like statues next to Yvonne.

She told me that if I did exercises they'd grow, and I spent an awful lot of time doing those exercises, and *nothing* happened. Then later she told me that they'd grow if I let guys play with them, and I did all that and *nothing* happened. I really tried to get them to grow, but they just wouldn't do it.

Hell, I was getting felt up *before* I had breasts! When I was about thirteen I once did it on a dare. A friend of mine bet me that I wouldn't let a guy who had been really diggin' on me, touch me. I'd been givin' him excuses for two weeks runnin'. I told him everything was wrong with me except VD, 'cause, hell, I was a thirteen-year-old kid and I didn't want to get fucked up. I've since learned that a woman has to allow herself to get fucked by one man so that he can protect her from getting fucked by all other men. I mean that's what happened. I had to be hooked up with *somebody* or else I would have been fair game for *everybody!* So one of the ways of getting hooked up was to be his "old lady," but then he'd have certain liberties, one of which was feeling me up. I didn't like it but I just gritted my teeth and submitted to it, and that was that.

That was a painful time for me. That's when I first started "getting into trouble." My mother would disappear and my father wasn't around. My brothers were all off in different foster homes, a jail, or a reform school, and I'd been taken downtown a few times—not booked, mostly to scare me. Finally I was placed in a foster home.

My foster mother bought me a bra—it was the smallest size you could buy. I had to put tissue paper in it and it was a *disaster!* But I thought if I put on a bra my breasts would grow into it. I was so proud of my bra I even went to sleep in it. After waiting patiently for about two weeks, when nothing happened I just threw the bra away.

I was sent by my white foster parents to prep school, which was a really strange, hippie environment, very blue jeans and country air and vegetarian atmosphere. It was very painful for me being thrown together not only with white kids, but with the ruling-class white—that kind of wealth. It was really strange.

I learned a lot about role-playing at prep school. I was a ghetto kid and I was *tough*—I couldn't be touched! One time a guy said to me, "I dare you to open your shirt." I said, "Yeah, sure, what's the bet?" He said, "I'll take you out to dinner." So we were sitting at the headmaster's dinner table when I did it—I just opened my shirt! And the headmaster said, "God, you've got some cute little breasts"—that's *all* he said! And I wasn't embarrassed or anything 'cause he handled it so well.

He told me later that right after it happened he went into his office and roared with laughter because I came there, such a hip, black, urban, street kid, and I played the role of a street-tough-ghetto-kid takin' no shit from nobody because I was so frightened. I didn't let anybody near me. And when I did something as ridiculous as open my shirt at the dinner table on a dare, he saw that there was a little teenage kid under there that he could reach, and that was the beginning of our friendship. From then on, whenever I'd get out of line, he'd say, "Open your shirt lately?"

●

When I was fourteen, my best friend became pregnant. I watched her whole body change during pregnancy, and one of the things that fascinated me were her breasts—they became enlarged and the nipples got darker. Soon after, I ended up getting pregnant, too, and had my first abortion. I've had a number of them since. . . .

My breasts always made it harder to have the abortions. It was easy for me to deny being pregnant since I could not see my child—the pregnancies were terminated so early. I would never know whether it was a boy or a girl, did it have a temper, or was it bright or was it artistic? But I *always* saw myself breast-feeding the baby 'cause even though my stomach was still flat, I could watch my breasts develop—you know, getting ready for the milk and for the baby. My breasts were telling me, "Hey, there's something growing inside of you."

After the last abortion was over and I had gone

back for the six-week checkup, my breasts were *still* making milk because they hadn't gotten the message that the pregnancy had been terminated. That was just so painful for me, because in every other way I could lie to myself and deny ever being pregnant, but my breasts said, "Oh, no, you can't." Like the time when I was taking a shower and I touched my breasts and they started making milk, and I just cried and cried and cried and cried.

There were times after my abortions when I'd get this really weird sensation in my breasts and then they would just drip milk. All of a sudden there would be two wet spots on my clothing where my nipples were. I wore jackets a lot 'cause I felt very guilty for terminating the pregnancy. Seeing the milk made me angry because I didn't want to be reminded of the abortions. Hell, if I'd been in a position to have a child I'd be breast-feeding it right now.

Children are a chance to start over. I want my child to start off knowing that he or she is loved so much! And I think with the breasts that's the natural way, when you can't sit down and say to a baby, "I love you!" And what does that mean, anyway? Just words.

I wonder how I will feel when I put the baby to my breast to nurse? And then years later, when he's in some bedroom at some other woman's breast . . . I know I'll wonder what he's thinking.

●

I only started enjoying sex recently. I was very sexually active before, but I didn't enjoy it. The man I'm seeing now was the first person who made love to *me,* and not to a particular part of my body. He made "love" to me, instead of "fuck-ing" me. He was really sensitive—we became sensual *before* we became sexual.

There were times we'd take a shower together and he'd just touch my whole body, and then I found out, "Hey! I like you touchin' my breasts. It feels good!" And he would pick up on that and just play that up without doin' anything else for weeks. We've talked about breasts—my having little breasts and how I feel about it—and he said the coolest thing. He said, "They're just right— just a mouthful—and I like that." And that was a really positive experience for me. I guess it's one of the reasons I love him. He took time and cared enough to find out what I was feeling. He's really done his work well, and now I feel that though my breasts are small, they are the most sensuous part of my body . . . and it makes *me* feel much better.

I adore dresses with a sort of V neck so that when I bend over my breasts show, and I like to wear the top button of a certain dress of mine open *because* of my breasts—I like them to show a little. I wore that dress to the university the other day and every black male I saw told me to button it up, which to me was a mind-fucker! It's this whole thing about the black middle class.

If white people say that black people are mor-ally loose, then most middle-class black people think we gotta be ten times more modest than whites are to *prove* that we're okay—that we're really not those sexual savages that run around loose and fuck everywhere.

●

I think that a lot of the message of the women's movement is teaching society that women de-mand to be experienced and treated as total human beings, and that their worth is not defined by the size of their breasts or any other externals. What women have been through and what black

DEAR ABBY

Some like 'em small, but not most men

By Abigail Van Buren

DEAR ABBY: How dare you perpetuate the myth that men prefer women with big breasts? In a recent column in which you offer men tips on how to make themselves more "loveable," you said, "If she's flat-chested and a 38-D walks by, pretend not to notice."

Abby, there are men who PREFER women with small breasts ("flat-chested," ac-cording to YOUR 38-D stan-dards) — my husband among them. He doesn't have to "pre-tend not to notice."

If you had done a little re-search, you would have known that men who prefer women with small breasts are more mature, intelligent and less chauvinistic than the big-breast worshipers.

Please stop trying to make me, and others like me, feel that we are inferior and unat-tractive, and that any man will slobber himself into a stu-por over a 38-D!

SMALL AND SEXY

DEAR S AND S: My apolo-gies. But in most surveys I've seen in which men were asked to describe their "ideal woman," the 38-D's were way out in front.

people have been through is very similar in a way, because when a white man was buying a slave, he wanted to know how big his muscles were. They even checked their genitals to see what they were like—that determined their value. Black people up on their slave block, like women on their pedestals, were not people—they were objects. What are his genitals like? How big are his muscles? Has she had any children? We outlawed that in this country and even now we can work up moral indignation that it ever happened. Yet this happens to women *all the time* in *Playboy* magazine and *Oui,* you name it. It's not what you are as a person, but what your measurements are! That makes me sad and I'll do everything I can to help women reclaim their bodies.

I think another lesson of the women's movement is teaching a woman to make conscious decisions about what she wants to do with her body.

There were so many times in my life that I had no control over my body—when I was growing up, when I was getting pregnant, and when I was having abortions.

I think women who have had children and whose breasts have stretch marks are beautiful, simply because there is so much history there. To me, because my breasts have a history with the making of milk and the interrupting of pregnancies and just being teased about them, *that* makes them beautiful.

Me and my breasts have been down the road together. It has been so painful to deal with them at times. The relationship I have with them now is like with somebody you go through a horrible experience with—we sort of have a mutual respect for each other now, even a love, you know.

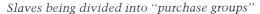

Slaves being divided into "purchase groups"

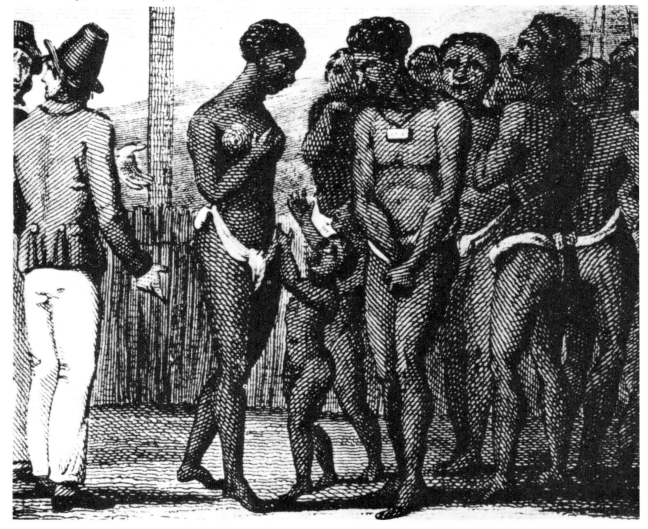

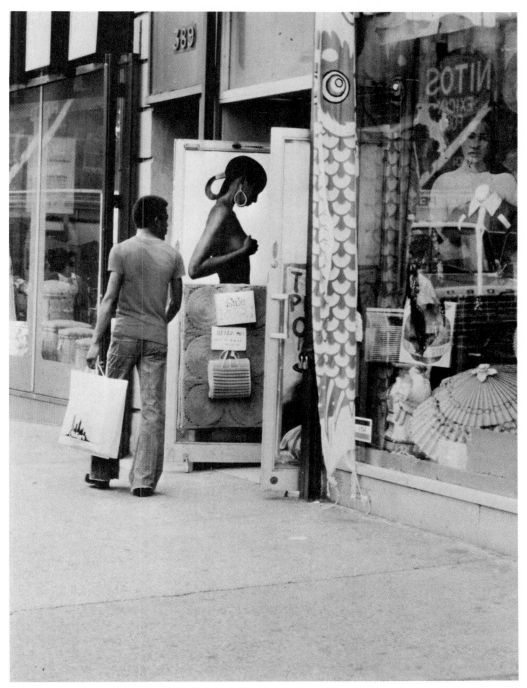

The gesture of covering the breast can be just as provocative and eye-catching as exposing the breast (No. 27 from the series "Tits Sell." I. J. Weinstock, 1978.)

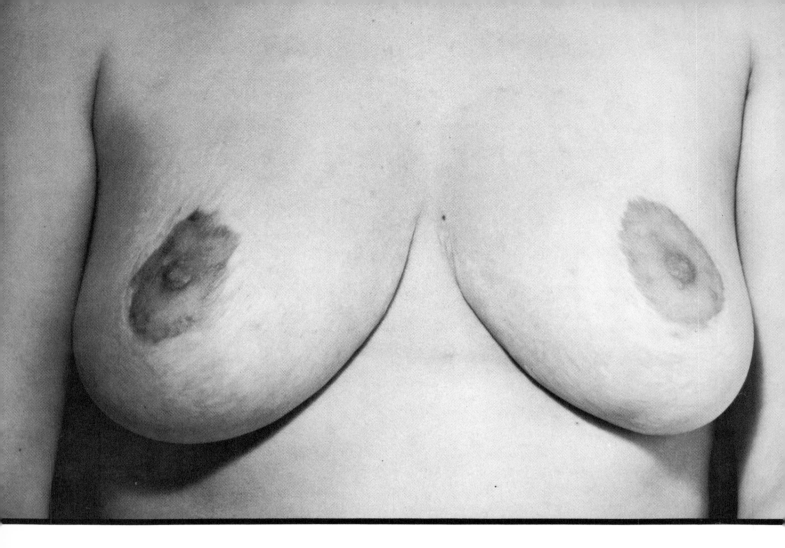

Linda   *Age 26 • Raised in the Midwest • Editor*

. . . As a child I had very large breasts, and at the age of fifteen I had a reduction mammoplasty at the suggestion of my mother, with a number of psychological repercussions. A couple of years of therapy, work in a breast cancer detection center, and a decent lover or two, put me in a somewhat better place.

I would be delighted to share these experiences with other women. . . .

—Excerpt from card sent to us by Linda

My earliest memories of my breasts are that they were a terrible secret. I noticed that my nipples stuck out more and they *hurt,* but I didn't tell anybody about it. I was seven—just a little kid. And I remember that I was scared to sleep on my stomach. I was afraid I would squish them or something, so I began to sleep on my back. They were like delicate fruits that I had to make sure not to bruise.

I was in the first grade and I didn't know what

was happening really. I was so young. All I knew was that something was going on and I should probably tell my mother about it, but I didn't want to. I didn't want to tell *anybody!*

I went to summer camp right after I got out of school and that was the first time I really began to *worry* about it. When I came back from camp I finally told my mother. She thought that there was something wrong, that it couldn't be breasts *yet,* but she was mistaken.

48

I didn't want her to tell my father, but she did, and I felt betrayed. My father is a doctor. She wanted me to show him my breasts and all I could say was, "Nooo!" I resisted it for quite a while. I wasn't going to show him, but eventually I did. I was very embarrassed.

How did doctors react to your breasts when you went for physical examinations?

After I got breasts I stopped going to the pediatrician. I went to the *other* doctor, the grown-up doctor, and he didn't really say anything about it. My mother had started early and my grandmother had started early, so it was a hereditary thing. It was just "me and my genes." I think he made a remark like, "You're Mediterranean and that's what happens." He was Italian, too, so it was very normal to him.

My mother explained to me everything that was gonna happen. She said, "Children might tease you, but you shouldn't listen. They're silly, and they're probably jealous and don't understand, or maybe it scares them." And she told me that breasts were for feeding children, though she didn't breast-feed any of us, and she also said, "You know, when you grow up your husband will like your breasts and when he wants to touch them you'll really like it, too." I didn't want to hear that at age seven. That was embarrassing! "Your husband will like them . . ." She was implying that breasts were *sexual.*

Getting breasts was something that I had no control over, and that other people would notice even though it wasn't my fault. That's what my parents conveyed to me more than anything—that people would notice and that there were certain responsibilities that went along with that. Bad enough to have them, but to be responsible for them, too?

Besides, it was the first time that something had happened to me that wasn't predictable. I felt as if my body had snuck up on me and done something unexpected. I'd never before had a real illness as a child, but suddenly *this!* It was uncontrollable. So it was very spooky and frightening.

My parents were worried about me. They were embarrassed by it, too. They didn't know how to handle it, or what to think about it, or what to *do* about it. So that was a very big part of the embarrassment I felt.

My mother had also started getting breasts early, so she should have known how to handle it with me. But she remembered her early development as a horrible thing. I remember her saying, "I know how you feel because I hated it. It's hor-

rible! When I was ten I had big breasts and I always hated it! I thought it was terrible and it *was!*" I was also aware of the fact that my mother felt that her breasts were getting bigger and bigger and bigger with each successive child, and that she didn't like it.

By telling me her feelings she felt she was sharing the burden with me or something. And though I think she meant it sympathetically, I just took it to heart. She made me feel like having breasts was a bad thing. For me there was no joy in "becoming a woman."

Nobody at school ever said anything about my breasts; nobody teased me. Maybe they were too young and childish and it was too spooky or something. Even in first grade I was never really childish because I had so many younger brothers and sisters whom I took care of.

At home I felt that I had to hide from the curiosity of my brothers and sisters. It was *my* secret, and I didn't want them to know *that* about me, or anything else for that matter. I was a particularly closed-in sort of child. I never told anyone anything, especially *this.* Forget it! I just didn't want anyone to know.

When I finally got a brassiere, the summer between first and second grade, I didn't want my brothers and sisters to know about it, or my fa-

Puberty, *by Edvard Munch*

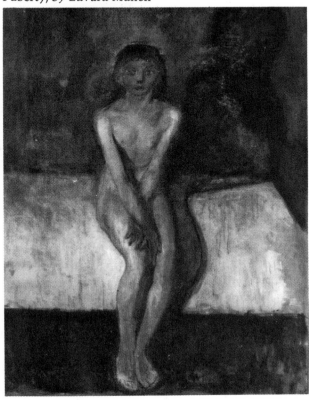

ther, or *anybody*. I didn't want my mother to talk about it. I refused to discuss it. She did end up telling my brother about my breasts even though I had specifically told her not to. When I realized that she had spilled the beans I was *furious!* "How could you?"

My brother didn't tease me or anything, but I knew he knew because he asked me, "Now are you going to look like a lady? Are you going to look like one of those people who's out to *here!*" He was about six years old. He wasn't ashamed to ask because we had been pretty sexual children up until then—prebreasts that is. After, *no way!*

Then I think my brother told my cousin. She's the same age as I am and was starting to get breasts, and I imagine her little brother was curious about it, too, because I remember him teasing me about it. So it was really getting around. It was all over town.

I remember always wanting to hide myself from my younger sisters. I shared a room with one sister so I would get dressed in the bathroom. She was very curious and wanted to know what this was all about. She'd always want me to show my breasts to her and I wouldn't. She'd say, "Oh, come on," and I'd say, "Oh, noooo!" My brother never expressed a desire to see my breasts—I think he was too scared.

By the time I was nine I *really* had breasts—like a C cup—and I was fairly short 'cause I was still a little girl, still a little person. Both my grandmothers are Italian and both have *enormous* breasts, *huge,* and they're both very short. So when I started wearing a C cup my mother would say, "My God, I hope you're not going to end up looking like your grandmothers," and then naturally I also hoped that I wasn't going to look like them. Before that I had always thought my grandmothers looked fine.

Whenever my mother and I went shopping for clothes, we would no longer pick out anything with a belt. (*Laughs.*) It started to be very difficult for me to buy clothes at all. I was still too little to fit into teenage or subteen sizes, but I had these breasts so I didn't fit into children's sizes either. It was always a big trauma to go shopping, especially whenever there was a holiday that I had to look nice for. Consequently I hated holidays and I started looking very dowdy, wearing just whatever would fit. I never wore tight clothes or ones that just fit well, they always had to be baggy. And for years I'd always go out wearing at least two shirts—*layers*—and a sweater over that. Even when it was warm out. *Always!*

Just *because* of my breasts my parents were afraid that I might start going out with men—at nine years old! (*Laughs.*) They were afraid I would be taken advantage of, since I was too naive to know any better. My mother started to say things like, "People are going to think you're older than you are. Older men are going to find you attractive and you're going to have to really *watch* it. They may want to feel your breasts. You don't let 'em!"

That was very hard for me to take at nine years old. It really was. I didn't want to hear that. "Don't tell me!" My parents' reactions to my breasts always seemed negative. I felt very vulnerable and ashamed. Once in a swimming pool some boy grabbed my breasts while I was underwater. I was so *ashamed* that I just left. I cried all the way home and I wouldn't tell anybody what happened—not even my mother.

It was weird to be a child and have the body of a woman.

The first time I discussed my breasts with anyone was when my best friend started to develop. She was around nine. I found out because her mother told my mother and my mother told me—"You know, it's really hard for her, just like it was for you. You should talk to her about it"—but I didn't want to. Eventually, we did get around to talking about it, if you could call it that. She'd ask me, "Did it hurt when you were first starting?" And I'd say, "Yeah . . ." I do remember a feeling of rapport with her.

Apart from that incident, I didn't discuss it with anyone. And as I got older I just sort of became a misfit. I became very studious. In school I hung out with the marginal types who didn't fit anyplace or whom nobody liked. I was one of them.

I remember thinking that my breasts were the reason I wasn't good at anything. I had been good in gym the first couple of years of school, but when I got to be fairly good-sized, I wasn't anymore. Probably it was just my being awkward and gawky when most girls weren't yet. And I was also very ashamed of my breasts and that inhibited my freedom of movement to some extent. I became rather anxious and tense because I didn't want to call any attention to my breasts, so I wasn't too graceful.

Despite my embarrassment about them, I continued wrestling and fighting with my brother as I'd always done before. But my parents would say, "You're getting too big for that now. You're becoming a woman so you shouldn't be wrestling with him. You don't want to hurt yourself." I think they were afraid of sexual contact. I remember once he tried to cop a feel. He grabbed one of my breasts and put his hand on it and I ran into the bathroom. That was when I was a little older and I was pretty big. It's hard to remember exactly *how* big I was by then. It seems like I *always* had enormous breasts, like there were no stages at all. It just *happened.*

By the time I reached sixth grade, my father started to get even more concerned about things that I did. He didn't want me to wear makeup, and when the other girls started to wear nylons my father was adamantly against it. "She's only in sixth grade! How can she wear nylons?" I did anyway, but he didn't like it, and I don't think he would have opposed it were it not for my breasts. He felt that I didn't need to look any older than I already did.

I couldn't *stand* having people look at me . . . *at all!* I *hated* being looked at on the street because I thought they were always looking at my breasts. Whenever I walked down the street all the men would look, and every look was a leer. I always felt vaguely ashamed, as though *I* was somehow responsible for creating their leers.

We lived in a city and there were always catcalls on the street—"Wow! What a pair!"—and that kind of stuff. If someone looked at me, I would either turn around or stare them down. I also developed a very mean sort of face. I'd scowl! When I got older, I began to yell back at the men. I'd scream, "Oh, shut up!" but still felt very bad when that happened.

By the time I got to high school I developed a lot of mannerisms that people called to my attention—shielding mannerisms. Whenever someone talked to me or looked at me I would somehow manage to have something in front of my chest. If I wasn't clutching my books, I'd be fooling around with my hair or my face. People would say to me, "Why are you always touching your face?" "Why are you always playing with your hair?"

I remember that when people mentioned these things to me, I was kind of angry about it and I thought, But they don't *understand!* I was pretty old by the time it occurred to me *why* I had these mannerisms—that I was trying to hide my breasts. I was about nineteen when I became conscious of it. By then things were very different—I didn't have those big breasts but I still had the mannerisms. I *still* do to some extent.

Because I was always trying to cover up, my shoulders became rounded. I never stood up straight—*ever!* In addition, I kept my shoulders raised up all the time. My bra straps were digging into my shoulders anyway, but when I kept my shoulders up it pulled on the straps even more. As a result of the pressure I got headaches. I had dents on my shoulders—worse than just dents, they were actual *sores!* I *still* have the dents, they haven't completely gone away. They're just deep enough so that a strap will never slip down. Actually that's pretty handy. (*Laughs.*)

I remember my breasts as being sort of long and skinny and coming down to my waist—that may or may not have been true. They seemed very big at the top, sort of tapering down like upside-down summer squashes. With clothes on, it was like having something so big in front of me that I couldn't see down past them. They felt like half a watermelon sitting horizontally across my chest—that kind of bulk. They threw me off balance so that I waddled from side to side, the way pregnant women walk.

●

As I got older, the attention my breasts got might've made me feel attractive or sexy, except by that time I had developed a curvature of the spine—supposedly from the weight of my breasts. One day my mother noticed that one of my hips was much higher than the other and that I was walking crooked. So we went to see the doctor and he said, "You better do something about it now or else you may not be able to walk when you get older."

I ended up having to wear a back brace. I got it the day that Kennedy was assassinated. I was eleven. I had to wear it for four years, from seventh grade until the beginning of eleventh. So around the whole time when other girls were noticing boys and stuff, I had it on. The alternative to a brace was spinal surgery, so everyone told me I was very lucky and I should be so *delighted* to have this. But I wasn't delighted at all. I hated it!

The brace was very noticeable—I couldn't conceal it. It was so big that it made my breasts . . . uh, not insignificant, but now, more attention was focused on the brace than on them. In fact that was the biggest reason I hated the brace. I hated being looked at *period!*

People didn't really know *why* I had the brace on—that it had *anything* to do with my breasts. God forbid! At first my brothers and sisters asked me some questions about it, but I would never answer them. No reference could be made to it because I would just clam up. I wouldn't talk to anyone who was so crass as to mention it, and that was pretty effective. (*Laughs.*) I wish now I could have been more open about it.

Naturally, it restricted my movement a lot. I couldn't bend from the waist or neck or hips without making major adjustments.

Since I couldn't move around very well I kept to myself and read books all the time. I didn't have much to do with kids my own age. I did get into a "mother" relationship with boys in my class—they would confide in me. I was like an older woman and they were like little brothers to me. I didn't date or make out with boys until much later, and by then I felt as if I'd missed the boat. I felt like I was older and it was too late. . . .

I've never heard the straight story about why my spine *really* curved. It was not a congenital thing. It just happened. They felt it was related in some way to my being so short with such enormous breasts that were supposedly weighing me down at such a young age when my body was trying to grow tall.

Do you think it was because of your breasts?

I'll tell you, it's something I've been very confused about. Either the brace was put on because my breasts were indeed pulling me over to one side, or else my spine curved in the process of growth for some unknown reason, unrelated to my breasts. The fact that my breasts were used as an excuse was perhaps more of a reflection of my parents' ideas about it. Somehow I always felt that that explanation was an outrage that was perpetrated on me. Intellectually I knew that the brace was a beneficial thing—I had to have it, blah, blah, blah . . . But emotionally I thought about it in terms of things that were being *done* to me!

Wearing that brace for four years was hell! I was fifteen before I got it off, three months before I had the operation for my breasts. . . .

●

Breast reduction surgery was my mother's idea. She was starting to think about it for herself, and by this time I was pretty disgusted with those big breasts. I was tired of all the trouble they caused me. At fifteen I was between a double D and an E cup.

As my mother presented it, the reason for having the operation was aesthetics—I would look better. When I didn't think that was a good enough reason, she started to refer to it as a health thing. The curvature of my spine had gotten better with the brace, but they were worried my back

was going to go bad again from the weight of my breasts. I suspected that my mother used my back as an excuse to convince me to have the operation. She might have believed that the operation was medically necessary, but it seemed to me that her concern was more for my appearance.

I'm not sure who wanted the operation more, me or my mother! At the time I wanted it—sort of. . . . I'd always wished that my breasts were smaller, and in that respect the operation seemed like a good idea, but for a lot of reasons I was ambivalent.

Because I knew that my mother was interested in having breast reduction surgery herself, I felt like a guinea pig. I would try it first and if it was okay, then she would go ahead and do it. I don't think she could really justify to herself having the operation, but if I had it, then it would somehow be okay for her to have it, too.

I ultimately had to make my own decision about the operation, but it took a long time. My mother said, "Whatever you decide. This is something we'll make available to you and you can have it if you want to." So I thought about it. Oddly, my thinking didn't go as far as the actual surgery. I was working on weekends in a hospital when I was fourteen, so surgery wasn't frightening to me. But I was still ambivalent. I didn't want to be the one to decide.

When I went to see the doctor, I was still trying to make up my mind if I really wanted to go through with it and I must say he didn't really deal with me very well psychologically. He took a lot of snapshots of my breasts, I guess to decide what he was going to cut and that kind of thing. That was horrible! I would just sit there and cringe! I'd pretend I wasn't there, that I was someplace else. I was *mortally embarrassed!*

The doctor told me about some things that might happen, like whether I'd be able to nurse my children if I wanted to. He said, "Probably sixty to forty percent you will be able to nurse and most likely more." I didn't have any response to that—I mean, what fifteen-year-old is already planning whether or not she'll nurse her kids? I was bashful that he'd even *say* it. Now, ten years later, I'm really worried that I won't be able to breast-feed because I'd like to.

And then he also said, "You might have some reduction of feeling in your breasts." I know it seems funny now, but I was *really* embarrassed about him saying that. (*Laughs.*) Another thing the doctor said was, "There might be a chance that you'll have some scarring." I guess I felt so bad about my breasts already that I thought,

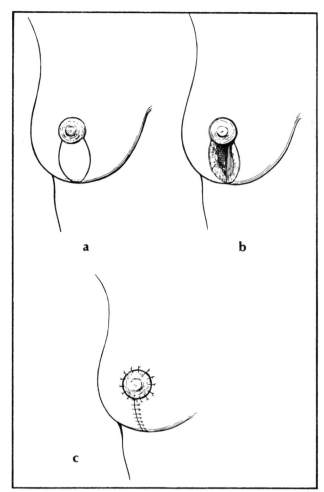

BREAST REDUCTION
In breast reduction, a keyhole-shaped flap of skin is cut (a), some tissue removed (b), and the nipple is reset on the smaller breast (c).

That's okay. I don't care. I don't care if I have scars. I don't care if I don't have any feeling. . . . What I really felt at the time was that it couldn't be worse than it already was. All I could think of was the end result, which seemed to be relatively good. But I wished that I could just wake up in the morning and they would be smaller—the idea of tampering with the body seemed somehow shameful and horrible.

As far as *how* small the doctor would make them, I really trusted him. It's weird to think of it now, but I had no idea of *what* he was going to do. *Nothing!* But I think the fact that the doctor mentioned all the bad things made me trust him. I felt that he wouldn't have mentioned the bad things if he wasn't trustworthy.

One important thing that he explained was *where* he was going to put the nipples—that's a big factor. He told me he was going to put the nipples "up here." He said, "A lot of people think that's really attractive." But I couldn't take it—it was all just too *sexual* for me to handle. I didn't want to hear about that. At fifteen, I wasn't relating to my breasts sexually or to myself as a sexual being. In fact, I denied my sexuality completely.

What made dealing with the doctor so unbearable was the fact that he was a man. I couldn't have a dialogue about my breasts with *him!* I just couldn't discuss it. It probably would have been a lot easier had the doctor been a woman.

Since talking to the doctor was so unbearable, why couldn't you talk to your mother?

I did to some extent, but my parents felt that *I* should be the one to decide. I always thought that was a cop-out, that they didn't want to take any responsibility for this terrible thing. I felt that they were throwing me to the lions by *making me* talk to the doctor, and that they didn't want to have any part of it. The whole decision had been thrust upon me and I didn't think that I really *could* decide. In the end, I felt that I *had to* do it.

●

After the operation I had some kind of allergic reaction to the anesthetic, so I was really sick for a while. In fact, I was unconscious in an oxygen tent—the works. When I came to, I had no idea what had happened. I just assumed it was the next morning. Well, it wasn't. It was *ten days later!* That scared me. Then I became conscious of being in *tremendous* pain.

It took a long time to overcome the horrors of the actual surgery, I guess 'cause I hadn't thought it through, or I couldn't think about it before the operation. There was no way I could have imagined what it was actually going to be like. Afterward, my breasts were completely black and blue, and for a couple of weeks I had horrible drains in the incisions. That really freaked me out more than anything.

I don't think my parents realized how horrified I was. They had been very frightened that I was going to die—that a chance had been taken with my life—and they felt very bad. My father said, "Of course, you got very sick—it was a serious operation. You just have to expect that. You know, they removed as much tissue as if you had had a whole breast removed." That concept horrified me! They removed about half of what I had. I know I weighed at least ten pounds less after the operation, partially of course from being sick, but *still!*

My mother was feeling particularly responsible

and guilty because I was so sick afterward. She wanted to be reassured so she constantly asked, "Well, aren't you glad now? Don't you feel better? Aren't you happy that I suggested it?" . . . for *years* after.

We didn't especially talk about the operation, though my mother would occasionally ask me what it was like. And I always thought that she wanted to know for herself. On some level I was suspicious of her motives for asking or for any display of concern, besides which I didn't want to talk about it either. From my own point of view, I was on the run. I didn't want to face the reality of what I'd just been through.

After some time passed, my mother wanted to see my breasts, but I didn't want to show them to her. I'd say, "I'll show you later. I'll show you another time. Not yet." So she'd say, "How come? Why don't you want to show them to me? Are you embarrassed?" But I felt it was just too much of an intrusion on me. When I finally did show my breasts to her, I remember her saying, "Oh, they really look nice, don't you think? Aren't you happy?" By this time it was quite awhile after the operation and I was pretty much healed by then. You see, she hadn't asked to see them right away, when they were still all black and blue and icky looking.

It took about three months for my breasts to heal. The scars took a lot longer. Once everything was completely healed, I remember looking at my breasts in the mirror and thinking they did look nice. I started to get compliments about the way I looked. People would say, "You look a lot thinner, you must have lost a lot of weight in the hospital." (*Laughs.*)

I went down to about a C cup. The doctor thought I probably would go down to a B as I got older, which I never did. That's okay, you know. (*Laughs.*) I never really cared about the particular size. I was only conscious of not having all *that* out in front of me anymore! So at first, when things got back to normal, I was really happy—my breasts looked pretty nice and when I went shopping I could actually fit into clothes.

Before the operation, my nipples were on the bottom so I never got much of a look at them. I saw them now for the first time. The scars I had were very small and the doctor told me they would go away, but that never happened. Later I was told that when I was older I could have the scars erased with plastic surgery, but I'm not sure I'm going to do that. Now I'm frightened of the surgery and I'm also afraid it won't be successful. I mean there's always a chance for that. They told

me I wouldn't have scars the first time around.

My parents didn't tell my brothers and sisters or *anybody* else, so as far as everyone was concerned, it was just an operation. We managed to keep the specifics a secret by saying it was a back operation, but I know that my brother knew something. He was very upset when my parents told him about my condition just after the operation. He came to the hospital when I was in the oxygen tent and was really shocked, and I think my parents told him I had some cysts removed or something.

Now, one of my sisters knows about the operation. I'm not sure about the others. She has big breasts and she's even shorter than I am, so my mother broached the subject with her, too. She wasn't having any problems with her spine or anything, but my mother always said, "Poor Toni, everything she puts on looks *terrible!* If she wasn't so busty, she would look really nice." My sister still wasn't as big as I was!

The fact that my sister's operation would be purely cosmetic reinforced my notion that my mother had hated my appearance and that was why she had wanted me to do it. I was *very* angry with her for the nasty remarks she made about my sister and especially for suggesting the operation to her. My mother told her that I had the operation, but she didn't tell her I almost *died!* She even asked me to talk to my sister because "she might be interested." At the time, I was eighteen and my sister was fifteen—the same age as I was when I had it done.

By then, I was already feeling regretful so I didn't want my sister to do it. I didn't tell her any of the really bad experiences about the actual operation and the pain. I just said that I wasn't sure that I would do it now. I told her that part of the reason was because I had scars and I felt funny about them. That was about as intimate as we got. Mostly we talked philosophically—whether it was ethical to change your body—and she said she didn't believe in doing that kind of thing.

The ethics of tampering with your body was a big factor for her. She was a vegetarian and had that sort of a bent, so for her, appearance was not a good enough reason to do it. I told her that I had it done because of my back, and that I had questions about it otherwise.

My sister thought about doing it for a while, but in the end she decided not to. Then I began to wish that I hadn't either. I respected her for accepting the way she was. I sort of felt that I had, you know, sold out. And I started thinking that I really shouldn't have done it. I should have stood up for myself. I should have resisted. She resisted, why didn't I?

It was around the time of this incident with my sister that my mother had *her* breasts done. She had always been very embarrassed about having such big breasts, and the fact that after she had her fourth and fifth child, her breasts became *really* big hadn't helped any.

The only thing my mother said to me about the operation was, "I've had so many children that my breasts are sagging terribly and that's why I'm having it." It sounded like a health-medical reason and I was surprised that she never mentioned that she'd *always* been unhappy about them, complaining that they were cumbersome and terrible. She didn't even take into consideration the fact that I almost died. No one even mentioned it! So she went ahead and did it, and as it turned out, she was extremely pleased with the results.

My mother's very pretty and youthful looking, and people sometimes remarked that she had a perfect figure. Before the operation, if that happened, my father would say stuff like, "That's what those big bosoms will do for ya!" I wonder if my father was sorry to see them go? . . .

●

I started getting socially active and going out with boys for the first time after my breasts were smaller. A year or two later at age seventeen, eighteen, I began petting. It was my last year of high school. It wasn't just because of the operation that it took me so long, it was also that I'd never done it before. I don't think I was even kissed until I was sixteen and a half, so petting was a new experience. Whatever anxiety I had about letting someone touch my breasts was plain sexual anxiety. I didn't like petting especially. I wasn't even aware of any feelings in my breasts. They were still numb from the operation. I'd think, Well, I'll just let him do this. It doesn't bother me, but it doesn't do anything for me either. It's nice—I like the fact that he wants to do it to me.

By that time my parents were more liberal, so they didn't bother me about going out. The only thing they warned me about was getting pregnant. There was no mention on my mother's part of how to deal with my scars in the event that a boy might see my breasts. Ironically, I was relatively calm about that. I thought that if it happened, well, I'd just explain it to him.

I'd worked out how to explain it before it ever came to that. I planned to say, "I had some breast surgery for cysts," because I didn't want to get into the whole complicated story. I figured that if I liked somebody enough to let him *see* my breasts, then I would say something to him beforehand. Sort of warn him. I felt that my breasts looked fairly nice, so I was not very anxious about being judged. In fact, I was so naive I was pretty confident.

In my first few petting experiences, the boy didn't see my breasts because it was *dark*. (*Laughs.*) The lights were off. The scars weren't too obvious and I'm pretty sure that he wasn't experienced or sensitive enough to feel them. (*Laughs.*) And anyway, he was too hot to notice.

The first boyfriends who saw my breasts said, "Whatever happened to you?" I would just answer, "I had breast surgery," and then I would *hate* them for asking. They were sixteen- and seventeen-year-old boys and they were shocked. Ten years later, I still can't stand it when someone asks, "Where did you get those scars?" I just don't want it to be a conversation topic.

When I was eighteen I had a long love affair. The first time I slept with him was one of those spontaneous, passionate things, and it was dark. He tore my shirt off, and I yelled, "*Wait!* I have to tell you something!" (*Laughs.*) So I told him that I'd had an operation because of my back problem. He didn't seem to mind especially. He wasn't that curious about it—he never pressed me for more details—but he did not like the scars, and eventually that came out.

He used my scars as a *weapon* against me. It wasn't a pleasant relationship at all. He had an-

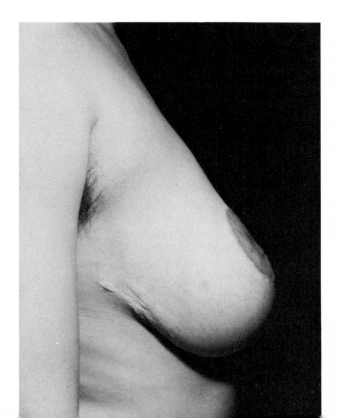

other woman on the side and when I found out, I started to make scenes about it. I would say, "How could you do this to me? Why her?" And he would say, "Well, she's better than you in this and better than you in that." Then he would say, "*And* she has nice breasts!!" He was really nasty. It made me feel terrible. He would *never* really fondle my breasts and I always wanted him to. I could never ask him to because I thought he didn't like my breasts. I just swallowed it all and I thought, You have to be understanding with him. It's not his fault—it's *mine,* never thinking, You son of a bitch!!! I felt terrible but not angry, just inadequate.

That's when I really regretted having the operation. I felt as if I would never be able to please anybody, that I would always be inadequate. My future was ruined! I'd never be able to get together with someone else. So I didn't leave him, and in fact we stayed together for over two years. He obviously didn't dislike me as much as he liked to make me believe. I felt as if I *had* to stay with him because no one else would want me. I don't know if that was a good enough reason for staying together so long, but it was a big factor for me. Finally, I broke up with him and ironically, *he* didn't want to split up.

I was so frightened of new encounters that for the next two years I was completely celibate. The thought of any sexual contact with a man was devastating. I was completely leveled by this last relationship—terrified of rejection.

Then I started to feel that it was *unfair* to have had the operation before I ever had any sex, before I had a sense of the importance of breasts to me or to men, before I had *any* idea what it was all about. If I were to consider having the operation now, I might not decide to do anything differently, but somehow it would be an entirely different thing.

At twenty-two, I got interested in men again. It was difficult at first. Because of my scars I wouldn't sleep with anyone as casually or spontaneously as I might wish—I didn't want to shock them. I remember kissing a guy and he had an erection. And then when he took my shirt off, he went soft and sort of muttered, "Oh, I'm sorry, I just can't go through with it" . . . and he *left!* In retrospect it's funny, but at the time it was a horrible experience for me. I felt so bad about it that from then on I would carefully explain in advance, often too much. I was overcompensating. I'd say, "You have to be prepared for this." But it never really turned anybody else off so completely.

These were basically short-term lovers—usually I slept with them only once. I either imagined that they recoiled when they saw my breasts or else it really happened. The men didn't touch them very much or look at them really, and that was probably more out of politeness or shyness because I had made such a big fuss about them. But at the time I was positive that it was because my breasts were so hideous.

At first I felt really bad about it, and then I began to think that it was *their* problem. A big factor in feeling that way was that I didn't really care about these guys at all. I began to view having sex therapeutically, as a prescription to overcome rejection. I'd been without sex for so long that I really wanted to get laid! And I liked the idea that men found me attractive enough to want to make love, even though I wasn't particularly attracted to them. So I made myself do it and wished that they wouldn't sleep over, that they'd go home afterward.

Another reason I preferred one-night stands was because I didn't want any deeper involvement where I'd have to talk about what had happened to my breasts. It was weird, but I would sooner have fucked somebody than tell him *that* personal a secret. It's as if fucking is less personal—at least it can be. There's just something about the operation that is so *personal.* . . . I don't know why.

At some point I got angry, and the anger was directed toward men in general. I went through a stage where I felt very, very sensitive to any slights from men, and I wouldn't *stand* for it. It wasn't a healthy self-acceptance, but rather a reactionary anger, and it turned to bitterness and rancor. It may have been the beginning of self-acceptance but I went pretty overboard.

Now I wouldn't *tolerate* a lover who didn't accept my breasts and like them anyway. Of course, I don't always react that rationally in those situations. I go up and down. I guess I'm mostly insecure about my breasts, even with my present lover who is really, really good about them. He asks how I feel about my breasts and he's very loving and gentle and all that kind of stuff. Over and over again he tells me, "You have really nice breasts. I love your breasts. I love to touch them. I love to kiss them" . . . blah, blah, blah. *Lists* of things that he loves about them! Even so, sometimes I wish that I didn't have these scars, and sometimes I wonder if he really *means* it, or if he is secretly wishing that I didn't have them either. I wish I could be certain—I want to know the truth.

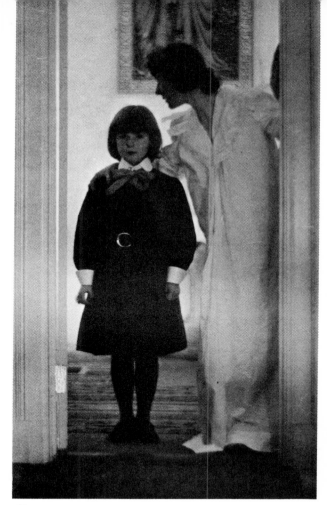

Illustration from card sent by Linda. "Blessed art thou among women," by Gertrude Käsebier

I was in therapy awhile back, and my therapist and I determined that because my mother is a very jealous person, her initiation of my breast reduction surgery was a . . . kind of castration. I was coming of age sexually and so she cut me off. Now I feel sort of silly saying that. I'm not sure if it's because my therapist was rather Freudian and I don't believe it . . . or I do and I'm just embarrassed to say it. (*Laughs.*)

I've thought of confronting my mother about her motives, but it would be too emotional for her. It would be pointless, unless I wanted to devastate her. I would never want to make her feel guilty . . . to make her pay for that.

She once said that I didn't have enough confidence in myself as a woman and that I didn't see myself as desirable, and then she said, "Maybe it's because of that trouble with your breasts." That's the only time she's ever referred to the operation: otherwise we absolutely never talk about it.

My mother's breasts look good. She has no scars at all. And I have to confess that in a way

I'm jealous. I feel it's unfair somehow. I know it's not her fault that hers came out better, but I do feel that I *need* them more! (*Laughs.*)

At the cancer detection center where I worked I got to see a lot of women's breasts, and then I began to feel more positive about mine. When I first started working there, seeing so many breasts was sort of stimulating. (*Laughs.*) I mean you never see breasts really. A large part of my job involved touching women's breasts in order to place them on the X-ray table. You had to place the breast just so, and I was very nervous. For the first day or two I didn't really want to touch these women's breasts. I was hung up about it, but that went away. After a while it became routine, even dull.

How would you describe your breasts now?

I'd say my breasts are average size. I don't know if that's true, but that's how I think of them because they were so big before. I have fairly large aureoles but really small nipples, which are quite high up compared with a lot of other women's. A lover once said to me that I have breasts like fried eggs, so I guess that's what they look like. (*Laughs.*) They're fairly firm. I'm only aware that I am sagging because the scars are getting wider. Most of my feelings about aging are connected with my scars getting bigger.

By now my breasts would probably be reaching my navel or *worse*. (*Laughs.*) So I'm glad I had the operation. However, I do wish I didn't have those scars. Apart from the scars I *think* I'm happy with their appearance.

Up until very recently my breasts weren't part of me, maybe because I didn't have *any* feeling in them. I couldn't define them spatially. It was hard to judge sometimes when I turned around. I would think I was going to bump into something and then I didn't! (*Laughs.*) After ten years I'm just starting to get acclimated to their size and that they are up here instead of out there. I've finally started to think of my breasts as being part of *me*.

Do you have any advice for women who are contemplating breast reduction surgery?

I would probably say, *"Don't do it!"* unless . . . (*sighs*) . . . unless you have curvature of the spine or something. I'm not sure that the result was so positive in my case. I still feel badly about the scars and about the fact that I don't have much feeling in my breasts . . . and about the rejections that I've experienced. Sometimes I feel like I've been having to adjust to my breasts *all my life!*

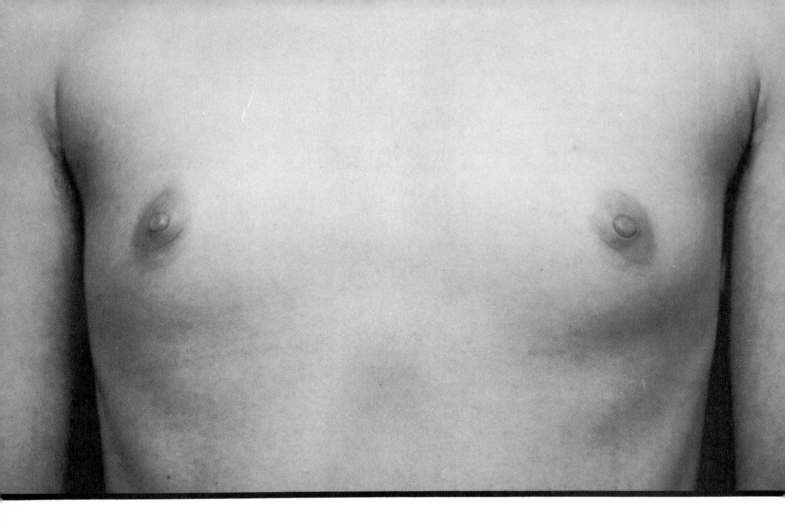

Doris

Age 24 · Raised in Brooklyn, N.Y. · Writer/Artist

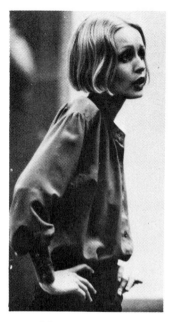

When someone asks me what I do for a living, I usually say I'm a topless waitress. I say it because it's impossible! Or if somebody makes a comment about my "condition," I'll usually explain it with, "Well, I used to be a topless go-go dancer but I shook it all away!" What I mean is that I'm so at home with my physical form that my circuits of righteousness and indignation have been blown. My response mechanisms—positive or negative—have been neutralized. I've exhausted the reactionary extremes of elation and depression. I've been through the ultimate or everything about it that I possibly can be confronted with. So it's gone! It's out of the way now.

I had to wait until Twiggy came to town before I was vindicated. (Laughs.) That was a big one—Twiggy's arrival on the cultural stage! But other than that, I wasn't considered a normal human being.

How did you consider yourself?

As a sportscaster! (Laughs.) Without breasts you couldn't participate in the dating game. I mean you're not playin', folks.

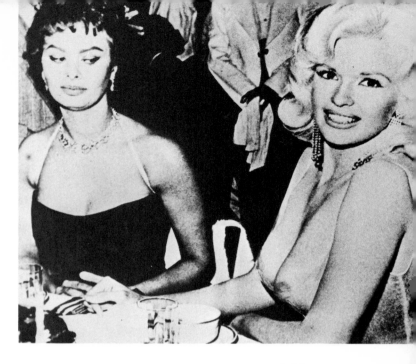

I just found out about a year ago that my mother didn't breast-feed me. I had come to realize that a baby is just so incredibly vulnerable, and that parents are responsible for every ounce of stimulus that the baby gets. So I asked her one day and she said, "No, I didn't want any part of that mess!"

I was born at a time when nobody knew about Leboyer birth methods. Instead, the media said, "Hey, maybe there's an easier way than the natural way, mothers. You don't have to have these milk stains on your silk blouses."

My mother was never very physical with me, except in a utilitarian way—like if I had clothing that had to be fixed. She wasn't a kisser and hugger. She's northern European—none of that overflowing tropical juice. I never remember touching or cuddling my mother's breasts as a child, but I do remember some of her friends doing that to me. Older people sometimes like to cuddle children, but I just didn't like the whole trip of a lady losing me in her breasts! (*Laughs.*) Maybe I just didn't like all that alien flesh. The physical relationship with my folks was so limited that when it came from strangers I really didn't understand it.

I think of my mother's breasts as normal—not a Rubens breast, not very robust, not like the ones in cartoons, but definitely breasts. I mean they're *there.* Yet I can remember comments about my mother's breasts being small because that was during the fifties and the ideal was *very* robust. Being small for the fifties ideal, I think she felt rather lacking because her posture was bent over, all closed up.

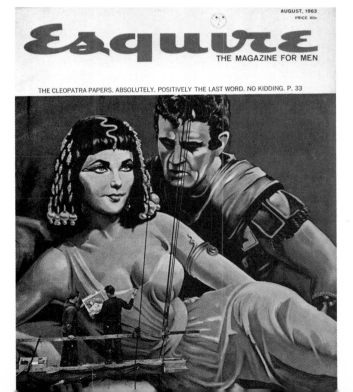

Whenever I thought about breasts as a child, it was because of conversation and media that I was exposed to, and then the more sexual aspect of them was usually stressed. I remember seeing a film with Anna Magnani and Burt Lancaster—I think it was *The Rose Tattoo.* She played an elderly woman and she had this cleavage. That's the thing I remember most—*cleavage! . . .* Ugghhh! The crack! (*Laughs.*) What's in there? What do they keep in there? The crack that goes beyond. . . .

And I remember that in movies women *always* put things into their cleavage. That seemed to be their tacit reference to the dark world that they knew all about. Women would hide money or whatever from their husbands . . . *down there!* (*Laughs.*) A super hiding place. I remember seeing that so many times in the movies, and my feeling was always that that part was bad. (*Laughs.*) It was so peculiar. What are these women *doing?*

I have compassion about cleavage now. I mean there's just a lot of things that happen to you if you have big breasts, okay? And you've got to have some sense of humor and awareness about it in order to cope. It's like being the rich kid on the block . . . a lot of stuff is gonna come at you and you're never gonna be sure why—if it's for you or your money . . . or your breasts.

As a kid I'd see women sticking stuff in their cleavage or notice a joke being made about a woman's breasts getting in the way of a table. And then maybe the woman would pick up her breasts and put them *on* the table to pander to masculine sensibilities. There just always seemed to be a negative cast to breasts and the way men related to them and even to the way women re-

59

lated to their own breasts.

I never saw breast-feeding going on; that would be considered obscene. So all I saw were the demeaning jokes and the images in magazines and movies—those big breasts just seemed to me like fat! *Flesh!*

I saw it all as a child—all this petty adult sex play bullshit—and I felt, I know those things go on but they're really ridiculous. I guess you gotta put up with them, but, oh, come on. Think of a new one. Why stop there? Why negate the limitless potential for majesty that's constantly presenting itself to you? I mean why just do your Groucho Marx imitations over and over again?

How old were you when your breasts began to develop?

They *never did!* I was somewhat pleased that I didn't have those vulnerable appendages. I was physically very active and just the idea of having weight there that would shift when I ran and moved was unattractive to me. I would hear women make comments about how they couldn't run because it hurt. And I thought, Ooooh, that's too bad. I think that another reason I accepted the way I was, was because people with big breasts obviously attracted attention.

I can remember a woman who had enormous breasts. She also had a very high-pitched, loud voice and the young boys on the block used to take thirty-ounce soda bottles and just hold them on their chests and they'd scream out her name real loud, imitating her voice. Now she was a woman in her forties and she had kids. I mean she was sacrosanct—a member of society.

Most of my memories of my breasts have to do with situations that made me feel a visceral reaction, as though some hand had pulled me back out of feeling good . . . *pffft!* . . . into embarrassment, *total embarrassment.* Embarrassment has always been a great factor in my life. How powerfully it can race through your body to the point where you just can't even *talk!!*

I have a vague memory of being very, very young and having my bathing suit on and really feeling like *hot stuff* 'cause I was going swimming, right? And I was walking down to the dock with my towel slung over me like a cape and suddenly somebody came along and screamed, "Hey, you! Don't you have your bathing suit on *backwards!*" Oh, God!! . . .

I can remember standing in the classroom one time when I was twelve, handing out a test paper. As I looked down at the names, two boys started giggling 'cause one was reaching forward with a pencil trying to touch me right *there.* It was some kind of ritual to try and touch a girl on her chest, but I didn't know how to react. I thought, I think I'm *supposed* to be embarrassed, right? I think that's considered a violation. I think I'm supposed to be incensed, indignant or something, but . . . so what? I don't understand. *(Laughs.)* What's going on, folks? It just blitzed by me like a lot of other adolescent psychodramas because it just didn't apply to me.

Bras never fit. Somebody gave me their daughter's clothes that she outgrew, and included with them were some tiny bras. So I tried one on. I even imitated my grandmother, bending over and lifting my nonexistent breasts into the bra! *(Motions slipping into a bra.)* Hey, 32A doesn't fit! Okay then, there's a 32AA. . . . Hey, you know, that doesn't fit either. They don't fit. "But you have to wear a bra!"—my mother. "What do you mean?"—me. "It's just done!" So I said to her, "Okay, fine," and I thought to myself that maybe it was to sop up sweat or something. I don't know. *(Laughs.)*

Those bras didn't have padding, they were just soft material. And they didn't make me *look* bigger, they were just *there.* That's why I didn't understand them. But my mother insisted that I just participate in the ritual of growing up and getting a bra.

I actually know of some women who brought their daughters to priests to ask them, "Do you think she can have her first bra yet?" The parent was really saying, "Do you think it's time for me to bestow this level of maturity upon my child? Do you think this child is responsible enough to handle *(sighs)* this explosive item?" Wow! And for the kids it was like, "I got it! I passed that one!" The first bra was a demonstration of power. It was a scalp! Amazing! And I'm sure the priests had a real good time with the whole scene.

I remember once in my teens I had a white outfit, and in order to make it fit, I was given a bra that was padded. I wore it once, *(laughs)* and I said to myself, Whooa! Hey, this is a *lie,* folks. This is just a great lie. I can't deal with it.

And bathing suits. They always, always, *always* had weird foam cups in them that kept me up in the water! I hated it. I'd complain, "I don't wanta wear this. It's *embarrassing,*" because if I wore one of those and went to swim on the first day of summer, the kids laughed like hell. And I felt, Wow, this is what they *gave me!!* It's not part of my body and it feels very "other" and it gets heavy when it's wet. It's just yeeech!!! The world was not making provisions for me.

As time went on I waited. I figured *something*

was supposed to happen because I took a couple of lateral glances and I couldn't help but notice that everybody was "busting out all over" and things were happening, but *nothing* was happening to *me*. I didn't know about physical growth. I didn't know what to expect. So, I figured, Hmmm? I wonder what's going on? (*Looks down at chest.*) When is that gonna happen? (*Pause.*) When *is that* gonna happen? This went on from age twelve to fourteen till I finally said to myself, Hey, I guess *nothing* is gonna happen? *Ohhh!!*

I come from a tight-assed Catholic family and I went to Catholic school for eight years. My folks obviously didn't give me too much information about what was going on there. They told me *nothing.* Even later, when it was obvious that I wasn't developing, they didn't say anything. They were embarrassed. They don't know how to deal with that subject even within themselves, so they weren't about to deal with it in me.

But I didn't really think that all this was too important because at some level I recognized "bare facticity." I mean a chair functions as a chair. Or if you're a cripple, you're not expected to get up and walk. Well, *I* don't have breasts!

My being "flat" was used to ostracize me. Girls would say all sorts of nasty things to me while walking home from school. It was like I was a pariah! It seemed like they were saying, "I'm having this experience. My body is going through these changes, and *you* . . . Ugh! You're just not makin' it!"

I remember breasts being used as some sort of hierarchical thing to establish your standing within the peer group, to attain power and influence within the group. It seems to work that way in terms of breast size. Your size definitely affects how you relate to your associates.

And I can remember that breasts were used by my peers as a sign of being a woman, of being "mature." Having breasts was some sort of signature—an ID—'cause everybody looked at comic books for their ideals of body proportion. So on the basis of that I can remember being morphologically alienated.* You failed! You aren't a woman! You aren't a *woman!*

In high school, every Friday there would be dancing in the gym. They'd open up the partition between the boys' and girls' sections, and the girls would walk, or rather *parade* past the boys for

* "Morphological" describes the form of a thing and is a very abstracted way of speaking which very literally describes Doris's "alienation"—a state of being withdrawn or isolated from the world.

inspection. We'd line up and march over. Meanwhile the boys would be sitting in the bleachers and as the girls walked by they were *assessed!* And the boys would say, "Hey, I want this one!" "I want that one!" "I don't want *that* one—that one doesn't have any *tits!*"

It was devastating! I remember so clearly the visceral flashes that went through me as if the wind had been knocked out of me—"Ooooh!"—and how my temperature changed. I just wanted to cringe—to *disappear!!* But you can't cringe in front of them, so I just kept on walking. That sort of morphological rejection simply put me on the sidelines. But I don't think I dealt with it in the best way I could because I completely ignored the social game. I wonder if I didn't take the lion's leap into the abyss . . . what that isolation really did to me?

I avoided social situations because whenever I went somewhere where kids were sitting around, the first comment I'd get was a tit joke. And I'd sit there and think, You're just showing me what a scab you are because you're not giving me the grace of recognition as an equal human being. Well, uh . . . how long is it gonna go on, folks? Would you like to have a *look?* Let's look at the stump, okay? . . . and now *what?* The majesty is gone, folks. I was forced to turn inward.

If one's whole process of being involves trying to develop one's faculties coherently, then to me it was much more worthwhile to write and draw and deal with the contents of my mind. Going into somebody's paneled basement and listening to records for five hours and making out with a boy could never equate with the majesty of creating my "spontaneous presence" . . . a splash on a page.

I didn't have any expectations of dating boys and petting, but that was okay because I really didn't want to be a piece of meat. I never wanted to get grabbed, *never!* I never wanted to be handled like that. The whole process of petting was just alien to me. It was all for somebody else. It was always a violation and never something for *me* because I knew the boys weren't considering me. Petting was like a treasure chest that the boys opened and they'd just ransack through you.

All through puberty I wrote about things in the world that I couldn't have, and they were physical things. I wrote that somewhere there must be people that don't behave like this—I knew it. The world couldn't possibly be just made up of animals.

If I really thought about it, I'd probably be immeasurably pissed that I had to spend so much time enduring various levels of alienation, rather than just being completely able to dismiss them and get on with life. I couldn't talk to *anybody!* I wasn't in a position to relate to people because they thought I was "strange."

I thought a lot about not being part of the gang. I'd say, "That's not my life." But it was sad because I was alone. Even though they were manifesting a particularly pernicious, disgusting level of being, they were still having a good time. And I still wanted to be with other people and belong to a group no matter how high or low a level it operated on. I wasn't having a good time. And the truth is, you really *need* people.

So how do you deal with that? What do you do? Do you sort of "get down and boogie" with the crowd? I just couldn't. Then I started to get these hints that I'd better learn how to reconcile my alienation or go crazy. So I saw that I had a couple of choices: I could either be a criminal or an artist.

If it had really been a choice at all, I probably wouldn't have been an artist. There's easier ways of living . . . nicer ways of living. But it's what I had to do, so I did it. Hopefully, I won't lose my demon and I'll keep doing it. Your demon is like your fire and your reason to keep going on. And whether you have breasts or not, well . . .

So I was rockin' and rollin' and gettin' bruised by my peer group. Because I was physically shaped a certain way, I found myself on the fringe, not really knowing how to link up with other people's lives, or whatever that process is by which people become friends.

I suppose, in a sense, the alienation really helped me out—in terms of funneling my energies away from the meatball and toward self-development. My prime concern became my work and my thoughts, and that was the barometer of everything. I tried not to let all the stuff outside . . . all the programming . . . touch me. So I pulled out of the world and back within myself.

●

What's interesting is what my experience with my breasts did to my posture. My chest just started to close up—really close up. I didn't even notice it happening to me. It's like something deep inside grabs you sternly and just *pulls* you back in, away from the world, hiding and protecting you. But when that happens you block energy in your chest, because you're closing up your heart center or heart chakra as it's known in Yoga. You really cut yourself off when that happens. It's *disastrous* what it does to you physically.

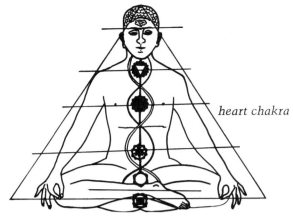

heart chakra

THE CHAKRA SYSTEM

Within that metaphorical way of viewing the body in terms of energy centers or chakras, your heart is your world connection and is related to the synthesis of emotional activities of the mind—in other words, what you feel. So fear, for example, is always experienced as a constriction, a tightness in the chest. My heart chakra just was pulled in away from the rejection—closed, hidden, and protected. In very fundamental ways I withdrew from the world.

I went around bent over long after puberty. That's how I faced the world. I carried that around with me for *years* until through yoga I started to learn about the body and what it really is.

It took me two years of yoga practice to physically open my chest up, to straighten out, and that was due to specific exercises I did. Your chest can structurally close and open, and the significance of that closing and opening has to do with self-esteem—how good you feel about yourself.

Before, my armpits used to perspire a tremendous amount from anxiety. I mean *tremendous*—just sort of like drip, drip. Not anymore! After I straightened out my body and opened my chest, that all fell away like a scab.

I know I haven't *really* opened my chest yet. Structurally I've opened it, but I haven't gotten the heart center really open and I haven't made it all alive yet. When your heart center is open and alive, you can feel the energy flowing through that part of the body. It's a beautiful feeling, like singing—the experience of your voice and its resonance within your chest. Singing opens your heart up and really connects you, and the vibrations are like a massage. When you're really quiet and relaxed, you can feel the energy flowing there, moving in and out with your breath, and if you're scared or tense, you feel that in there, too. It's so delicate. Now, with me that feeling only comes and goes.

Are your breasts sexually arousing?

Well, they're part of my body and, gee whiz,

they do all the things that contractile tissue does when it's touched. I like to think of the sexual interaction as an improvisational dance, and in that sense I don't have specific requests to my partners that they spend X amount of time stimulating that area. I might just find that someone touching my *elbow* might be enormously arousing under certain circumstances!

The last time I wore a bra was around age nineteen. I wore bras for a long time to disguise myself, until I became more enlightened and educated about the body and acknowledged what I'd instinctively known all along—that this contraption just wasn't necessary for me. Up until then the culture (and my mother) made me feel that it was *necessary,* that it was part of the protocol of being a young lady.

How have men related to your breasts?

It always seems very important for men to tell me they like my breasts so I don't feel inferior and insecure—it's *always* stressed—and that's just based on their assumption that *I* don't like 'em. But my attitude is, "Like 'em or not, folks, that's the way they are and *I* like 'em. My body's okay, really, and why are you in a space where you *think* you have to let me know I'm okay? I would be in a bad way if I were really dependent on your approval."

I just flashed on a relationship with a particular gentleman. After a certain period had elapsed he suddenly commented about what I had breast-wise, and I found myself having to say, "You'd better go out and get yourself a grown-up now," because of what he wanted and how he *expected* a "grown" woman to be formed. So no matter what you think you are, you're physically culture-bound. And no matter how much you think you've overcome things, the culture is always

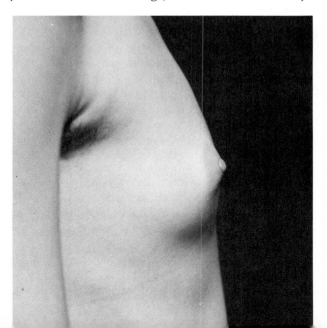

reinforcing everyone's preconditioned expectations. The culture is *always* there despite your efforts, it really is.

Most men react to me in an "androgynous" way, although I don't function androgynously by any means. I can remember a gentleman saying to me, "I don't mean to insult you, but it's just occurred to me that you're probably more used to sexual contact with women than you are with men." I had to explain to him that I didn't find women's bodies attractive sexually. I *am* a woman and I'm attracted to men.

With some men I've often felt as though I was fulfilling some sort of lecherous scoutmaster's homosexual fantasy. (*Laughs.*) No way, folks! I don't like being expected to be a man for another man just because they don't see breasts on me.

I was walking down the street the other day and there was a gentleman who was somewhat inebriated and in an advanced stage of disillusion . . . a bum, right? He was standing outside a bar and as I walked by he said, "Let me suck your cock," 'cause when some people see me they think I'm a fag. They scream at me out of cars, "*You Goddamn faggot!!*" (*Laughs.*) Or they'll peer over the grocery counter and say, "Can I help you, sir?" And then when they get a better look at me it's, "Oh, I'm so sorry, miss." (*Laughs.*) It seems like my gender is always in question.

You know, I remember when my breasts were just starting to change—becoming soft or *whatever* the change was—my father would come over and go, "What's *that!* (*imitates father laughing*). Hey, you're getting knockers!" (*Cringes.*) Now, not only do I not have knockers, but I'm twenty-four and I'm not married and don't have any children . . . and he's trying to figure out whether he's the father of an android or what?

I think my breasts will definitely change *if* I ever have a child. That's a whole other space that I don't entirely understand, being a mother, and I know that it would be a one hundred percent turnaround. If I went through that, I'd do it as organically as possible. I'd experience the whole thing—I'm talking about breast-feeding.

Some people have tried to lead me to believe that I wouldn't be competent—my breasts, that is. I can remember one man, in the middle of a conversation about nutrition, looking at my chest and saying, "How are *you* ever going to sustain a baby?"

Men's doubts aside, *I've* never been worried about that. I really have faith in my body, implicit one hundred percent faith that my body'll come across. Why not?

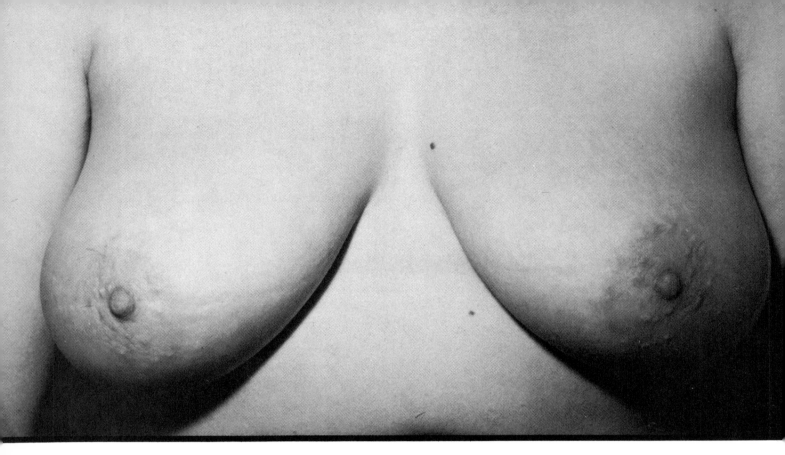

Jeanette

Age 27 • Raised in the Midwest • Artist/University Instructor

Our whole family didn't relate to sex and nudity very well. They didn't admit that people have "things" between their legs, or "things" which hang off the fronts of women or anything like that. Being a Quaker is really good in many ways, but we are raised so that we are ashamed of our bodies and we're not allowed to get pleasure from them. And, boy, I'm still battling around with that, too! I'm really pissed off that you can't just dismiss those ideas which are given to you at a very young age.

I was probably a very horny little girl just like everybody is, but I was told I wasn't supposed to look or touch. So I used to draw lots of dirty pictures—breasts and stuff—and then rip them up. And as an adolescent, I touched my body all the time and had lots of fantasies about my developing breasts. Even now, sometimes I catch myself thinking about sex and then telling myself that I am not "supposed" to think about that. So tits are on my mind a whole lot!

I was raised "by the book," my mother said, whichever book she was using at the time. I think I was breast-fed some, not a whole lot, that's for sure—probably not any longer than "the book" recommended. It wasn't fashionable to breast-feed after World War II. It was the birth of the nuclear age. There was a tremendous advance in technology—food was beginning to get more and more processed, TV was just beginning. It seemed as if progress and technology had saved the world and promised miracles if we molded our lives accordingly. So at the time it was "modern" to bottle-feed babies on a schedule, rather than breast-feed on demand, which was old-fashioned. In fact, the avant-garde way to raise babies then was in a Skinner box, invented by the psychologist B. F. Skinner.

My mother wanted only the best, so when I was born my parents built a Skinner box for me. It was a waist-high box measuring thirty-six by thirty-five by thirty-six; it had a glass door and a glass top and the baby didn't wear diapers because it was a temperature- and humidity-controlled environment. It was also soundproof, so the baby couldn't hear, but could see everything that was going on in the room.

Skinner's own daughter was raised in a Skinner box, dedicated scientist that he was. She was so pissed off when she found out that he'd experimented on her when she was a baby that she is presently suing him for malpractice. It seems that as a result of her upbringing she's turned into an artist. Coincidentally I am also an artist and I find it all very interesting. I sort of like the symmetry of it, the whole pattern that it sets up. From Skinner box to artist—I really relate to that. I think artists are not the happiest people individually. That Skinner box didn't do what it was supposed to—create healthy bodies and healthy minds. In fact, it created a bunch of little maladjusted bambinos right after World War II.

When my younger sister came along a few years later, my mother was much more relaxed. Maybe she raised my sister by another "book." But she didn't keep her in the box all the time. I resented the fact that I was raised in a much more constricted way. I am paying for all of that now—for not being fondled and breast-fed more and all that kind of stuff. I have what is known as an "oral fixation." I'm always chewing gum and biting my fingernails. Here I am being interviewed and I am chewing on ice cubes. (Laughs.)

Ironically, as modern as my whole family tried to be, they were not too public about nudity and things like that, particularly my mother. There are some people whose backbones are extremely straight and rigid—she is a rigid, upright person. She lacks a certain softness, and I don't think she's any softer now than she was then. You walk over to her and kiss her and it's like kissing an ironing board—she doesn't give and flow and I was conscious of that all the time.

As a child I couldn't touch her and I couldn't watch her crap, dress, or undress—no way! We weren't supposed to do any of that. If I did see my mother's breasts, it was always by accident, somehow inadvertently. When I walked in on her, although she never turned away, I had the feeling that she was cringing emotionally. She would stand there with her tits hanging out and face the music, 'cause she knew that was what an adult does when a child walks in the room. But she was embarrassed and you could just feel it coming through her skin, so there was a lot of pretense.

When I was about seven or eight I remember my mother wearing a purple sweater and I thought that her breasts were the most beautiful things in the world. I wanted to touch her tits but I didn't want her to know. So I put my arms around her neck so she couldn't get away, and then I shyly put my cheek up against her breasts. It was so taboo that I remember being extremely turned on. And then I became embarrassed by it! Of course, she knew why this horny little kid was doing these things, but she pretended not to.

I was never taught that breasts were "dirty," I just knew that they were taboo and that someday I would have to conceal them in a bra. For my mother it was not a topic that she could handle too well. She burst into tears when she tried to show me how to work my training bra. I couldn't figure out how to put it on. I got upset and she got very upset and burst into tears. She wasn't being sentimental; I think she just didn't want to have to admit that breasts are really there and you have to deal with them. Her sentiment wasn't that her daughter was getting a bra—wasn't that wonderful. It wasn't like marriage tears or anything; it was pure embarrassment. She was embarrassed to death!

When I started to get genuine tits, my mother was so embarrassed about having to buy proper underwear for a fifteen-year-old that she avoided it completely. She made me wear hers, which were Maidenform elastic "cross-your-heart" stuff. They got all wrinkly and puckery because there was nothing in the cups—I couldn't possibly fill the bill. When I got old enough and brave enough I bought my own.

As an adolescent I was a beanpole—flat-chested, string bean, straight up and down—and I wanted to have big breasts. At the time, I tried to gain weight because I knew that if I did, I could have big tits at the expense of having a little bit of fat elsewhere. I got tits on me quite late, but once it started it all happened within one year.

Hell, I was proud as punch about getting breasts. They represented something very symbolic about passing into an accepted condition—you're a real teenager now, not just a pseudoteenager. In the beginning I would kind of run around and let them jiggle up and down because it was such a neat new thing to be able to do. Later, when they got a little bit outsized, I got embarrassed about them.

I found it very difficult to remain an athlete because these tits were fairly heavy and they bobbed up and down and crashed into things, and I couldn't run as fast as I used to be able to. I was kind of shocked by this turn of events. I continued to play varsity hockey and lacrosse and all that kind of stuff, but I would go bumping up and down the field, and I would be very embarrassed about it. I began to be very conscious of my breasts as a liability. And it was so ironic. I had wanted them so badly and when I finally had them, I didn't know whether I liked them so much.

I was embarrassed by all the attention, too. Even though I had started my menstrual period years before, people didn't treat me differently until I got those outward symbols of having turned into a real adolescent. People only recognize that you are turning into a woman when you get breasts. Men started to treat me differently.

I remember being embarrassed when my father's friends came to visit. They looked at me and leered and oooh I'd be so *embarrassed!* I got touched some at parties by my father's rougher friends, but I would always laugh hysterically and brush it off and pretend that nothing happened.

For some reason, in high school, it's implied that if you have big tits you're fast. That's what I always felt from the boys—"Oh, she has big tits! Let's try her out and see if she's fast." Well, even though I had big knockers, I was a shy person, so what good did they do me? My body created expectations that I couldn't fulfill, and that was too bad because my tits didn't make me feel as good as I'd hoped they would. Everybody felt cheated!

I knew that I wasn't supposed to acknowledge my breasts and be proud of them, and yet people called attention to them, so what was I supposed to do? I *had* to be embarrassed about them! I was in a bind. I went full circle—first I was embarrassed because I didn't have breasts and then I was embarrassed because I did.

The first time I had a sexual experience with my breasts, I was making out in a car and the guy had his hand on my breast. I was still a virgin. He said dirty words like "breast" into my ear and I thought that was the horniest thing I had ever heard. I was so turned on I could hardly stand it. He was rubbing my nipple through the fabric of my dress and I loved it, but that's about as far as I would go.

When I was in college, before I was "devirginized," my boyfriend used to suck on my breast a lot, and he had dreams about getting milk. I think

he had trouble with his mother, but I liked it. He was obviously pleased with me—my body—and that felt good.

●

Men have described me as "big," but I would say that my breasts are just "full" and slightly pendulous, with large pink nipples. They look like soft, round forms instead of pointed or flat forms. If the *Playboy* kind of breast is high up, mine tend to hang a little bit.

I like to look at the women in the magazines and I always compare their bodies to mine—like, "Oh, look at her tits! I don't look anything like that." But there is no such thing as an ideal breast and I know that for a fact.

A few years ago I did some artwork, the object of which was to take something which can't be permutated and permutate it in a grid formation. The concept of "permutation" [presenting something in many variations] was real hot stuff in the art world at the time, and it seemed that all you had to do was take something and permutate it, and that was art. It was being done to *everything!* My purpose was to draw attention to the silliness of that concept.

I wanted to permutate something that was round, in contrast to the straight lines of the grid. So I chose breasts because they do come in many varied forms and shapes. Also, my choice had everything to do with the fact that breasts are taboo subjects. They are something you are not supposed to take photographs of and stick up on the wall in that kind of cold, permutated sense.

I intended the work to deal with art issues so I was really shocked to be labeled a "feminist artist" at the time. I thought I was taking the female form, something artists have always dealt with, and, by putting it into the male grid structure, I was drawing attention to how silly the idea of "permutation" was. Truthfully, I was more interested in pointing out the silliness of that idea than I was with the subject of breasts.

I sat in the cafeteria of the art school, and to almost any woman who went by I would say, "Hey, can I take a picture of your chest?" Or depending on the person, "of your breasts." I was pretty uptight about doing the project and fifty percent of the time I got a flat refusal. But the other fifty percent of the time, women said sure as if they had nothing better to do and were just having some coffee and why not? So we went next door to an office and they peeled their T-shirts off and *none* of them wore bras! I began to realize, as I was taking the photographs, that *I* was tied up

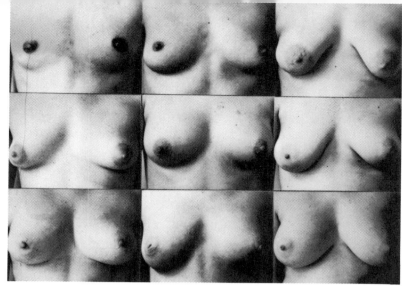

"Breast Forms Permutated"

real tight in a bra and no one else was. It came as a bit of a surprise that almost everybody else at the art achool was very loosey goosey. So I began to inspect myself as a result of working on this project.

The reason I was nervous about doing the project was because I was asking people to do something which they only do in front of lovers or mothers, and then I was recording it, which was worse. One of the women was extremely nervous. She was shaking so hard—visibly trembling—that I practically couldn't take her picture. As it turned out, she moved to New York and became a successful artist. Some of the women who were much less uptight about having their picture taken have flapped off to the country since, and are plowing fields and raising horses or something.

It seems like there were two sets of attitudes: a very laid-back attitude about your body—you're not ashamed of it, just hang it out, and if somebody wants to take a picture of it that's fine. And then a very, very uptight attitude. But I think that the woman who was so nervous didn't have a logical reason *why* she should refuse. She just couldn't think her way out of it fast enough and I got her before she could.

I photographed twenty-one breast "forms" and then selected nine. The "forms" ranged from flat-chested to pendulous across the top of the grid, down to conical, and catty-cornered to round-spherical, and the so-called "perfect set" was in the middle.

I thought the piece was fairly amusing. Interestingly enough, a lot of men liked it a whole lot, but for the wrong reasons. They thought that these were all the *possible* breast forms! They didn't get the joke. Female critics have understood the piece. It has had a very good reception. It's one of my works that has really succeeded and in fact, in that fiscal year, it was the only piece that I sold!

Whenever people saw it, they asked me who was who and I wouldn't say. And they also inevitably asked me which one I was and I'd say, "Why, the 'perfect set,' naturally." Of course, I wasn't! In the photograph that I made of myself, I was very surprised and upset to find that my tits were unequal—extremely unequal. I tried to fit mine into the grid, but they were so unusual that they didn't fit in this beautiful diagram of permutations I was making. There were conicals, sphericals, pendulous, but mine were just *lopsided!*

I think I have fairly good-looking breasts, but I think that the whole body affects your self-image. As an adolescent I was embarrassed about the combination of being long-legged and short-waisted and having big tits and square shoulders all at the same time. It seemed to be awfully cruel to be stuck with that body. That was a very big blow to me because I thought that your body had to look good for sex to be satisfying, and I felt I would never enjoy sex because I did *not* have a beautiful body!

For a long time I was into looking good in bed, and I thought that if your body wasn't perfect, your underwear might as well be. So I had very beautiful underwear—with underwiring and lace all over, really sexy and "battleshippy"—to make up for my "shortcomings." I just couldn't look beautiful on my own credits . . . *I* wasn't enough.

Nowadays I'm getting a lot more satisfaction out of my sex life since I found out that you can enjoy sex and not have a beautiful body. You can enjoy it a whole lot and look perfectly awful in *Playboy*/Hollywood terms. That's been a very satisfying adult experience for me. I'm relatively happy with my body because I'm old enough to appreciate it, but it didn't do me too much good when I was younger. It seems like these rewards come to you when it's too late to appreciate them!

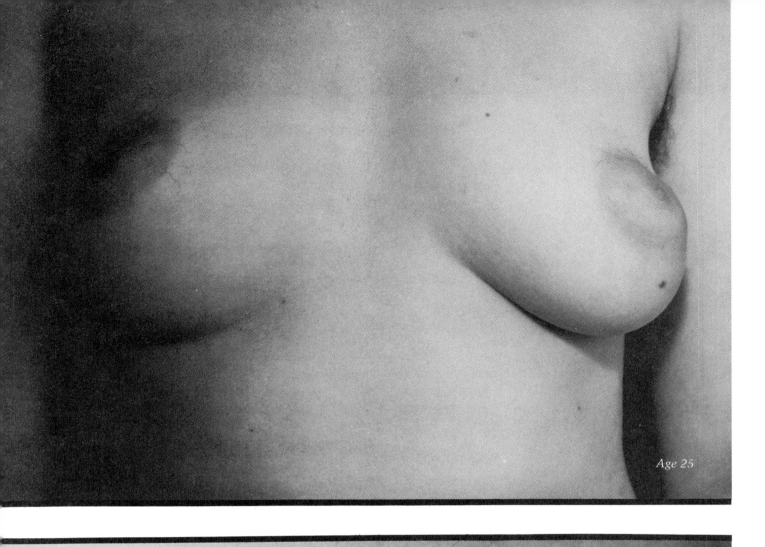

Age 25

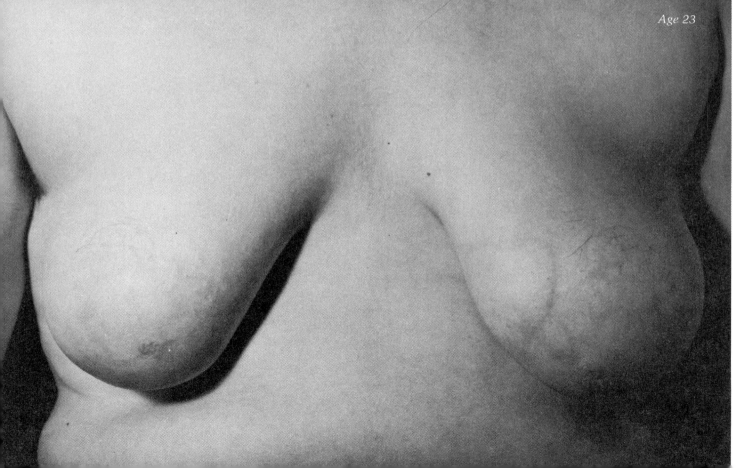

Age 23

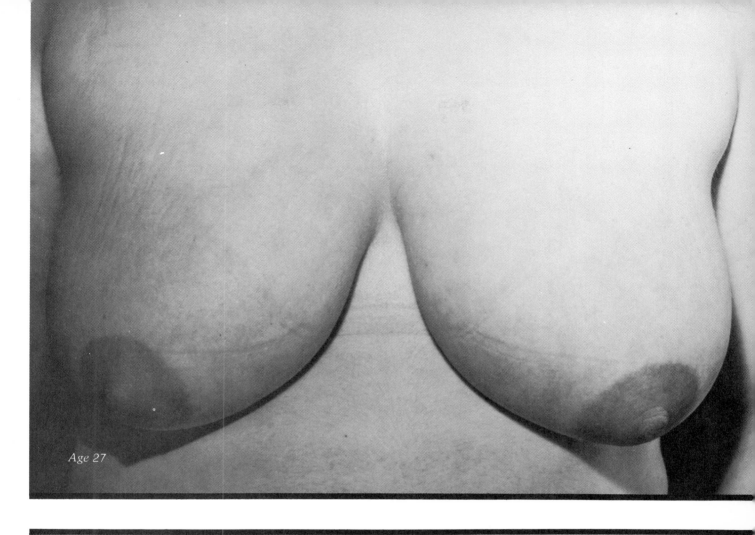

Age 27

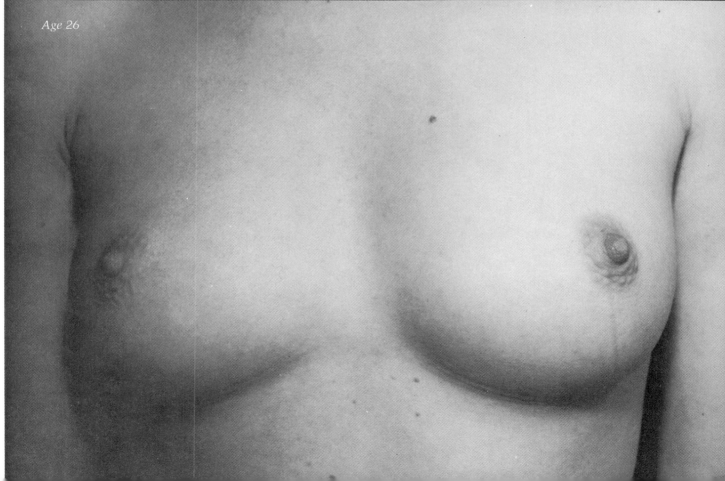

Age 26

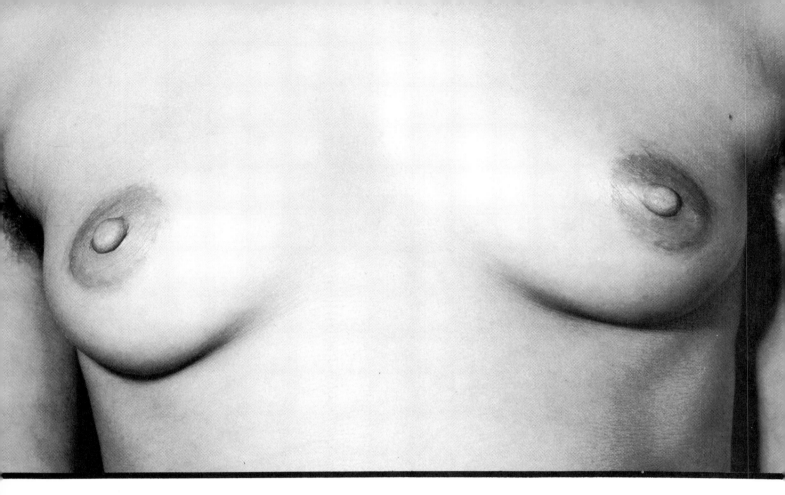

Terri

Age 26 • Raised on East Coast • Kindergarten Teacher

When you told me before that a really large percentage of women aren't turned on sexually by their breasts . . . well, that just made my day! Because I always thought that I was the only woman. It has always upset me that my breasts aren't a turn-on. Even my dearest friend in the world said to me, "Every woman I know gets turned on by her breasts," and I keep hearing it from everybody! I have a friend who comes just touching her breasts, and I just don't understand it.

My mother is really a crazy lady. I mean, she's the crazy lady from the Bronx tenement who's not quite normal. When we were growing up, she had a really nasty habit of going, "Oh, look at your titties growing today," and she'd grab them. It was horrendous! She'd do this in front of the neighbors—like she'd show us off. My mother is like an animal, a more instinctive kind of woman, and so to her it meant her young were growing up and it was neat. She was proud so she wanted to share it. But meanwhile, I'm thirteen and there's this woman! She would even do it to my friends.

I can't pinpoint the time when I grew breasts—it just feels like one day they weren't there and

the next day they were. I know their development was gradual but my memory of my breasts is *these.* (*Indicates by grabbing her breasts.*) They feel as if they've been like this forever.

I was always waiting in line for my sister's old bras which never fit. We didn't have a lot of money, so my mother would give me my sister's bras and then stuff them with cotton. It was horrendous!

My sister is the feminine one—she always played with laces and dolls and I was always in jeans. As our breasts started growing, she really got big ones, I mean they were huge, and it was obvious that I was never going to get there. My sister had an incredible figure and I was always like a stick. My mother was huge, too, so I became the family joke. I was my father's favorite and he always introduced me as his "son." I wanted to be big like everyone else in the family, so my father made jokes all the time like, "You must have been the last one in line when they were passing them out."

Wow! I just remembered a very heavy story. When I was ten or eleven years old I was still a tomboy, still wrestling around with the guys. Most of them were younger than me, except for one guy, my next-door neighbor, who was more like fifteen. One day . . . God, I remember it so clearly. I had on a yellow T-shirt; I remember that. It's so strange, I haven't thought of it in *years!* . . .

One day I was in the yard playing football or something and we were all in a tussle on the ground. I saw my neighbor coming toward the group, and you know how you can tell just what's going to happen sometimes? Well, somehow, I knew. Maybe because of the way he had been looking at me for the last couple of weeks. He sort of got in the group and there was a lot of tumbling around and suddenly his hands were *under* my T-shirt. The other guys were younger and wouldn't have even thought of that, but I sensed it was going to happen from the moment I saw him coming toward us. It was kind of psychic. I couldn't get away because all those little kids had me tackled on the ground and he was . . . Oh, he was horrible, really *horrible!!* (Terri cried hysterically as she remembered the trauma.) And I couldn't get away, I couldn't get away! . . .

●

Before I understood how a baby is made, I thought that if you let a guy touch your breast you got pregnant. I mean we all had our little myth. To me it was crazy, because everyone wanted to feel me up and I knew there was a huge taboo on that and I didn't get off on it anyway. So I used to wonder why it wasn't taboo for him to rub my *elbow.* Since touching my breast didn't feel any different from touching my elbow.

In my teens, my breasts were little things but I was content with them. I just wondered why they didn't get turned on. Now I sometimes wonder if the whole experience that I got all hysterical about before didn't do something to me . . . somehow change my breasts.

Over the years my breasts were always a joke. I had a routine when I was in college—I called one Fred and one John or Charlie or something (it's funny that I named them after men), and I was the most open person in the dorm. Everybody else just cleared their throats (*clears throat*) at the mention of sex, but I never felt that way. I had little dialogues in which my breasts talked to each other, and I painted faces over the nipples, so it was always a funny attitude. They were obviously *never* a sexual thing.

I like touching my breasts. They just feel real warm . . . real, real warm. I touch them all the time. I could sit here all night and touch them. It's not a sexual feeling; I don't feel like jerking off when I do it because my breasts have never been a real hot part of my sexual body.

Men I've gone out with used to pinch and squeeze my breasts and I hated it. I wondered how those son of a bitches would like it if I did that to their cock! I got so pissed!

A lot of men were turned off by the fact that I would push their hand away from my breast because it didn't do much for me. But the man I'm with now thinks they're great—he thinks they're aesthetic—and we just blend together and everything about my breasts is okay with him.

The first night I met him he did something that nobody else had ever done. He was sitting behind me and there were candles and it was all very romantic, and we were reading a pornographic novel together out loud. . . . Then he slipped his hand under my shirt from behind and just touched the outer rim of my breast very, very gently . . . and that was a totally new sensation to me. No one had ever done that, *ever!* He's a very soft man . . . and I just fell in love.

●

Lately, since I am thinking of having a baby, my breasts have changed. They change depending on what I'm going through in my life. It's as if they feel excited, "Oh, we're going to get to do it now!" They're probably gonna get big. When I'm pregnant my whole body is going to grow and change.

Whenever I look at nursing mothers' breasts I envy them. It's a whole new experience. There is no question about nursing—how can there be? I was breast-fed and it has always instinctively felt right to me. After breast-feeding, I think I'm going to dig my breasts a whole lot more. I think I am going to have a whole new relationship with them and I think it's going to be a good one.

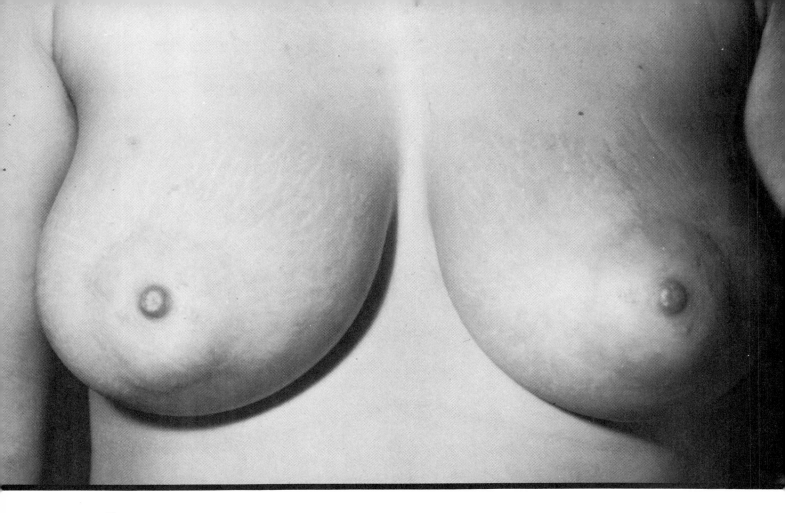

Susan

Age 27 • Raised in New Jersey • Writer/Dancer (Topless)

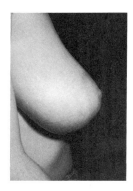

A lot of people think that women who dance topless are victims, and that may be true sometimes, but personally I've found it to be a very positive experience. Of course, it depends on how you feel about yourself and what kind of consciousness you bring to it. But people always impose their judgments and you have to be careful. No matter how liberating dancing is for you, if enough people tell you over and over again that you're being a "victim" . . . Well, it kinda gets confusing.

When I was a little girl, I used to *love* to watch my mother powder under her breasts. (*Laughs.*) I think breasts are an incredible "construction"! That they're made the way they are. They really are lovely. I can see how men get so involved with them, plus all these "mother" things about them. They are really quite *amazing!*

I really liked my breasts when they happened, and I thought they were decorative. That's how I relate to mine even *now.* I loved that they were growing! I looked at them *every* night . . . sometimes *twice!* I would look at them *all the time!* And I could see changes from week to week. I even told my father about them. He said, "That's wonderful! What a big girl you're getting to be. You look beautiful."

I was amazed by everybody else's breasts, too. I remember there was a black girl who lived up the street and she had breasts like *cones!* They were wonderful looking, but honestly, I didn't think so then. I thought they were strange and kind of sterile looking—they were so sharply defined! My mother's and my grandmother's seemed cozier, sort of mushing together. And I couldn't believe that *that* was a breast and *that* was also a breast. I used to wonder how come there was such a *difference.*

I have to admit that I touched my breasts a lot while they were growing. I felt the shape of them . . . the outline . . . the nipples. I liked to feel where my body went out and then in. I wanted to have big breasts and I wanted them to be round, and I wanted my body to be all curvy.

When I got dressed, my grandmother would say things to me like, "Oh, you make a nice line on the dress—that's a good line. You're very lucky!"

At the time my breasts were growing, I thought they were the most beautiful part of me 'cause I *hated* my face. I would sit and stare at my breasts for *hours* in the mirror, and at the same time I felt guilty that I was getting such a *kick* out of them.

It was okay for *me* to like my breasts a lot, but I didn't know how to handle the fact that boys liked them. They'd look straight at them.

I used my breasts as an excuse to keep boys

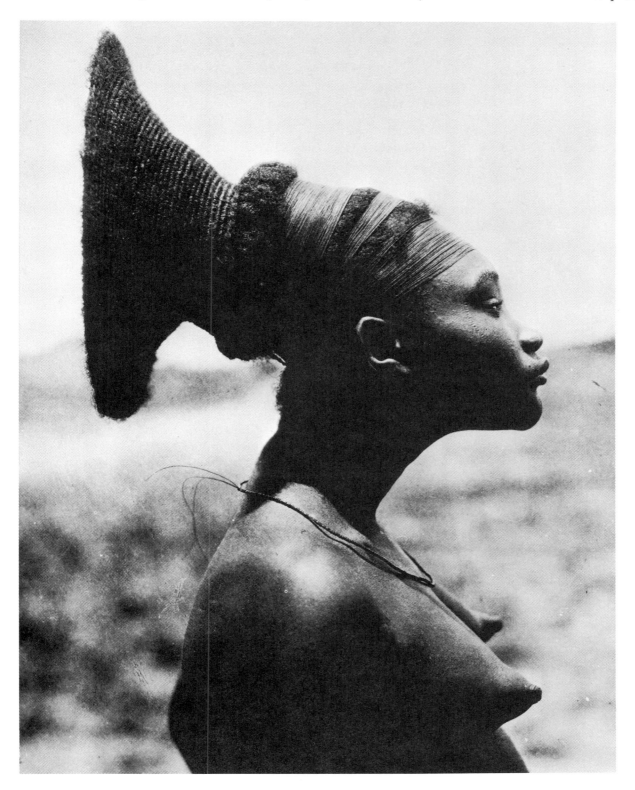

away. I thought to myself that they just wanted to be with me to touch *them.* Somehow it was worse and low and *carnal,* and it made me a shitty tramp. So my breasts made me very uptight and self-conscious with boys.

In junior high school I got an award for having the best figure. (*Laughs.*) At the same time, I had braces on my teeth and I felt really *ugly.* So I felt, why don't I have an angelic face to go along with my body to justify all this attention in some higher light? Since by *body* won that award, that was somehow embarrassing. It was not my face, which wouldn't have embarrassed me if it had been unusually attractive. It's silly but it bothers me to this day that the principal of my junior high school remembers me mainly because I won that award. My great achievement! (*Laughs.*)

I guess I asked for it somehow. My self-image was very tied up in my body, and yet I was terribly ambivalent about it. I liked my body but I didn't like *other* people liking it. See, I didn't know if I liked anything else about me, but I knew my body was good! I sort of felt that at least I have *this* to hold on to.

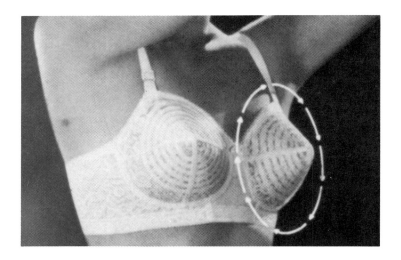

For a while when I was a teenager I wore Hollywood Vasserette bras with the circular stitching—the kind that come in thirty-two colors and make breasts pointy and high. So my mother would come around and push them *down,* which

I felt was a hostile act. I felt that I was being negated.

Anything I put on looked very sexy, just because of the kind of body I had. But my mother was trying not to see that. Whatever I wore she'd say that it looked too old for me.

I always felt I was being *cheated.* My mother tried to cover my breasts up, telling me it was more ladylike. She wouldn't even let me wear two-piece bathing suits because she felt my breasts were too . . . you know. And I thought, Why should other girls go around wearing little flimsy tops and I can't? Well, too fucking bad if it causes a sensation. It's *my* body—I can't change it. I have large breasts and I'm gonna dig 'em!

I was a romantic teenager. Sometimes I thought I was being very nurturing to a guy I was with, because I had large breasts and could give them to him as a gift. There was one time I actually let a guy touch my breast and I really remember it vividly. It was an *incredible* feeling! It sort of made my stomach contract. It just went all through me and I *loved* it.

It could have become a habit after that, but it didn't happen much. A lot of times I wouldn't let guys touch my breasts because I thought they were just with me because they wanted to touch my breasts. I was ambivalent, so I wouldn't let myself get into the fact that *I* liked it, too.

Now I get some nice feelings from my breasts, but not as much as I once got. I really like it when the nipples are nibbled and licked . . . and I like the whole breast licked.

●

For a while I dressed to hide myself like my mother wanted me to. My whole attitude was to wear loose things that looked fine, and then when I got undressed a man would say, "Wow! I never knew you had *that* kind of body." I didn't like having my body as the basic attraction, never have. I was afraid that it would get in the way of me being related to as a human being. But worrying about it just made me defiant. I realized that wearing smocks negated that voluptuous, womanly part of me. So I started dressing differently, more to reveal my body and my breasts. I wore sheer, clinging things—I really got into it.

One time I went to a bar with the guy I was seeing and I wore a gray chiffon dress. It was pretty transparent, but this was a loose place and a lot of friends were there. I felt good, like this is my body! And as I walked through the crowd to the back, everybody looked at my breasts. So my friend said to me, "You don't need to do *that* to get attention." He couldn't quite get the idea

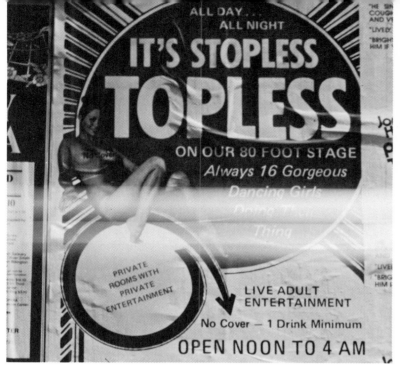

Detail from sidewalk billboard

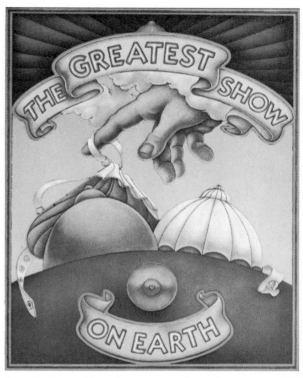

Illustration from National Lampoon

through his head that maybe, just maybe, I thought it was a great *freedom* to be *able* to do that.

I have had to deal with similar misunderstandings when I dance topless—*my* feelings about what I'm doing and *other* people's reactions. You know, just because you act certain ways, people objectify you. They figure you're acting out of their reality rather than out of your own, which might be completely different.

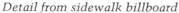

I wasn't attracted to topless dancing at first. (*Laughs.*) I was studying—taking dance classes, writing poetry, the whole bit. A friend of mine told me that she was dancing topless and she was gonna make a thousand dollars really quickly, and why didn't I try doing it? I thought, Are you kidding?! I couldn't do *that!* That's like a fantasy. That happens in movies. I always thought of myself as more serious. I couldn't see myself up on a stage with no top on.

Well, a few weeks later when I was still broke, she said the same thing to me, so I went to see the owner of the club. I danced *once* and he fired me immediately! (*Laughs.*) He said something like, "Honey, you're just not cut out for this. You should go back to school." I was the *only* one he ever fired. Well, that bothered me a little and then I thought, Wait a minute—I *still* need money! So I pleaded with him. His biggest complaint was that I didn't move enough.

Actually, I didn't move at all. My eyes were

practically closed. I couldn't bear it! I thought, What am I doing in this role? It seemed so strange. Even though I had spent a great deal of my adolescence looking at my body, when it came time to exhibit myself, I went, "Me? I can't do *this!*" And I was very frightened and *rigid* like a statue.

I kept thinking, What am I doing here taking off my shirt and dancing in front of a bunch of strange men? My breasts are making me money?! I just take off my shirt and make money?! (*Laughs.*) What is this? It just seemed so very, *very weird!* I mean there were people coming into a place to have a few drinks, but mainly to watch my breasts being *exposed! This* was a form of entertainment? To watch *them?*

Pretty quickly, though, my attitude changed. Once the shyness left I felt fine about it. It was like—"You guys wanta sit here and pay money to see 'em? *Great! '*Cause I need the money!"

The size of your breasts always determined how many bookings you got. There are a lot of dancers whose agents will say, "Oh, your breasts are little—have silicone," and they just *do it.* I think it's so weird. Why would anybody want to do a thing like that? Couldn't they get into the fact that they're really nice the way they are? I've seen some bad silicone jobs, too. I've seen woman mutilate themselves for that image in the movies and magazines.

The first dancer I met had beautiful, small, lovely-shaped breasts. Then she had silicone shots and got great, big, beautifully shaped

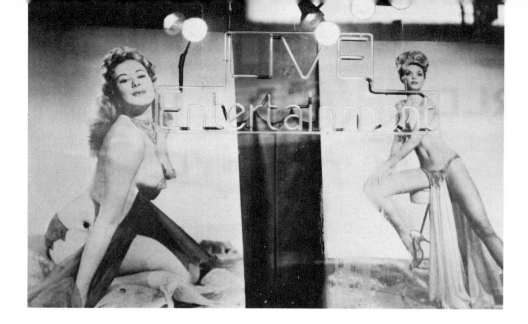

breasts, but they were hard like rocks—they weren't like breasts at all.

I've used all different kinds of pasties. There were kinds with sequins, and the beaded ones with the tassels. I've sometimes made pasties out of live flowers because that gives you a feeling that you're one with nature, and it's very nice to augment something that's natural *with* nature. In some places you have to use pasties by law . . . and if you didn't *have* to, that meant, "We want to see *more.*"

It's strange. Sometimes when I wore pasties, men would say, "Hey, that's not *topless!*" So I said, "What do you mean—it's not topless? What the hell do you think *that* is," and give my breasts a squeeze. Weird—if your nipples don't show, they think you're covered.

I was once dancing in a place where they didn't want us to wear pasties, but we had to completely opaque out the nipples with some kind of makeup. I remember catching a glimpse of myself in a mirror. There I was with a breast-shaped breast, but no nipple—it was all one flat color—and that was the most *bizarre* thing. *That* freaked me out worse than bras or pasties or anything else. It was the *official* regulation of that city. And they thought *I* was weird dancing topless?

Some of the other dancers let people touch them—they sell them a "feel" of their breasts. Or they tease and play with the guys who are really shy, the ones who aren't likely to cause trouble because that would give everybody else a laugh. The women poke their breasts in the men's eyes or shake their breasts at them and try to embarrass them or make them show eagerness.

I was never *that* raunchy, but if I was dancing with pasties which had tassels I would do tricks. I would make my breasts move independently of each other, turning them in different directions and reversing the directions.

After a while I tried to downplay my breasts because I was afraid that too much jiggling would encourage them to fall. Besides, my breasts hurt after shaking them around so much. I became very concerned about protecting my breasts and not doing anything that would damage the muscle or tissue. So I studied some belly dancing, because I was interested in the stylization of the dance. I worked out a system so that my breasts stayed in one place and the rest of my body . . . *everything* around them . . . did the moving. From then on, while I was dancing topless, I was supercareful. For every moment of going without a bra, I'd do exercises to make up for it.

I took a lot of pride in my dancing. I became incredibly ladylike in all my dance acts, and so unraunchy that it was amazing. People would give me money and say, "I'm doing this because you have *class.*" (*Laughs.*)

Sometimes I would touch my breasts in a "Penthousey" way as a spontaneous response to what was happening between me and the audience. As a performer, that interaction was very important to me.

Occasionally, I'd dance in a go-go cage with bars on it, and I worked up a bit where I would dance with a bar between my breasts. The crowd *really* went for that—their eyes popped out of their heads! And they just loved it if I picked up my breast and pretended I was sucking my nipple. The men would literally groan, kind of egging me on. There was tremendous communication then between the stage and the audience—very intense. I could literally feel the temperature in the place *rise.* I really was in control . . . and they loved it. Then at a certain moment, they'd throw *money.* It was like an automatic reaction—it seemed almost Pavlovian! (*Laughs.*)

Excerpt from article, "I'll Cry Tomorrow But I'll Strip Tonight," by Victoria Hodgetts (a journalist who tried burlesque):

Do you ever feel demeaned by this?
"No I don't feel that. . . . The only thing that messes up the flow is if you start to *care* about the audience and what they think of you. When you are tuned in though, when you see it from a high perspective—then you see that women are created like Venus Flytraps. They're supposed to attract men. So when the energies are free-flowing and it is supposed to be a sexual turn-on, then you get the energy *back*—you are connecting."

_____

When I'm feeling good, I'm a pretty spiritual and adventurous person, and so at those times I felt as if the dancing was a way to raise my consciousness . . . and *their* consciousness, too. It's like belly dancing—once it was a sacred dance with lots of meanings. Well that's kind of what I wanted to do. I wanted to communicate men's *projected* fantasy back to them . . . plus my own narcissism and freedom, you know, the fact that I *liked* doing it and that I considered it an art form. It was a performance using really "bare" props to communicate this pinup fantasy or archetype theatrically.

And when I danced, I assumed that the men knew it was a fantasy, too. I never doubted it for a moment. I guess I was naive. It was a rude awakening to realize that some people actually thought about women in that way. It was really a shock. Like who was exploiting who, you know?

The only reason I could dance topless before was because I had an incredibly strong sense of myself, and to part of me this topless dancing really was a big joke.

But then I talked to the men at the bars, and they told me how they felt about their wives. A lot of them were working class and they'd say, "I just keep her around to take care of the kid. I'm being nice to her." They couldn't understand that maybe their wives had an identity of their own— they just *couldn't* understand that. And that woke me up. I thought, This is *amazing.* I can't believe it! *They* really *believe* this fantasy—they think it's reality. For a long time that confused me about *what* I was actually doing.

_____

Once you get it in your head that you might strip, all the moral questions fall away. (Is this sexist? Is this exploiting women? Is this exploiting men?) Instead you worry about whether your stretch marks will show. Are you too old? Are you too fat? . . . And [I had] a fear that on the one hand I would not be able to turn them on, and on the other hand that I would. That I would find them drooling, animal, faintly contemptible and disgusting.

—Victoria Hodgetts

_____

Despite my ambivalence about it, topless dancing was an incredibly liberating experience for me—just one myth after another exploded. There's so much camaraderie between the women, and not because we were all banding together as "victims." It's that we just keep being amazed that these guys *pay* to see our breasts.

When I was dancing and still feeling good and proud about it, before I began to question it, I really wanted *other* women to see the *performance* of it and that it's not just *me.* I wanted women to pick up on the *celebration* that was happening there. I thought it would be very consciousness-raising and for some friends of mine it was.

_____

The object of the game is to get so in touch with your own seductive energies, with all your demon forces, all your power, that your own 20-minute statement is a pure and perfect statement of yourself. . . .
On a whim I took along a brown paper grocery bag stuffed with foam-rubber eggs and breasts that I just happened to have on hand. (In my militant Feminist artist days I once did a kitchen for a place called Womanhouse which was all flesh-colored—ceilings, walls, and floors—and which was dotted with foam-rubber fried eggs gradually metamorphosing into milk-filled breasts. There was a certain irony in my creations serving me equally well as Feminist or Stripper; this pleased me very much.)
. . . And then the music started. I came on. . . . I began to empty out my shopping bag. The men all waited. An egg. A fried egg. A fried egg with a pink yolk with a nipple! And then a breast! And more breasts! This was fun. The music played. I took off my coat. I danced. I tried on one breast, then another, a child out playing with her mother's falsie. I threw the breasts out to the audience. . . . They were very pleased.
And then slowly I did my strip. . . . And it was not like I expected—nothing like that at all. I rather enjoyed the dancing naked. I didn't really mind showing them my body (at swimming pools I often strip without compunction; ironic that there men should have to pay for what you get for free in all the backyards of Beverly Hills and Hollywood.). And the men were not contemptible. The men were . . . *sweet!* I had expected that they would save the foam rubber breasts for souvenirs, but they dutifully returned every one to the causeway, like good little mother's boys. One man slipped a dollar tip surreptitiously beneath one tit!

—Victoria Hodgetts

_____

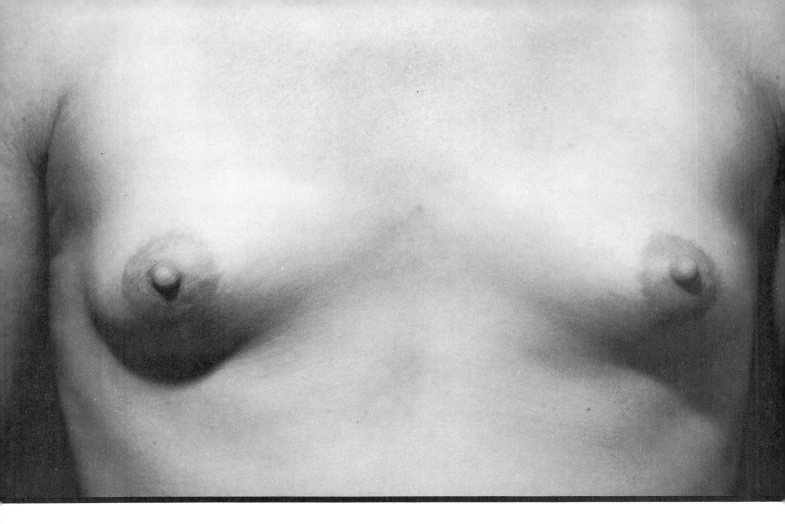

Alice
Age 26 • Raised in Pittsburgh, Pa. • Dental Assistant

My breasts are small and firm—big on nipples, small on breast. Sometimes I think they're beautiful and sometimes I think they're ugly. I like them least when they're warm and puffy because then the nipple protrudes much more—it's definitely out of proportion to the breast. So when they're cold and tight, my breasts are much more beautiful to me. I feel that my nipples dominate my breasts.

My breasts seem to me to be the part of my body that is the most out of proportion. When I took the pill, they were slightly fuller and seemed more in proportion. I have a small frame, but a big waist and big hips, so that when it comes to fitting clothes, it's always the breast that needs to be altered. Ready-to-wear fashion certainly dictates what the ideal size breasts ought to be . . . which just isn't fair. If I get something that fits me in the waist and hips, then it's too big in the breast. Or if I get it so the breast fits, then the waist has to be let out. (sighs) You begin to feel like you don't fit in! (Laughs.)

When I was younger I always wanted to be larger. It's something that I still feel sometimes. Even now, I wouldn't mind being larger, but I'd never try to change them because it's only a fantasy. It's easy to want something, but to pursue it? That's another matter.

My mother's breasts were generally hidden. As a child, in the few instances when I did see her breasts, which I remember vividly, I was surprised that she was so small. Her breasts were small compared to my conception of what breasts *were* according to my brother's magazines.

I also saw my neighbor's breasts. I mean some of my girlfriends' mothers were much more open about their bodies—one mother in particular. This woman had back problems, so she spent a lot of time in her bed, flat on her back. And sometimes when I'd walk in, she'd be nude on her bed with a sunlamp on or something. In fact, I do remember from a very early age that her breasts were much bigger than my mother's. My mother's bras were padded, so I had the sense that she was lacking.

Did you know why women had breasts?

Sure, I knew they were for milk. I saw a neighbor nursing, but it was like all other dirty things that you caught a glimpse of. You weren't supposed to take advantage of that glimpse and *watch,* or it would be taken away from you—you just take that glimpse and file it away! It was a privilege, more or less, to be *allowed* to see such a thing, and I understood it to be an "adult" thing . . . a "dirty" thing.

As I grew up, my friends and I were vaguely informed that we were going through changes that would affect us and we were going to have breasts and that we would then be more responsible and grown-up—everything went together. I was feeling very anxious at the time, and very eager to start becoming what every child wants to become—you know, "grown-up." Of course, I was intrigued by the idea of getting breasts, waiting for them to grow, watching them day by day.

What was most important to me was that while I was lying down in the bathtub my breasts would stick up highest. I remember lathering my chest and drawing designs on it—like a vest with buttons and buttonholes—because that was the flattest surface for artistic work in the bathtub, right? I would go under the water and when I'd come up, year after year, I would watch and wait for the time that my nipples would be the first thing to break the surface of the water. (*Pause.*) And *it never happened!* I was thirteen when they started.

As I was developing, my uncle was constantly feeling my back to determine whether or not there was a bra strap there yet. I was just as anxious to have that bra there as he was. I didn't resent him doing *that,* though he took much greater liberties at other times.

Wearing a bra was something I wanted to do very much—I looked forward to it for many years. My mother denied me a bra—she refused to recognize my going through puberty, and I didn't have any money, so I had to *steal* a bra. I *shoplifted* my first bra! There was only one store where I could find one that was small enough—it was in a small-town five-and-ten. It was a 30 double or triple A!

I didn't get caught shoplifting, but when my mother first saw me wearing this bra she went into hysterics because she thought it was so funny, so ridiculous. She was reacting to the fact that I thought I *needed* a bra. I had such tiny little breasts! She was laughing so hard . . . but I can only remember the humiliation I went through. When I finally had the breasts to fill the cups of the bra, I was very proud of myself. (*Laughs.*)

From age fourteen on I started letting boys feel my breasts all the time! The first time was just groping in the dark, more or less, along with necking. Of course, there *were* certain limitations. Whether it was my nude breast that was touched or whether it was over the clothing depended on how new the relationship was, how much I liked the boy, how much money he had spent on me, or how many times he had taken me out. If he was somebody who wanted to meet me all the time, maybe he wasn't worth as much as the guy who wanted to take me to a movie and *then* feel my breast or something.

●

When I was in my teens, I had one younger girlfriend who was always in despair because she developed more slowly, of course, and she always compared *me* to the Playboy bunny. That was the *one time* in my life that I was complimented on my breasts.

My father once made a comment about my breasts when I was around nineteen. He told me that he had hoped I would get his sister's breasts, but unfortunately I hadn't. His sister's breasts were rather generous. I wonder what that says about his acceptance of my mother's breasts? After all, she's small, too.

How do you relate to the term "flat-chested"?

Well, I don't find it offensive. As a matter of fact, I see my being flat-chested as a potentially great gift. Should I ever have to disguise myself as a boy, I think I could do it quite easily. I always see that potential. Who knows? (*Laughs.*)

I've found that sometimes small breasts can be a blessing. When the whole movement was toward taking off the bra, I had a couple of friends who tried to do that and found it painful to walk about and move around with any speed. For me it just meant freedom. Before, bras were very constricting and uncomfortable because they confined me in so many ways—my front, back, and shoulders. Hell, it was like being harnessed!

Once I stopped wearing a bra, I started joking about having small breasts because I was no longer as uptight about it. I was nineteen then, and though going braless was the thing to do, I wasn't influenced that much by other people. Several of my friends said, "Go ahead and do it, but you won't catch *me* doing it!"

The strangest reaction to my going braless came from my mother. When I told her about it, she said she used to wear Band-Aids or adhesive on her nipples so that they wouldn't show. I don't know what the fashion was when she did that, but for a long time she had gone braless, too. And she told me that it was *very important* to keep your nipples from showing and that wearing adhesive was a good way to do that. I tried it once or twice, but I found out that *removing* the adhesive was not easy and not very pleasant.

It's curious that now, when going braless has become acceptable, my mother wears a bra. And I feel no need to try and convince her to take it off. I'm sure she doesn't even *consider* it. It's like wearing underpants to her—it's something you do, *period*.

My breasts never developed as fully as I wanted them to . . . as fully as they were "supposed" to, so I think I am lacking in ego and in self-confidence somewhat. I think most men are attracted to breasts and sometimes judge women *by* their breasts. I suppose I've been judged many times because of my breasts and that I've been dismissed once or twice—or maybe even more—*because* my breasts are so small.

As an adult, I've been teased about my breasts by men and it's probably had a bad effect on me. Men have said things to me about the fact that I have "small breasts." It's not that one breast is different from the other, or that the nipples are inverted, or that there's anything unusual about them. It's just that they have been considered "somewhat lacking."

My husband used to joke constantly about me getting breast implants! That was until recently when he saw a "60 Minutes" program about implants on TV. Well, now he realizes that there are dangers and that you don't always get the results

that you want, and maybe it's not worth the procedure anyway.

He's a "breast man" all right. His idea of perfect breasts is even *larger* than most people's! We've talked about his relationship with women's breasts, particularly his mother's. His mother has very large breasts and I like to think that he's never been weaned because he's so hooked on breasts—it's an obsession. I've asked him if he was breast-fed and he's *afraid* to ask his mother!

He would definitely prefer to be with a big-breasted woman, or that *I* had big breasts. And I'm sure that plays a role in my secretly wishing that I were larger. But then, of course, if it weren't my breasts it would be something else. My breasts are just the most obvious target if he wants to find me lacking.

For a long time, when I was still a virgin, I was very uptight about exposing my breasts to a man because of their size. I wouldn't mind if my lover would feel them or kiss them, but I really didn't like them to be exposed. I would rather have kept my breasts under the blanket . . . or under my blouse . . . or under *anything!*

Now if a male friend walks into the room and I'm changing my shirt, I only hesitate about him seeing my breasts if my husband is there. He is just *very* uptight about me exposing my breasts, so I have to be sensitive to his uptightness, see, because *he* gets embarrassed if someone else sees my breasts. I don't know why—I think it has to do with his feelings about modesty. If he's not around, I'm not embarrassed. I don't flaunt my breasts, but I don't run for cover, either!

In the past couple of years my husband and I have had a lot of people around the house, and when he's there I behave one way, and when he's not I behave another way . . . as far as changing clothes and sunbathing and things like that. Of course, it bothers me because I don't like to have to change the way I behave because of the way *he* feels. There've been many, *many* incidents where that has come up. I mean *every time* it happens, it's an *incident!*

There've been many times I would have gone sunbathing topless, but I didn't because I was with him. I mean he's even uptight if I'm lying on my stomach and I undo the top of my bathing suit so there's no line across my back. And sometimes I do it anyway. We fight about it all the time . . . *all the time!* But don't get me wrong, If there's nude or topless sunbathing anywhere on the beach, he's the *first one* to take a walk and check out all the breasts, you see. He just doesn't want anybody else seeing *mine!*

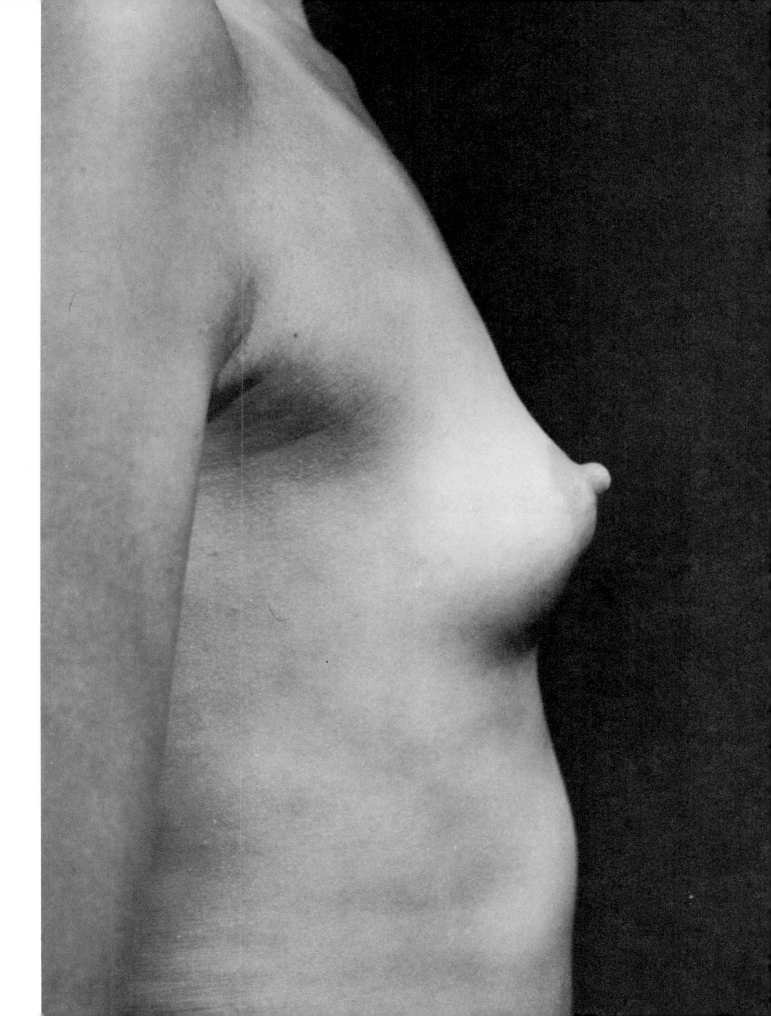

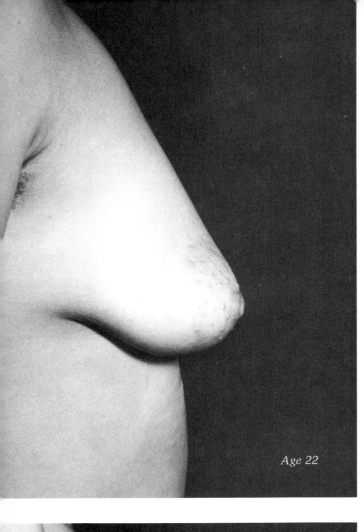

Age 22

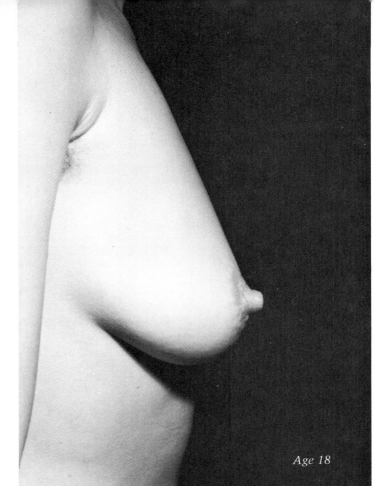

Age 18

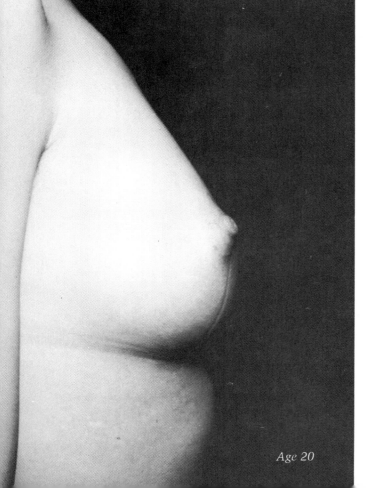

Age 20

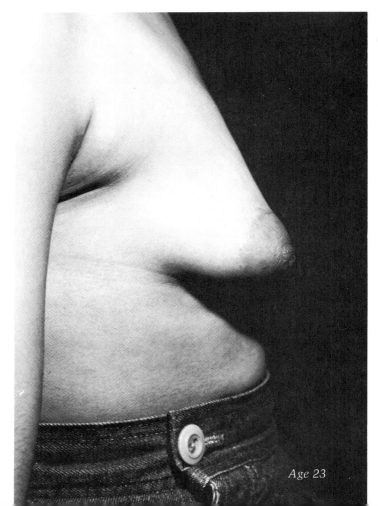

Age 23

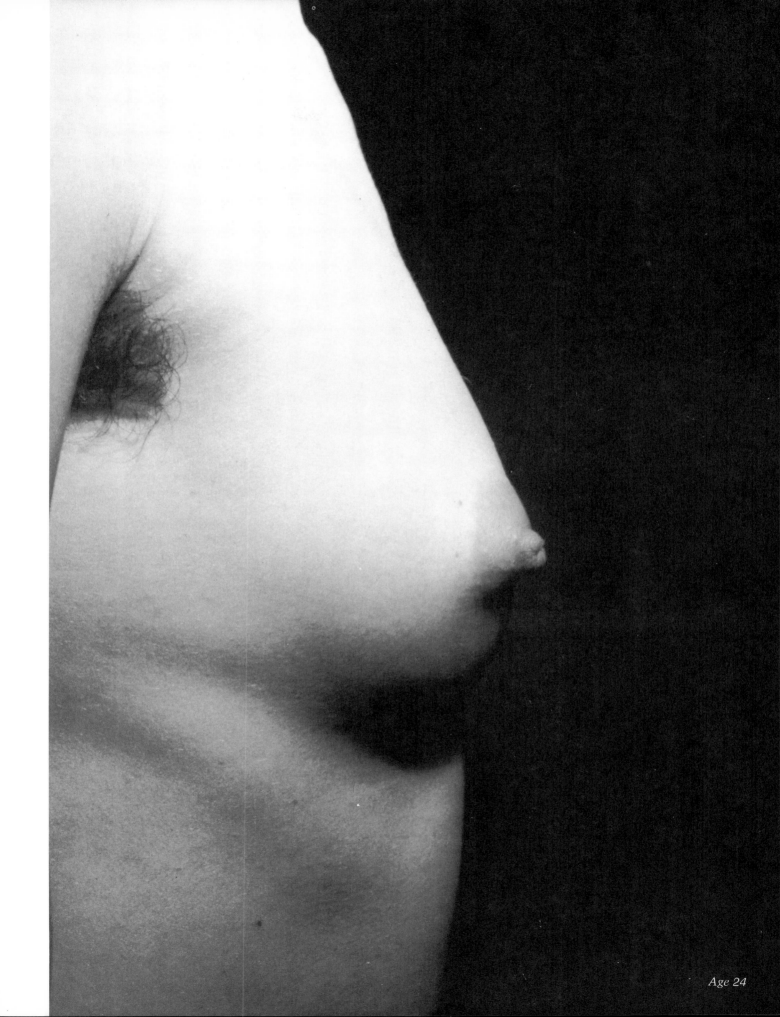

Age 24

Barbara
Age 24 · Raised in Colorado · Topless Dancer

My boobs are real important to me now—they're my income! A while back I was havin' a rough time findin' a job. I needed money really bad! Someone told me about these topless dancing contests—that it was easy money. So I went to see what the whole situation was. I had my swimmin' suit on underneath my clothes. I really liked the sound of the music they were playin', so I just went up on the stage and danced, and for the last song . . . I took my top off!

I didn't win anything, but it felt kinda good, you know. (Laughs.) Well, I didn't really know how it felt 'cause I was kind of tipsy. But it was okay! *I came back and started doin' it. I wasn't winnin' at first. I was losin' quite a bit. . . .*

I was scared at first, but drinkin' helped me loosen up. Then I wasn't dancing that great—I was really uncoordinated! So I watched what the other girls were doin' to win—playin' it straight and not having to get loaded when they danced—and that's when I started winnin'. I started to think of myself as a dancer, not just a pair of boobs up there onstage . . . shakin'! See, that's what scared me the first time I got up there—I thought it was really perverted! *(Laughs.) But now, I don't.*

When I was a kid nobody ever mentioned *any-thing* about boobs. My brother's the one that brought them to my attention. He'd sit by the pool and try to run into the girls' changin' room and see all the chicks. I didn't know what he was interested in until one day I saw some lady come out of the shower with *nothing* on! I was about ten years old and I thought you're not supposed to look at 'em—you're not supposed to be looking at older people with boobs! My mom always wore high 'jamas and turtlenecks. That's why I'd never seen hers.

I never noticed mine until they started to grow. It *hurt!* I was pretty grouchy. I didn't like material rubbin' against me—it irritated the crap out of me! And I didn't like anybody bumpin' into me accidentally and hittin' me in the boob. I couldn't *stand* it! And sleepin' on my stomach hurt! It just *basically* hurt and I got really *upset* with *them* havin' pains!

I kept askin' my mom why they were always givin' me pains and she said 'cause they keep growin' all the time. She was always givin' me a hot water bottle, and tellin' me it would feel better and it would stop when I got older. She said, "You hurt the worst when you start and as soon as the growin' stops, or when you're twenty-one years old, they'll subside." So I kept thinkin' that it was gonna stop sometime—the worst was over—and then it really wouldn't bother me as much. Sometimes, I'd massage my breasts because they hurt so much. All I remember about that time is feelin' the pain was so bad—them growin' pains!

I can remember when I used to try to look at other girls' breasts at the swimmin' pool and stuff like that. My older sister and me and my next-door neighbor would crawl underneath the shower stalls in the locker room and look at the older girls. And they'd get really pissed at us!

Now that I'm older, I see little girls doing the same thing to us, and they look at you like, "Oh! Look at *that!*" They're really in awe of 'em. And I look at myself now, and I say, "Oh . . . big deal. . . . You know, you'll be that way when you're older." But back then, we were fascinated by boobs and we felt kinda . . . *guilty* lookin' at 'em and stuff. And I don't know why.

When I first got a bra, those ole bugger boys would come up behind me and go "pppppttttpt" and snap it! That was the one drawback about wearing bras.

And my brother! He was constantly tryin' to hide in my closet or break in on me to see my tits—*all the time!* It got so I would booby-trap the shower with mops and hot water, and when

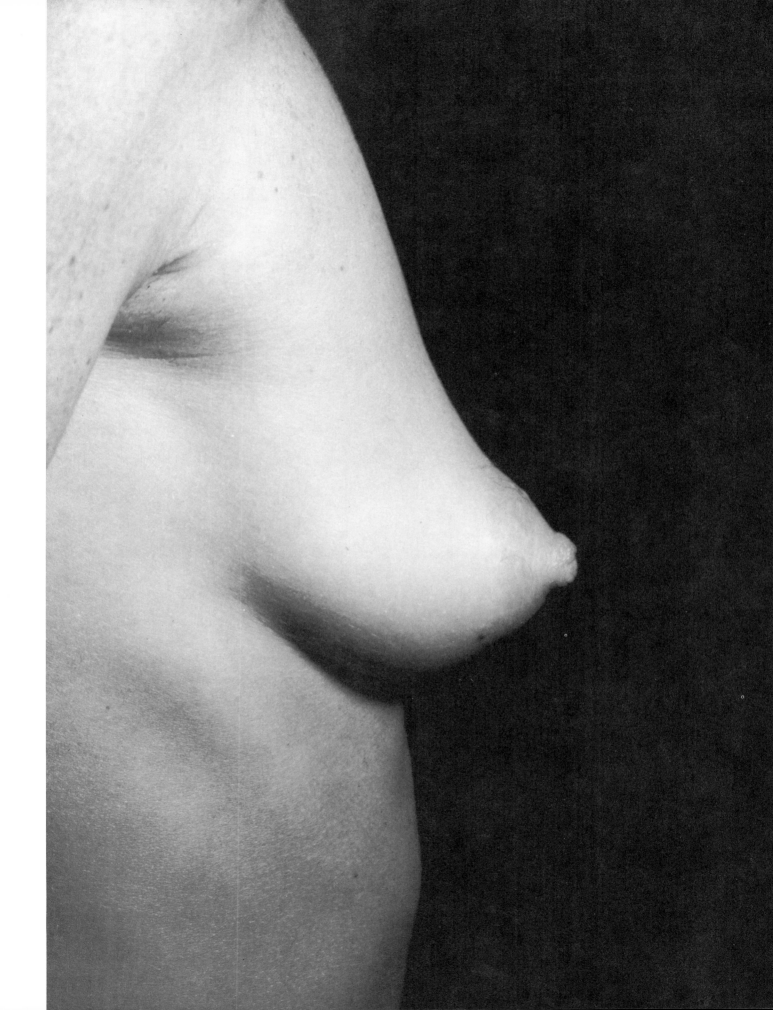

he opened the door, the mop would come crashin' down on his head and he'd step in the bucket of water! And he was always tryin' to look at the girl across the street with *binoculars!*

I couldn't stand my father—I hated his guts!! He embarrassed the hell out of me one time. I didn't want *anybody* to see my breasts, but one day I wasn't hurryin' up fast enough in the shower and he came burstin' in on me and told me to hurry up and get out of the shower. Well, here I was all *naked* and he started slappin' me! It just sorta warped my mind. I was screamin' 'cause I was so *embarrassed!* And I was tryin' to hide behind the shower curtain, and he was just slappin' at me and hittin' me more to get *out.* I thought he was bein' perverted, and it sorta turned me off guys after that.

Also, my mom started scarin' me by saying, "You're not supposed to let 'em touch you," and all that shit. So havin' breasts made me sorta stay away from boys.

My memories of the first time a boy touched me is kinda hazy. It was in tenth grade, and we were at a drive-in, you know, where the guys are *constantly* tryin' to lift up your blouse and touch you and stuff like that. And I said, "Don't do that! Quit it! *Don't do that!!"*

It really didn't turn me on at first because I was too *scared* to relax and enjoy it! My mom had scared me shitless that I'd get pregnant if I got touched or kissed or whatever.

The first guy to really touch 'em—the first real one—was my next-door neighbor and he was married. He touched me and it really felt good, so I let him do it. The next day I came back. I was sittin' there and he did it to me again and I felt embarrassed. I felt like I shouldn't be doin' that. So I told him to stop it, and he started laughin' at me!

●

Back then I was wearin' wire bras and I didn't like 'em because when I raised my arms those suckers came clear over my boobs and they'd catch me in the middle and they'd hurt. I'd be walkin' down the street, constantly tryin' to pull 'em *down,* and I just hated it.

When I was still livin' at home I went without a bra sometimes, but my mom and dad would call me a slut and say, "What are you gonna go out there without a bra for? You really look like shit." And I just ignored 'em because I liked goin' against my parents. You know, I guess it was like sayin', "Up yours! You wouldn't let me grow my hair long, so I'm gonna go without a bra whether you like it or not." I was about nineteen. My boyfriend doesn't like me goin' without a bra either. I guess he doesn't like anybody else lookin' at 'em.

Goin' braless felt pretty good at first—I really liked it! Well, it was a fad, and I thought I'd try it and see what it felt like. But then I saw some chicks that should be wearin' bras and their breasts were kinda long. And I looked at 'em and I thought, Ooooh, I hope *I* don't look like *that.* That makes me wanna go home and put a bra on. I think I look better with a bra because it pushes me up. My breasts feel funny when they're not supported, and I don't like the way my nipples protrude through the shirt.

●

The women I dance with now always look at you to see if you're big, or small or saggy or if you've got lines on your tits and stuff like that. At first I was embarrassed, but now I don't care. Before I couldn't even get undressed in front of my girlfriend without really being shy. And now, being thrown together all the time, it's nothin'. You get completely undressed in front of the girls when you change your costume and they really *look* at you. They check out the competition to see what size breasts you have and what shape you're in. (*Laughs.*)

I constantly observe the other girls to see if they are goin' down. That's why I don't want to work in a topless place too long, I'm afraid my tits are gonna go *kerplunk!!* . . . Pfft!! . . . . And one thing I don't want is *long skinny tits!* There's a cartoon in *Playboy* of this little old lady who's got knockers clear down to her *knees,* and it just kinda freaks me out! I hope I don't have boobs that hang down to my kneecaps. I remember I used to visit my grandmother in a nursing home, and I'd see all those little old ladies with *things* down to *there!*

Dallas started goin' down from workin' here. She's just been droppin' and droppin'! And she musta come back with exercises or somethin' because she's gotten a lot firmer. One girl was on the pill and she was quite firm, quite big up in the chest. Then she went off the pill and she lost her tits! They went like pancakes—just flattened against her chest. That's what scares me about gettin' off the pill, 'cause it adds a little bit more. Sorta firms 'em out a little bit—before the pill mine were really *narrow.* I call 'em "ski slopes" (*laughs*) because they go down and then sorta curve out. They could stand some improvement—like everybody else's. I'd like to have 'em bigger, firmer. I like 'em, but I'm not really thrilled.

One day I asked Tulsa, "Were you born with those big knockers?" And she said, "Yeah, I was born with them, but a lot of people think that I've had silicone shots." And she *hasn't!* But there's one new chick who came out the first time with these *things* stickin' straight out, and we were all hopin' that they'd fall down to her stomach when she took her bra off. They didn't. They just went *straight out* in front of her. They looked like miniature watermelons! Everybody told me that they could only be that way if she had silicone shots, but I'm not brave enough to ask her if she had the shots or not.

I've been tempted to get a little bit fuller by silicone shots, but they tell me it's dangerous. I'll be real tempted to if they drop down because I don't wanna have long, skinny ones. Sometimes I really get upset the way they slope down and narrow out—sorta like bullets. (*Laughs.*)

Since I've been dancin', I always watch for stretch marks and I take care of 'em a lot better than I used to. Before, I really didn't care about 'em that much. Now, I use lotion so I won't get stretch marks.

How do you think men feel about women's breasts?

Nothing! . . . They just think they're somethin' to look at, that's all. Somethin' to look at or play with like little kids. My man ignores 'em.

Once in a while, I'll be without a bra or somethin' and he'll just reach over and "cxxccxzzzkkyiii"—*squeeze.* It irritates me when he does that. I just don't like it. I tell him, but he don't care—he just does it anyway.

I've also begged him *millions* of times: "Will you *please* pay more attention to my breasts during sex because I really *like* it. It really turns me on! Will you please do it?" And he goes, "Okay, okay. . . ." And the next time, he just touches 'em for a couple of seconds and *that's it.* But *I* don't want it for just a couple of seconds 'cause I really like it. It really makes me feel bad and pisses me off!! I wish he would do more with 'em, instead of ignoring 'em like they were just two pieces of meat hangin' off of me. I'm so *tired* of the male sex ignorin' every part of your body except for the main thing!

I've sometimes had dreams about other women, but I haven't done anything. I think that maybe one of these days I will. But right now I'm too shy. I'm gettin' so tired of men ignorin' every-

thin' except *their* business. I figure that if I ever make it with a woman, I *know* what she wants and she knows what I want because we're both women.

I like my breasts to be touched right on the end—the very end, the part that stands up. It's part of the nipple, I guess. To be sucked on gently and have somebody run their tongue around it, instead of chompin' down and bitin' and pinchin'. Just really bein' gentle, 'cause the other way it hurts and it doesn't turn me on at all. Touchin' the outside part of the breast doesn't really do much for me. Except somebody told me that if they play with that part, you get bigger. . . . (*Laughs.*) I don't believe it.

●

The guy I'm livin' with doesn't like me to show my tits to all the other guys, but I don't see my dancin' as just showin' my tits to somebody else. I feel like I'm entertaining 'em, you know. I don't like the reaction I get from most guys when I tell 'em that I'm a topless dancer. They think that means I go to bed with *anybody.*

When I dance topless, I see the *way* the guys look at me, and I . . . uh . . . sorta get this thing inside of me that says, Hell, I'm teasin' *you,* and you can't touch *me!*

And I've *never* really been able to do *that* before without someone callin' me a dirty name for teasin' 'em, or for just bein' affectionate toward 'em when they thought that I meant more. And this way, I really like doin' it 'cause I can tease 'em and they can't touch me. It's a real power trip—it is! I don't know if that's wrong or not, but that's the way I feel about it.

●

. . . I remember thinking that it was like rape, only backwards. The women got to violate the men. There was something angry in these dance-seductions. The women tried to get the men as hungry and turned on as possible. Then they left them hanging. They could do nothing. Nothing but sit there in exquisite frustration, eager guilt. It was revenge on all the times that men put their greedy fingers all over women. It was striking back.

—Victoria Hodgetts.

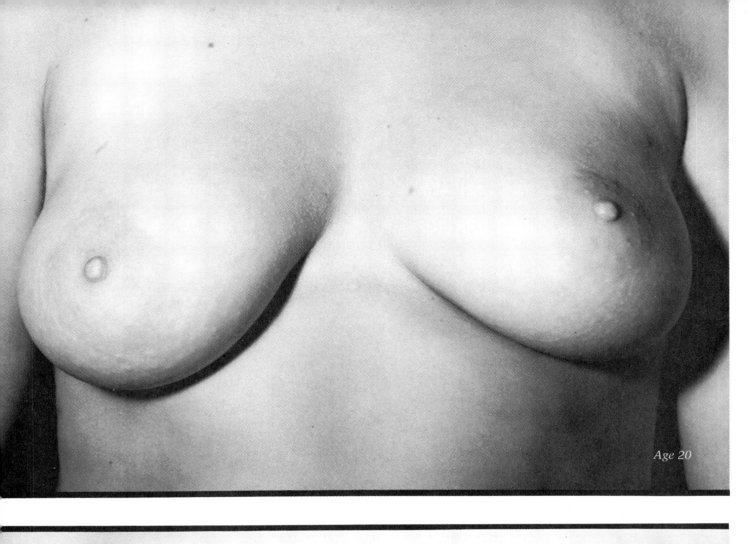

Age 20

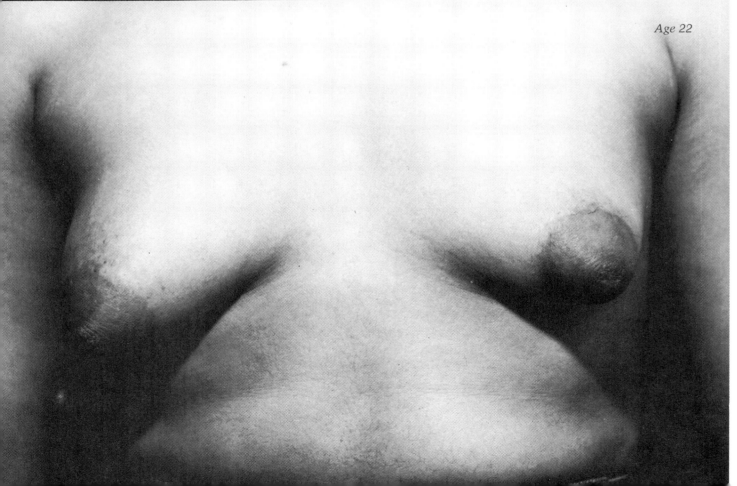

Age 22

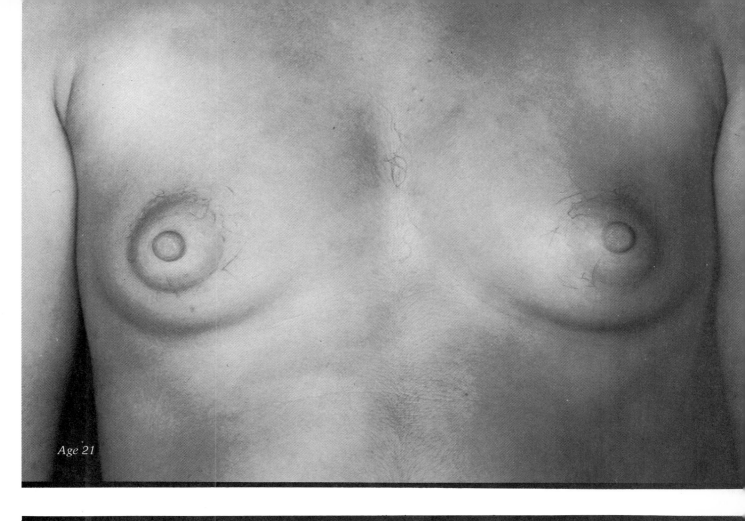

Age 21

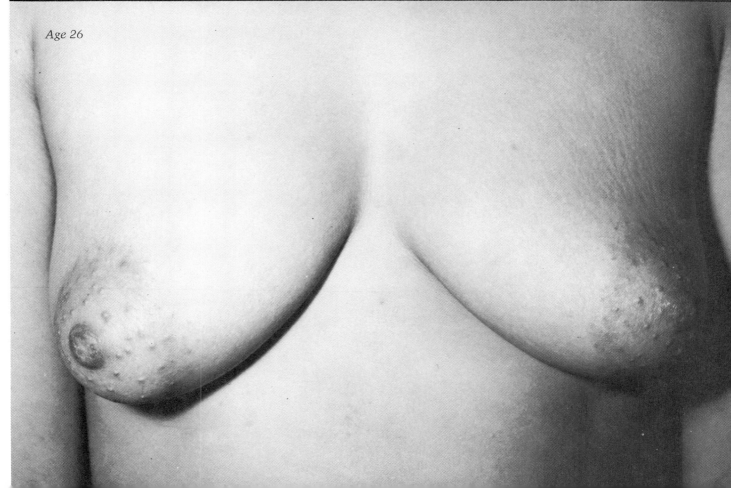

Age 26

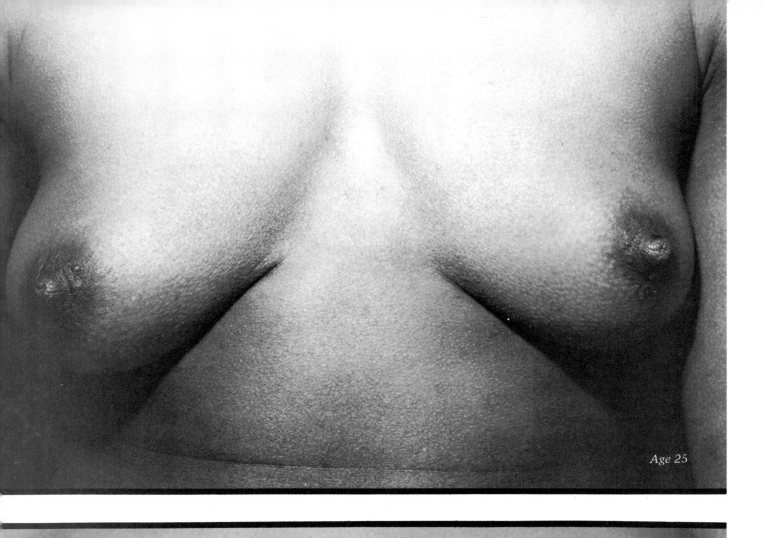

Age 25

Age 24

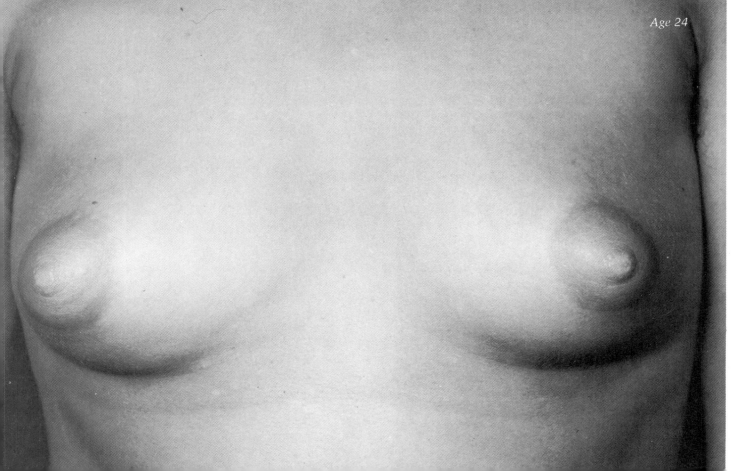

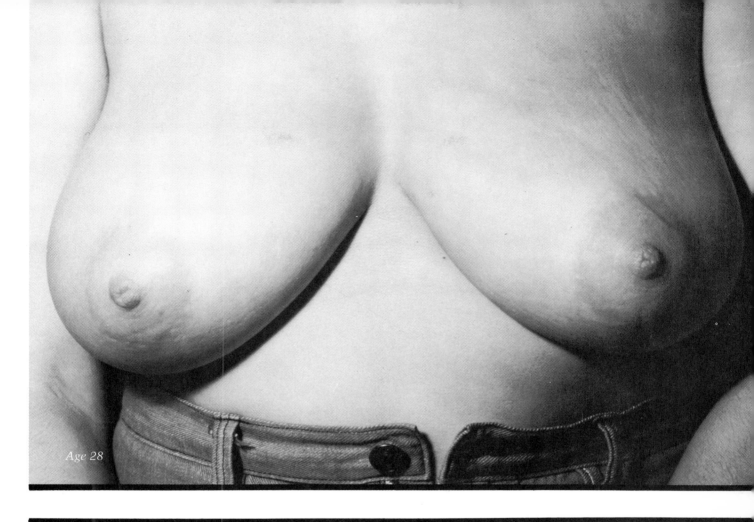

Age 28

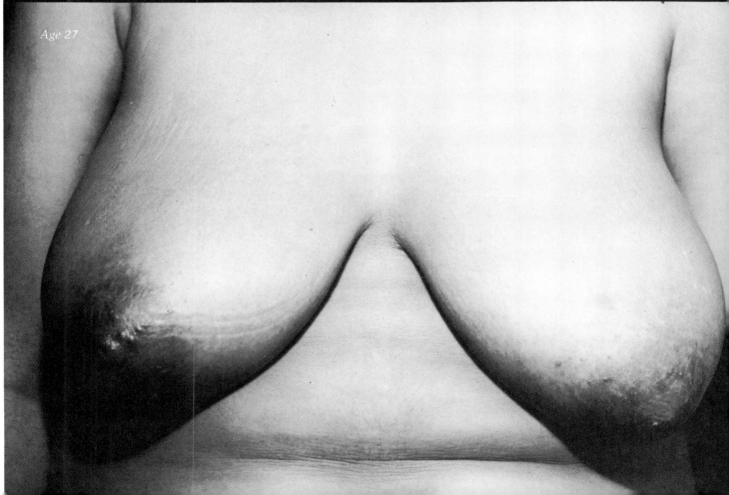

Age 27

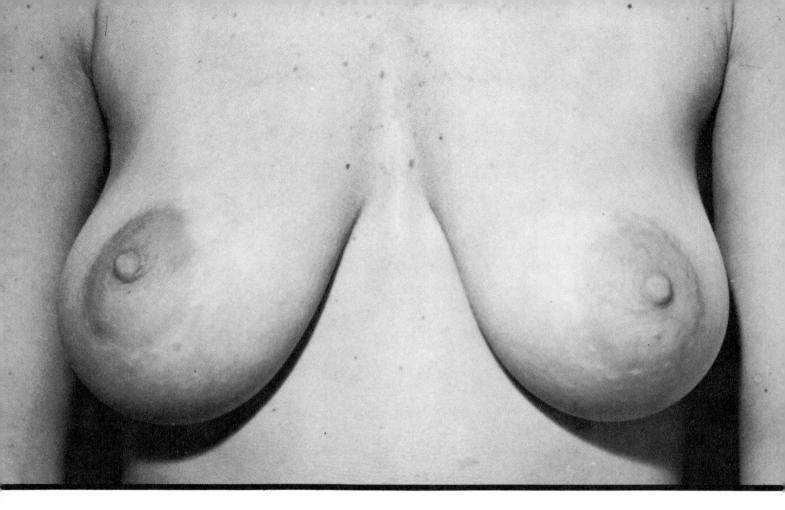

Sherry

Age 22 • Raised in New York City • Model

My tits look better with my arms up (laughs), straight up in the air! That's the only way they look like they're not on my belly button. That's the way I feel most comfortable about them, and that's the way photographers usually position me.

Sometimes I'll pretend that I'm manipulating my tits or touching them, you know, while I'm really holding them up. They're just too low in comparison to the other photographs of nude women that are selling. So, the photographers pose me in positions where I'm holding my tits up, always! . . . Always!!! (Laughs.)

Once I was photographed for an article that was going in a magazine which was supposedly written by a girl who had really big tits, about her trials and tribulations with them. For that story I was photographed from my neck to my belly holding a silver tray with lettuce on it. My tits were held up by resting on the tray, so it looked like I was holding a salad, offering my "tomatoes"!

When my tits first started growing, nothing showed, but I was aware that there was something happening inside. I was the last one to start growing among my friends, so I was really relieved.

In the beginning I really wanted my bras to

show. I remember wearing white shirts and sitting in class bent over so the guy behind me could see that I had a bra on. It was a *big deal* to let a guy know that you had a bra and I'll never forget it.

The first time that I ever was aware of my tits as a turn-on was with a girlfriend of mine—this was in eighth grade. When I think back on it, it was the first time I ever felt horny or had any sexual feelings at all. At the time I had no idea what was going on. We were really good friends and somehow we ended up in the bathtub together. We began to talk and we were fantasizing that some guys were gonna pick us up for the weekend and what they were gonna do to us. We began to play with each other's breasts and really got horny. It was really neat to touch another person's tits at the time, but I haven't done it since.

It was fantastic the first time a boy felt me up— I'd been looking forward to it and I got incredibly excited when it finally happened. I was already fifteen. It was my first initiation into sex. I was aware of *that* before I was aware of my cunt at all. I could've ended up a *puritan* the way my mother is, but for some reason I never went through any sex hassles.

I went on the pill when I was seventeen, and all of a sudden I was a D cup. It was really horrible! I hung out of my bathing suit. I just looked awful! I was doing fashion modeling at the time and walking all over the city, and I constantly got comments. That just grossed me out so I slouched—I still slouch a lot because of that. I could never walk tall because I just never wanted them to stick out. About a year ago I went off the pill because my breasts were so big. I couldn't stand it anymore! I was finally able to get down to a big but normal-looking size.

My tits are nice and friendly, but they're large, so they're *there,* if ya' know what I mean. They affect me 'cause they're a part of me that I'm so aware of, and so are other people. They look a lot of different ways at different times . . . they're just really fascinating. Sometimes they're beautiful and sometimes they look funny. Men like them because they're large, and for them it's an extra goody—like the prize in the Cracker Jack box. Yet *I* could take them or leave them—I'd feel just as good with smaller tits.

●

(Continued on page 98)

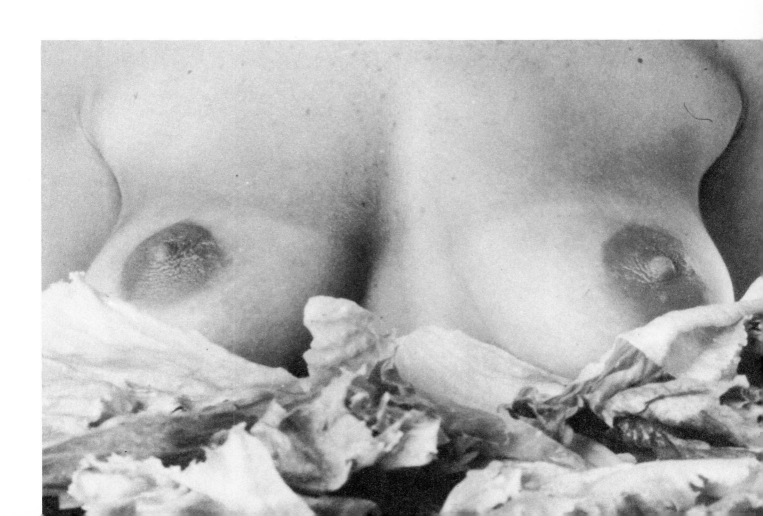

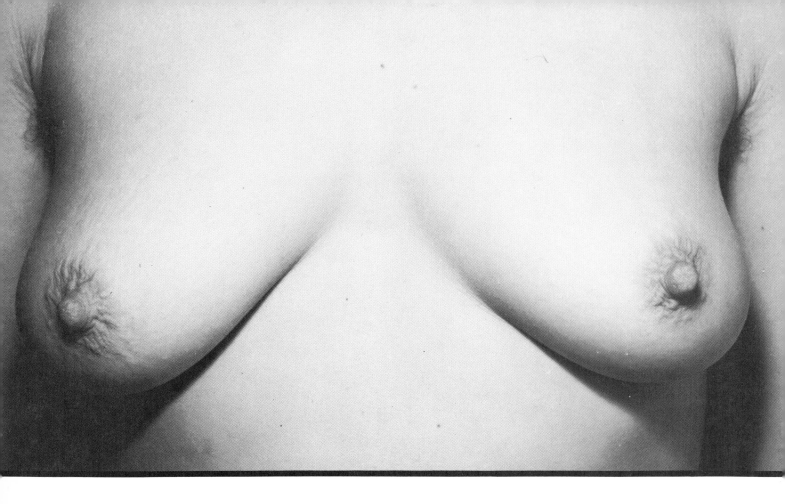

Jackie

Age 27 · Raised in New England · Model

There are certain little "tricks" that a model uses, ways of posing, that supposedly "improve" her breasts. They are very subtle and the man in the street doesn't pick them up. He sees that her breasts look full and that they're uplifted, but he doesn't know what is doing that.

When I'm being photographed, I'll often hold my breasts and play with them, especially in certain poses. You see, a model may not be playing with or fondling her breasts, but she can draw attention to them just by how and where she positions her arm. A model may be running her hand up her leg, or she may be posing as if she were masturbating or something like that, but at the same time she's got her arm pushed up against the side of her breast so it makes her breasts look fuller than they already are.

Another trick is to fondle each breast with your hands and at the same time hold them up, so it looks like your breasts really stand up. When a man sees that picture he thinks to himself, "Look what she's doing to herself! She's fondling them and they're so full...."

The men that buy these magazines are in a fantasy world. They look through the magazine and see the kind of women they figure they can never have. This is a total fantasy trip for them! So in the fantasy, the magazine has got to create the ultimate in perfection for the male.

You never see any blemishes that show real life, like a pimple or stretch marks. Most women have stretch marks if they have breasts at all, and the women who do nude modeling don't exactly have little bumps for chests. I've had stretch marks on my breasts ever since they blossomed so suddenly after my freshman year in college. With lighting and camera angles, they can be obscured. It's easy.

I was a late bloomer, so developing breasts was something I expected. As a matter of fact, I couldn't wait! All year long through eighth grade I sat next to the girl who had the biggest breasts in the room, and *me* without a bra! I was still in T-shirts and that was absolutely devastating to me!

I never really had a fabulous social life in school and part of it had to do with my lack of sex appeal, that is, breasts. But after my freshman year in college, all of a sudden they grew! I mean they just ba . . . lossomed! I was barely in a B cup and suddenly I was spilling out of a C!

I didn't really think about it until one day I went to the beach. There was always a big crowd of kids who hung around there every summer, and until this time nobody ever paid much attention to me because I was just a skinny kid. Well,

there was a lot of bantering and talking, and as usual nobody was paying attention to me. Underneath my shirt I had on a swimsuit that had underwires, so it pushed my breasts up like two bubbles peering over the top! Well, I took off my shirt and all of a sudden everybody immediately shut up. Complete silence. I was so embarrassed! I knew exactly what everybody was looking at, and what they were thinking—Wow! Where did she get *those?*

After I recovered from that initial shock, I thought, This is great! (*Laughs.*) I loved it! I began to view my breasts as a . . . symbol of sexual power, I guess.

●

(*Continued on page 98*)

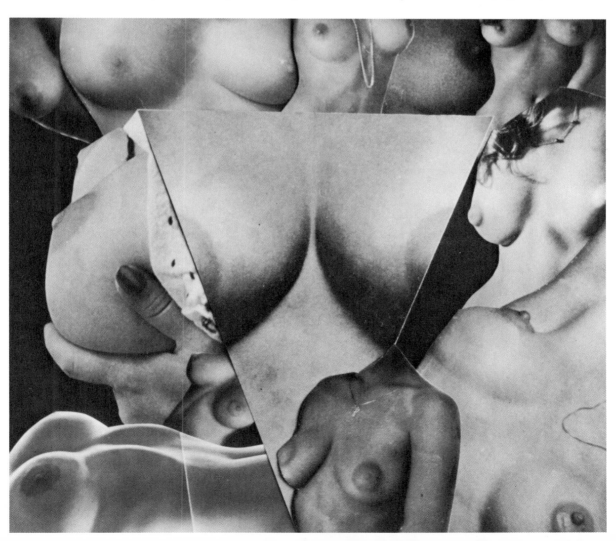

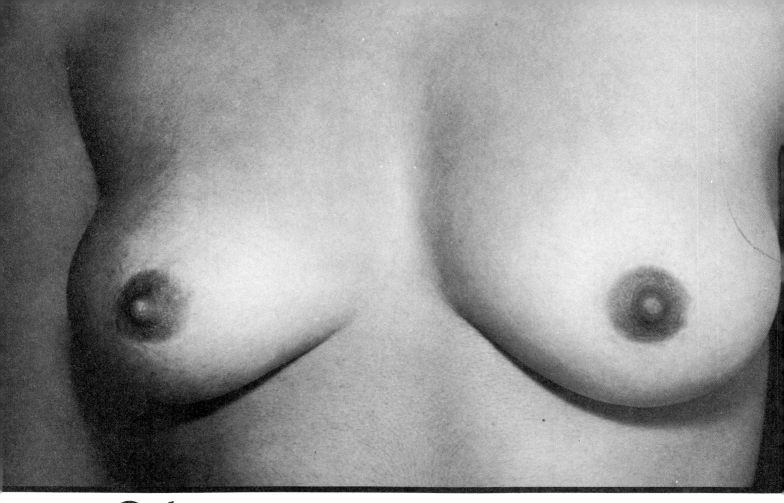

Gail

Age 26 • Raised in Ohio • Model and Actress

Occasionally, they put light pink stuff on my nipples. Oooh! I really hate that! They look like strawberries instead of nipples. (Laughs.) I think makeup like that is stupid. They look nice enough without it, and I don't think they should try and glamorize the body. When they ask me to do that, it's hard to complain, so instead I've made jokes about the nipple makeup. But the photographer can't be bothered to talk about it. He doesn't really care, as long as he gets the shot done.

There are some good photographers who don't bother with makeup. They just shoot a woman the way she is and don't care about flattering positions, because just the body itself is nice, whatever shape it takes, and there is no perfect idea of what it should look like.

But Playboy *magazine is different, you know. They want the best positions possible—"Hold in your stomach! Stick out your chest! Stick it all out!" And that's not really what women look like! It's not very realistic, is it?*

I don't remember not having breasts or being completely flat-chested. I only remember wearing a bra. For some reason I've blocked out a lot of my childhood.

My mother never seemed to acknowledge the fact that she had any breasts or a body. She's very uptight. Never told me about my period—nothing!

96

I've done nude work. You know, it's strange—my mother knows about it and she has seen it, but she doesn't comment on the fact that I am nude. She's either oblivious, or pretends that she is. It's all very strange! She really wants me to have a giant career, so I guess she feels that if the exposure might help me, it's not bad. (*Laughs.*) She was always uptight about boyfriends and if I'd had sex or whatever, so her not being upset about my doing nudes is very contradictory.

I vaguely remember touching my breasts one time when I was maybe fourteen, and my mother came in the room without knocking. Well, I was so shocked, I literally fell off the bed! She didn't acknowledge the fact that I was "exploring" myself. Oh, it was as if I was just reading a book, only she was very mad. I could tell by the way she said, "Wash up for dinner!" She never mentioned it, but it made me feel very dirty, especially when she said "Wash up." You only wash off dirt, right?

My sister was very large-busted but in terrible shape. She was very saggy and I felt sorry for her. It was kind of a turn-off for me to see her getting dressed or undressed, and I always hoped that wouldn't happen to me. I was the attractive one in the family and there probably was some jealousy from my mother and my sister, but I was unaware of those things.

I wasn't very popular in high school. I was pretty introverted and suppressed. I think people thought of me as a snob and aloof, but I was just shy.

I had the same boyfriend from about thirteen to seventeen. It was a year before I allowed him to touch me. I thought petting was *evil* (*giggles*) but it sure felt good! Yeah, evil because I was brought up in such a straight fashion that anything related to my body was a little racy . . . which, now that I think of it, might have even made it a little more enjoyable.

My second boyfriend I met when I was seventeen. We used to go to bed in my parents' bedroom when they went out. (*Laughs.*) And when we saw the lights pulling up the driveway in the front, we'd get dressed real fast and he'd run out the back door. I almost had a heart attack every time, because we could have been caught so easily. And why I didn't do it in *my* bed? . . . Uh. (*Laughs.*) Well, maybe I secretly wanted to get caught. Then again, maybe it just added to the excitement.

●

(*Continued on page 98*)

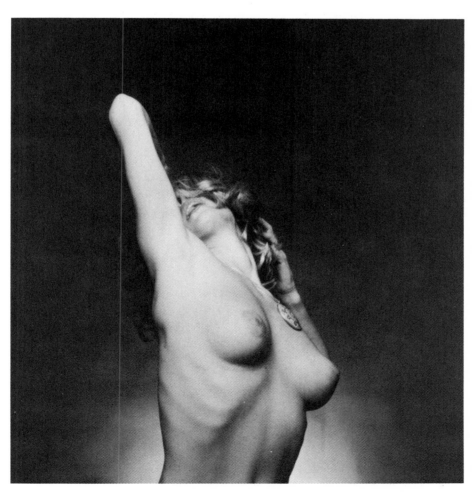

The Models

The responses of *Sherry, Jackie,* and *Gail* to questions about their careers modeling for men's magazines appear together here so that they may give a more complete picture of that experience:

How did you become involved in nude modeling?

SHERRY—I was doing some fashion modeling and always meeting photographers. I met one man who was photographing mostly for men's magazines, and at the time I needed some money badly. I didn't feel that I was degrading myself and I wasn't living out any sexual fantasy. It was just a job.

GAIL—As an actress I had never dreamed of doing nude modeling, or *any* kind of modeling for that matter, and I never thought I could. It just happened. It was a complete accident. I never even thought of myself as being that attractive! The main thing that it's been to me, and always was since the beginning, is money. Modeling meant some security and that was really important because as a struggling actress you don't make a lot of money.

JACKIE—It was a quick way to make money—the Big M—at one throw.

What was your first nude modeling experience like?

JACKIE—As it turned out, the first time wasn't difficult at all. It was four hours of shooting, constantly going from one outfit to another and then gradually taking each one off. It was very hard work and *very tiring,* especially since I didn't really know the *moves.* You can't just step out of a pair of pants like a slob. You've got to take them off alluringly and *slowly* with the right moves.

GAIL—I was never really uptight or worried about posing. What was strange was that when I was actually doing the photograph I didn't feel self-conscious, but I had been when I walked onto the set—while I was still *me.* And afterward, in the dressing room, I remember I was very aware of the fact that someone might see me . . . that I should shut the door because someone might walk in. Yet I had just been totally *nude!* When I was *myself,* I didn't want anyone to see me. It's a strange thing.

When I'm modeling, it's like nudity is my costume—it hides me. I can completely divorce myself because people don't make comments and it seems very antiseptic and asexual. Despite the fact that I do nudes, I'm not that comfortable about my body, and I'm fairly modest in my per-

sonal life. I would never walk around the room nude in front of a girlfriend.

SHERRY—My first job was for a book called *The Naughty School Girl*—you know the kind. It was a shot of me wearing a skirt and I had no top on, but only the back of me was being shot. It was the first time the photographer saw me without my clothes on, so when I walked down to the set, he and his assistant started cracking up and laughing at me because my tits were so big! And when he was shooting my back—this schoolgirl's back, right?—my breasts were sticking out from the sides. I was terribly embarrassed and self-conscious.

Are your breasts an important part of your modeling image?

GAIL—Yeah, I'm considered "voluptuous" in the business. Some might say I have a "nice pair." I think my breasts are average. They're nice and firm, but there's nothing *really* unusual about them.

SHERRY—The perfect fashion modeling size is 32B—that's standard—and I never was. It was always a drag that my tits were so big because I looked funny in a lot of clothes. I always wore bras that were too small and hid my tits under loose sweaters. Most models are really flat, but I had big tits and I lost a lot of work because of it. It made me uptight about them, but with the nude work it's definitely been an asset! My breasts are a big part of my photographic image just because they're bigger than, uh . . . I don't know if "normal" is the right word . . . but they're bigger than most models'.

JACKIE—Breasts play a large role in *any* nude model's photographic image because they are a sexual focal point.

Do you have to prepare your breasts in any way before a shooting?

JACKIE—Sometimes, especially if there's a blemish, I use a regular foundation makeup. Once in a while in a shooting, depending on the lighting and the film and those technical things, a photographer will ask the model to redden her nipples with lipstick or lip gloss just to give them a little shine and to make that particular area the center of attention in the photograph.

GAIL—Sometimes I've had oil put on me to make my breasts shine, and once for a shooting I had a painting on my chest which took nine hours to paint. The guy who was doing it was drinking martinis, so it took a long time. I've had to lighten up a suntan with body makeup. I did a nude one time and I wore lacy panties and a matching bra, except the bra was all missing. It was just the underpart and everything else showed. I've seen those advertised in Frederick's of Hollywood and they look silly.

SHERRY—Hard nipples are definitely considered a turn-on. That's what photographers think looks best. So the one thing I do to them is make them hard by putting ice on them or somehow getting them cold, and that's a *bitch!* Either my nipples get really sensitive or frozen or numb!

It's so weird to me. What's this myth about hard nipples that I'm suffering for?! I don't know why people always assume that you're aroused if your nipples are hard. Just hitting warmer or cooler air, any slight temperature change, will make a nipple go hard. Men have said to me, "You know your nipples are erect, you must be turned on!" They just don't understand that it happens with any slight stimulation no matter what it is—it could be the fabric of your shirt. It happens with men's balls also; it's the same kind of erectile tissue. When a man goes into cold water or cold air, his balls go back into his body for protection—they get all crinkly and tight. And when it's too hot, they drop down because they want to cool off. (*Laughs.*) It's true!

GAIL—Sometimes you have to cover up the nipples so that they don't show, if you're doing a semi-nude shooting. This applies particularly to ads. They can show everything but that little part. There's actually laws against that—you can show around it, but you can't show the nipple. It's so ridiculous. Just because they are a different color or shape, I don't understand why they have to be covered up and why the rest of the breast is okay. I mean the nipple is just a small part of the whole breast. Why is it obscene?

SHERRY—The guy at the newsstand where I used to live sold these magazines and wherever the nipples were showing he would take black tape and stick it on them. It was so funny to have black tape here and there. But they could get arrested for showing them in public to kids.

Have you made any observations about women's breasts as a result of having worked with nude women?

JACKIE—The thing that I've noticed most about other women's breasts is the size or coloring of the nipple. I never realized that there was any difference, so it's been quite a revelation to see how different they all are. And some women have the most incredible erections on their nipples, it's amazing! There was one woman I worked with whose nipples were so erect I swear that the center was at least half an inch high. Really! I was astounded.

SHERRY—One thing that I've noticed sometimes on other models is dark hair on their tits. The first time I saw that it freaked me out. I had never seen anything like it! I've got a lot of fuzz on my tits, but not dark hairs!

GAIL—I did a shooting with a couple of women and it was a strange experience. I had to touch one woman's breasts a little bit. She really had a terrible body and it made me sick in a way. The other girl had had a silicone operation—it was quite apparent—and that was a turn-off, too. I had to touch the side of her breast and it was *hard!* One of the women also had to touch *my* breast. Actually, it didn't feel weird—I mean, if I closed my eyes, it could have been a guy's hand. It didn't make me nervous; it made me more nervous touching them.

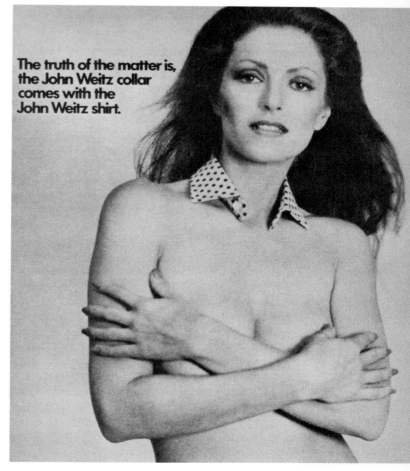

The truth of the matter is, the John Weitz collar comes with the John Weitz shirt.

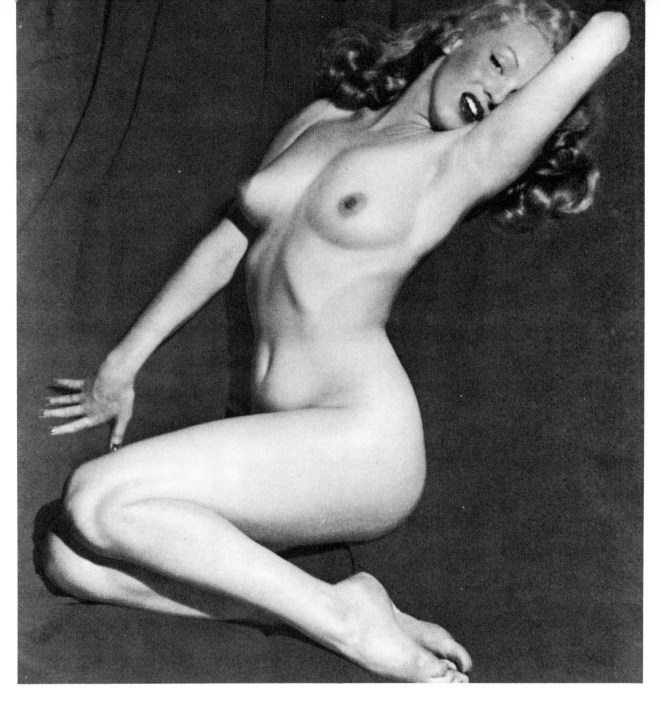

Has nude modeling affected the way you feel about your breasts?

JACKIE—I've become more self-conscious about taking care of my body better. Now I have to make sure that my breasts don't age or sag, so I exercise every morning. I have to be careful when I'm having sex with a man. I bruise very easily, and if a man bites my breast or handles me roughly, it leaves red marks. I can't go and do a nude shooting with these marks on my breast, you know, I mean really! Aside from not liking rough treatment, bruises and marks are something that makeup just won't cover, so I've got to guard my body against all that kind of stuff.

SHERRY—When I got into fashion modeling, I definitely became more self-conscious about my appearance . . . *definitely!* Just seeing how thin the other girls were. I always had big hips and tits so I was self-conscious of my body. I was never satisfied with how I looked. After I began nude modeling I became even more self-conscious of my breasts. I started feeling them more often, rather than looking at them, 'cause that's how I could tell if they were sagging.

GAIL—I don't worry about my breasts too much, but I don't want to sag. I should start doing exercises or something for the pectoral muscles just to keep 'em where they belong! (*Laughs.*) I've been taking advantage of the fact that I am pretty solid. I know girls that have been doing exercises their *entire life* and sometimes I feel that at my age I should probably do some.

But I'm not really afraid of sagging because it wouldn't affect my acting, which is more important to me than the nude modeling.

SHERRY—I know a model who had her breasts lifted. She always worried about sagging, so she had a silicone operation. Now she's *ecstatic,* you know, because she's not sagging at all. If anything, they're so upright, they don't look real!

GAIL—It's interesting . . . Marilyn Monroe, who was a sex goddess and who appeared to be so tremendously stacked and voluptuous, in reality had a figure very similar to mine, especially from the waist up. She had an average-size bustline and an average body, but they built her up. They padded her and did all sorts of things to emphasize her bustline. In her famous calendar pose, her breasts aren't that large, and yet whenever you talk to a man about Marilyn Monroe, you'd think they were huge! She really didn't have that incredible stereotypic ideal of what a woman's body should be like. I'm sure part of her unhappiness was that she never felt satisfied with what she had because they *never* left it alone!

JACKIE—Up until a year ago my breasts were very full but right now they have lost some of their fullness. I think it might be a hormone change in my body. The authorities, whoever they are, say that you can go braless only if a pencil will *not* be held up underneath your breast. Well now I fail the pencil test. But *I've* never been

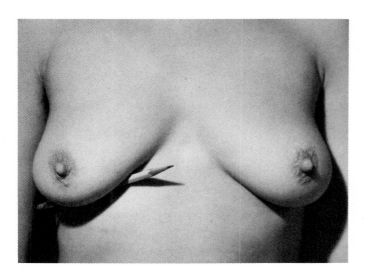

really displeased with my breasts. As a matter of fact losing some fullness didn't really upset me until the photographer with whom I work exclusively started complaining. There was a noticeable change but there was nothing I could do

about it. *He* thought I could get one of those bust improvers from the magazines and be a Raquel Welch—a bazoom bunny—in a week. Well, I said, "No thanks! No way!" But I did start to get paranoid about my breasts being smaller and saggier.

And then one day I sat down and really thought about it. This is crazy! I thought. There's nothing I can do about it—I have to live with what I've got. As far as I'm concerned, all those pills and potions and creams and all this crap to develop breasts doesn't work. They're just gimmicks to make money. The only thing that helps is exercising, which I've been doing faithfully every morning. Besides, *my* rules for beautiful breasts aren't that stringent. I don't think breasts have to stand up on end to be beautiful.

How do you think the image of the idealized woman portrayed in the magazines you model for affects people?

JACKIE—I don't think women like to look at voluptuous models because it reminds them of what they aren't. Most women just don't have that good a figure, especially older women. On the other hand, the really thin models aren't too representative of the public either 'cause there aren't many women who are that thin.

SHERRY—I think there are some women who get off on the magazines. I appreciate seeing a beautiful body. You know, there are some magazines that really are gross with gross-looking women, but the ones that have beautiful photographs of beautiful women, I get off on. I guess if I was fat or not as attractive as I am, maybe I would be intimidated by it or maybe I'd wish I could be that way. I can't say really.

GAIL—If you ask anybody what the ideal breast is, they'll probably say large and pointed up. In fact, very few women's breasts ever look like that, and when they do it's for a very short time. It's almost an impossibility. It's some ideal that doesn't really exist, and it must have a bad effect on women. Maybe it makes them insecure and perhaps promiscuous so that they are always seeking a guy who will make them feel attractive. And maybe they don't feel attractive simply because their breasts don't match this ideal.

SHERRY—It's probably true that if there weren't magazines like that men would appreciate their wives more. I can see women getting uptight if all their husbands did was bring home those magazines and jerk off, you know, instead of getting it on with them.

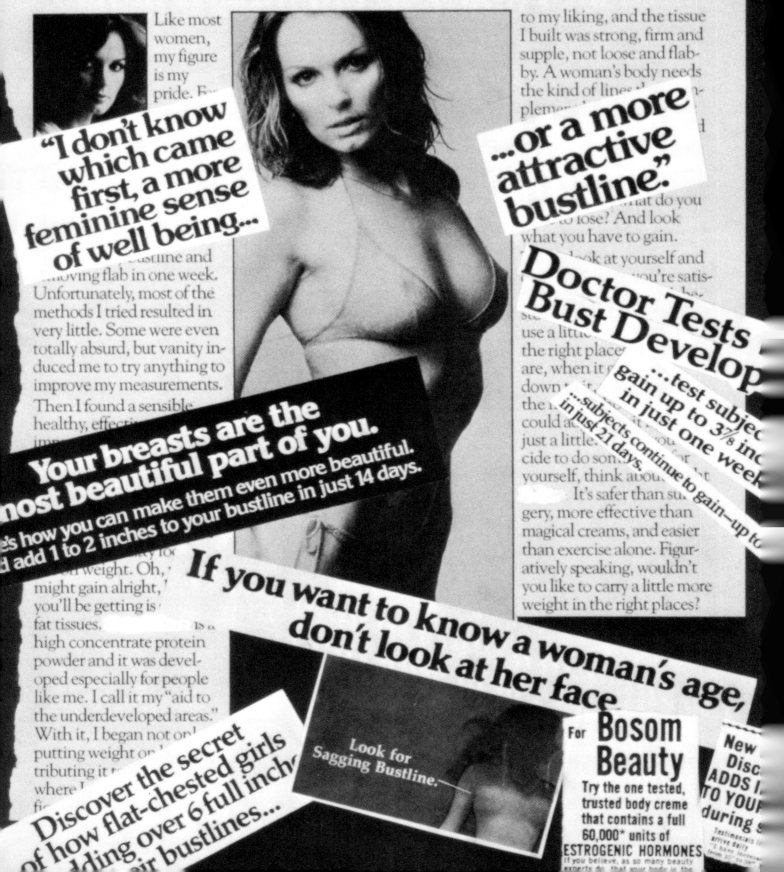

Measure Up.
Gain Weight In The Right Places.

Men relate to breasts too much for me to cope with. That's the *first* thing they look at—your tits. That's the *only* thing! You know, it's like they don't want to know *you* . . . they just want to look at your tits!

JACKIE—Most men I've met go for a really big-breasted woman whose breasts are out of proportion to the rest of her body. But I don't think it looks good. I think it looks ludicrous.

I think the magazines have affected men, too, not just women. Breasts are the biggest thing going in this country! I think it's because through the late sixties the nude magazines could not show a woman's crotch. *Everything* was centered on the breasts, so that men were brought up with a breast fixation. This censorship warped people and created a misplaced fetish on breasts. Men's big turn-on was *breasts* because this was what they always saw in the magazines.

GAIL—There's such an emphasis on breasts as the almighty symbol of *womanhood* . . . and it's really too bad because there are a lot of flat women that think they're *not even women!* That's crazy! I mean, a woman has sex down there, not up here!

I've known girls that are really screwed up because they're flat-chested. Some of them have had operations on their breasts and have gotten into trouble with infections and horrible things happening. It's sad that they base how they feel about themselves on their *breasts!* God, it's like nothing else counts! I guess a lot of that is from the magazines because they give people a false idea of what a woman's body really is.

JACKIE—These magazines make it look as though the only women who are beautiful are the young twenty- to twenty-five-year olds, and are the only women that men should be attracted to.

I was twenty-five years old when I started modeling and that is very old. Most girls begin at sixteen, and somebody once told me that *Playboy* has a rule that you have to quit at twenty-five. A time is going to come when I won't be able to model anymore. Some magazines have already rejected my stuff because they say I look too "mature" for a young girl. I resent this arbitrary cutoff because it's not only eighteen-, nineteen-, twenty-, twenty-one-, twenty-two-year-old girls that are great looking. There are a lot of women over thirty who look great—just super! And I'm sure there are many older women who resent it.

But I use magazines for my own ends. As far as I'm concerned, business is business. I make money from them, but for other women who don't look like young playmates they do a lot of damage.

Many women have complained that the models who pose for men's magazines are hurting women. How do you feel about that?

SHERRY—There will always be women who will do nude modeling. I guess most do it for money. Maybe a lot get off on doing it, too. It doesn't hassle me in any way 'cause I know those magazines are always gonna be around.

GAIL—There are more nude magazines now than ever before, and the news magazines are all folding. I don't think there should be so much emphasis on it but for me it's money—survival. I guess if I felt very strongly about it, I wouldn't do it, but I don't feel too guilty. I bought myself a fur coat even though I hate killing animals. But the coat was on the rack and the animal was already killed. If I quit modeling it won't stop every girl from doing nude modeling in magazines. If I thought I could single-handedly stop them, then I might consider it. But I'm not gonna lose out on money and be the one girl who's so selfless.

Are your breasts sexually arousing?

SHERRY—My breasts play a large role in my sex life. Sometimes I like them touched very lightly or sometimes I like them touched very hard. It goes from one extreme to the other, really.

JACKIE—My breasts are a very erogenous zone—they have always been. I really enjoy having them fondled. Right now I am going out with a man who is a doctor of psychology, and he is very experienced, well-traveled, and mature. He's no kid! A large part of our sexual experience is for him to watch me fondling my breasts and getting turned on to myself . . . which is fine with me because it feels great! The only way that he can keep himself from climaxing is to not touch my breasts. As soon as he touches them, he gets off—it's like lighting a stick of dynamite! It's incredible! (*Laughs.*)

GAIL—I haven't had that much sex, to tell you the truth. I've been seeing the same guy for seven years, which is like being married, and I don't really see anyone else. Uh . . . he's not that sexual and my energies are so concentrated on my career that, uh . . . you know . . . maybe once every two weeks . . . or three weeks . . . or a month . . . which is not very much sex. It's a little embarrassing, but it's even hard for me to remember whether my breasts turn me on or not.

Most people have the idea that girls who pose nude for the magazines have a wild sex life. The magazines try to promote the image that this is a woman who fucks like crazy, but it's a fantasy.

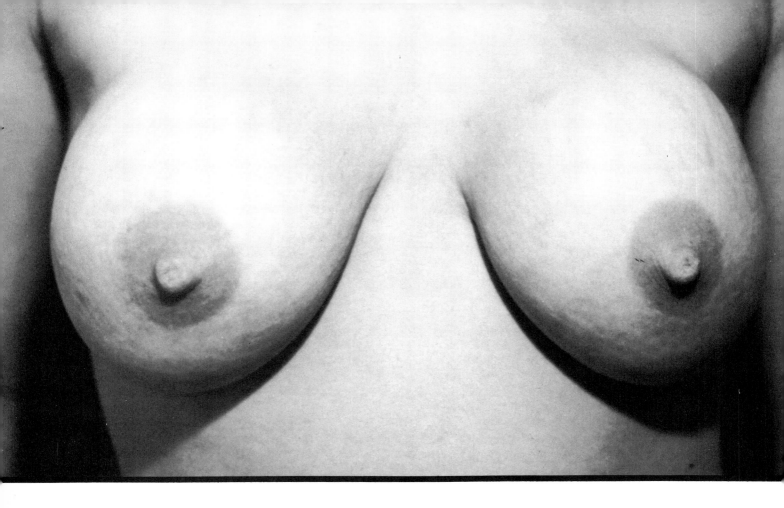

Carol   *Age 29 • Raised on the East Coast • Executive Secretary, Singer*

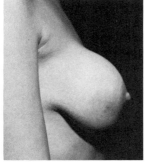

I was always considered to be an attractive, sexy, and fairly intelligent woman with a good personality, except that when I tried to get into show business, I suddenly realized that I had not developed fully enough for the people sitting out there in the audience—that is, according to the managers and producers and anybody who considered hiring me. And I kept finding that out over and over again.

Several years ago, I was doing a lot of dancing to support myself. Then you could make twenty-five or thirty dollars a night as a go-go dancer in a discotheque, dressed in white boots, a miniskirt, and a tight sweater. But if you didn't have big breasts, you weren't considered one of the better dancers. I happened to be very good because I had studied a lot of modern dance. So I could really see what happened if you didn't have an extremely big bust. There was always a girl with a flat ass, wide hips, and knock-knees, but as long as she was *big-chested*, she was put in the middle of the stage. And, of course, the middle was the focal point.

One time I tried out to be a Playboy bunny. The first thing they do is give you a one-piece-swim-suit-type outfit—the bunny uniform—and fancy black mesh stockings. Then they stuff your bra with cotton—just stuff, stuff, stuff it up, so that your titties are pushed up until they can't come out any more—till the nipples are almost exposed. You have to parade around the club wearing this "uniform," and people look you over and check the "goods" out. Finally, you go back and get rejected. That really broke my heart.

Another time I got a job working with a comedian. Part of my act was being his straight girl while he was telling jokes. A couple of the jokes

104

referred to breasts, with him looking down my dress, and all that. But when he looked down my dress, there was not that much there for him to look at. Personally, I didn't consider myself small-chested. I was a small 32B, but a B nevertheless. But one day I was informed by the management that if I did not put padding there, or somehow boost myself up, I was going to be fired. All on account of my breasts! Well, that affected me enough to consider *permanently* changing the way I looked.

I had heard about breast implants from a lot of the girls I was dancing with and from other people in show business and I decided that was my only hope. I had expectations that with larger breasts the world would open up for me—a career, money.

After the operation was over it was just marvelous, really wonderful! There were two tiny scars underneath my breasts, and I was two sizes bigger than I had been. You never really see the scars—you have to look for them. I had to stay bandaged for a few weeks until I was healed, but I wasn't in too much pain. The only thing that made me suffer during that time was the guy I was living with. He actually tried to *kill* me!

He had been very much against the operation but he never *told* me. Later I could see his reaction. He was just wiped out by it! He was always very jealous, and one night we had an argument and it all came out . . . he thought I'd had the implants to attract other men, not for myself or for my career. So we had a big fight about it and he tried to *strangle* me! I was in real danger because of the bandages. I couldn't move my arms, I couldn't fight back, so I just screamed and screamed and screamed until finally he let me go, and then I *ran.* That ended the relationship.

●

There is an afternoon TV program where wives and husbands are asked questions about each other. One of the questions the wives were asked was, "If your husband was on a panel for a beauty contest and he found out that the winner they'd chosen had had silicone, would that change your husband's opinion about her being the winner?" All the wives answered, "My husband likes everything *natural,* and he would definitely renege and pick another girl." Then the husbands were asked the same question and *all* of them said they didn't *care!* If the girl was intelligent and pretty *and* had silicone, it would not change

their attitude toward her. Those men just didn't care . . . and that's what I've found also. . . .

Before my operation, I found that the men I went out with paid very little attention to my breasts, which is something that really disappointed me in my sex life—that they weren't loved and fondled more. After the operation, I got more attention and fondling, and it wasn't curiosity either.

I've never felt anything with the implants that I haven't felt with my own breasts, except the implants cause my skin to stretch tighter over my breasts so I can feel sensations a little stronger. So I find myself being more turned on. My nipples, on the other hand, are so sensitive now that if my lover is not really careful, it disturbs me.

One of the things I'm unhappy about is the way "breast men" are attracted to me since the operation. I categorize them that way only because they insist on categorizing themselves. I know that they come on to me specifically because I have a certain attribute that they like which, in fact, is artificial. These men . . . would they like me if I had smaller titties? If the answer is no, then it's their loss and I don't really want to have anything to do with them. But I have my own double standard about "breast men" coming on to me—it's a kind of conflict which I'm not clear about.

Sometimes I'm attracted to these guys against my better judgment and I think it has to do with my father. I've always had certain images of him that I admire. He was in the merchant marine and he was an extremely, *extremely* handsome man. All of the women he ever had relationships with were very buxom and very beautiful—women that looked like Marilyn Monroe or Ursula Andress or Anita Ekberg. I am sure that has had a lot to do with my self-image—I know it has.

To me, having big breasts meant a whole lot of things . . . a career, sex, looking like a leading lady in the movies, social acceptance, confidence in myself, not being second to anybody with a big chest. It meant always having something *else* to rely on . . . a magic lamp . . . some secret power. But the thing is, once you've got the big breasts, is that really what you want? Because I'm older and a little wiser, I can say that no, it isn't. I didn't become Queen of the World! No man has come along on a great big horse to take me away. And still I didn't become a star!

Natalie

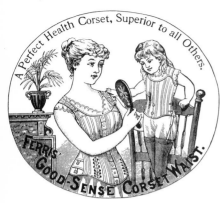

Advertisement, 1886

I'm just disgusted with my whole body—always have been, probably always will be! I'm one of those people who constantly exercise, diet, use every cream, go to doctors for injections . . . anything that I can possibly find.

It's a sin that women have to live this way, 'cause men don't! How many men do you know who really concern themselves with the way they look? They figure they don't have to—they've got it all and you've got to come to them.

But it was inbred in women that looks are crucial for our survival! From the time I was five years old, it was drummed into my head that you had to look after yourself. You couldn't let yourself go. You had to be gorgeous! Even if you weren't born with that figure, you had to get it! No matter how you got it.

I was totally demoralized by not having any breasts. It depressed me terribly. From the time I was a child, I was taught absolutely nothing about breasts except what I saw for myself—that every woman had them. But even then there was the advertising aspect—it was everywhere. You had to be beautiful! You had to be busty! Men liked big-busted women and if you didn't have them, there might have been something wrong with you.

My mother was a busty woman and she complained a lot about bra strap marks. She kept

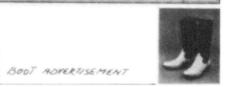

BOOT ADVERTISEMENT

drumming into my head, "Maybe it's great to have a big bustline when you are young, but, my God, when you get older, it is terrible! It's ugly!" She used to say to me, "Please be glad that you are small-breasted. Be glad, because when you get older you're going to hate the backaches and you're going to hate looking fat. You're going to hate *them!* You look slim now and everyone envies you for that." But I would cry in a store whenever it came time to try on a bathing suit. So she would cry with me. And I wouldn't go to the beach.

Even though I was so young, I was already very conscious of fashion—I just became an adult very early. So I started wearing makeup and hairstyles and dressing like an older person to make up for the fact that I wasn't "developed." I *had* to be the most fashionable person in my school. I read *Vogue* and *Harper's Bazaar* while everyone else was reading *Ingenue,* and I became the pacesetter for my class. I even started makeup trends and went to charm school—the whole bit. I would plan an entire outfit the day before—I had to dress better and look better than everybody else! It almost became a sickness, this whole obsession with fashion, but I felt inferior and it helped me compensate for the fact that I was "flat."

At that time it was also very chic to be thin, so I decided if I couldn't be voluptuous I would be as thin as I could get. It was just crazy! I cried like hell because I just couldn't get thin *enough,* and consequently I became ill. I was starving myself to death. By then I was fourteen.

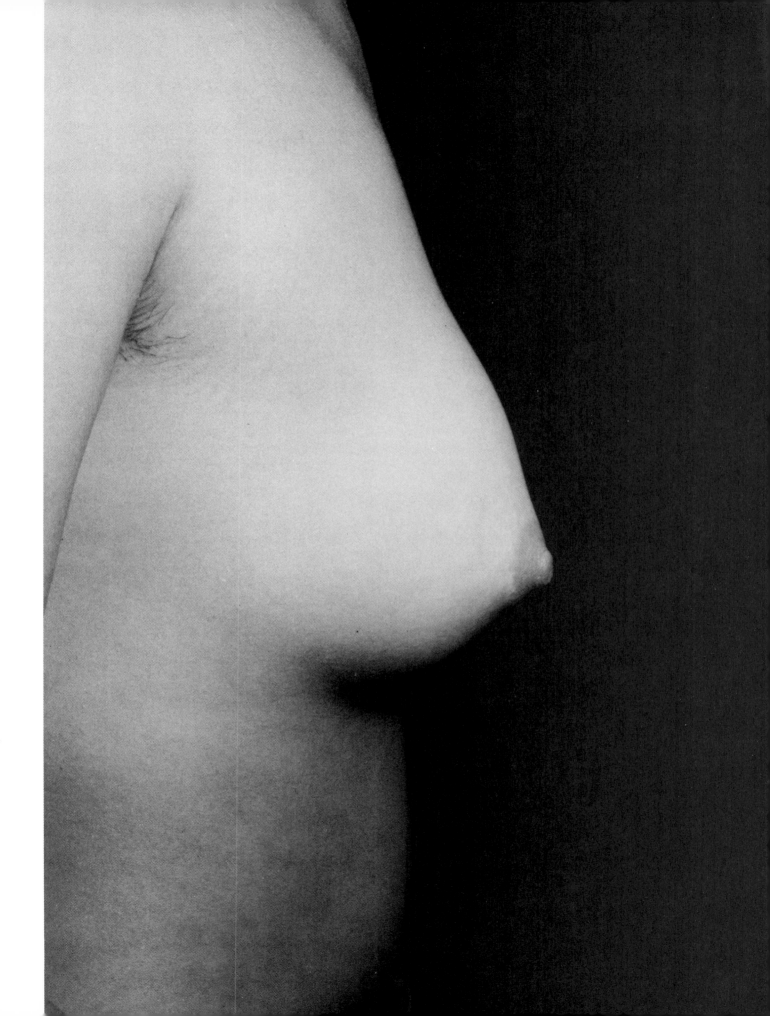

Before dieting I had really small breasts, but then I completely *lost* everything. They just *disappeared!* I had dieted so much that I became flat as a pancake and lost *everything,* even my menstruation cycle! I became terribly depressed.

Everyone in my family was extremely busty—at least a 38C—and I was the only one who wasn't! I couldn't understand it. I knew that breast development was hereditary, but I couldn't understand about *my* heredity—what made me different from both sides of my family? I was like a freak of nature!

Girlfriends, boyfriends, *everyone* would tease me. Even my father and my brothers would tease me because I was so flat-chested. If I didn't wear makeup and if I wore blue jeans and a sweater—I had very short hair—people would call me "sonny"! I could have passed for a twelve-year-old boy!

I didn't really start dating until I was fifteen. I guess I was terribly embarrassed because of my padded bra, and I was *afraid* they'd find out. I was going out with someone who was terribly young and very inexperienced. I didn't realize then that it didn't make any difference to him anyway. He could have been feeling a *chicken* and wouldn't have known the difference!

I didn't enjoy petting. I couldn't enjoy anything to do with sex because I was so conscious that someone would find out. I felt sexually incompetent and I approached sex and bodies from a technical standpoint. I was terribly intellectual, maybe because I was afraid to show emotion, to get close, to be touched.

When I was seventeen, going to college, and feeling very abnormal because I didn't have a voluptuous figure, I went to a doctor just to help my breasts, and he prescribed birth control pills. When birth control pills first came out they were very, very strong. Well, they helped my breasts all right, but the rest of my body got so fat that it didn't make any difference! My hips, my buttocks, my legs—*everything* became enormous! I was as wide as I was tall! My face was a barrel. I went from a hundred pounds to a hundred and sixty-five pounds.

I thought myself the ugliest person in the world! I wore a raincoat *all the time* to hide my body. I couldn't stand myself! I couldn't stand people! Wouldn't walk on the street! I cried all day long! I was constantly in clinics for therapy.

I ended up in psychiatrists' offices thinking that I was really going *crazy* and never knowing that it was the hormones in the pills I was taking. I

was so hung up on looks that I didn't realize that my mind had so much more to offer people. Women were not liberated at all then, so nobody gave me any incentive at all.

●

I've found that *most* American men I meet are breast conscious. They are absolutely propagandized into believing that the *only* thing that makes a woman is her breasts. They have been brainwashed to believe that the bigger the breasts, the more feminine the woman.

Yet I've found men from other countries are more interested in other things—women's legs, shoulders, neck, hair, eyes—sometimes even in the type of person you are. But I wound up getting married to a very young man who, as it later turned out, was *completely* caught up in women's breasts. When I'd complain about myself he'd constantly, constantly reassure me, "No, no, I love you the way you are. I don't care if you are fat, thin, whatever!" He protested so much, I should have known. And I guess deep down inside I just *knew*—I would see him looking at other women. . . . We would go to a party and I desperately wanted to be the belle of the ball, and I couldn't be because I was this fat, round *thing!*

I went to countless doctors to find out what was wrong with me—shortness of breath, all the symptoms of mono. Finally they discovered it was the hormones in the pill that the stupid doctor gave me. They were much too strong so I was taken off the pill. I starved myself and dropped twenty-five pounds, but when I got down to my normal slim self, I was absolutely flat as a board again.

Aunts and cousins made little remarks like, "Well, now that you're married and you have plenty of sex . . . ," referring to all those old wives' tales about sex helping to develop your breasts. Obviously, no one else thought I had enough either!

Well, sex didn't work so I sent away for those exercisers—the ones in the magazines—and I cried because the exercisers hurt so bad. It wasn't the pain. I cried because I knew it wasn't going to do any good! I didn't believe in them but I did try vitamins. I went on a whole vitamin kick while I was living in California with all the vitamin nuts. I tried *everything!* And people still made the same jokes like, "Why don't you eat standing on your head and maybe it'll settle in your chest?"

I'd gotten into the whole hippie syndrome in college. I was trying to get away from being the materialistic, fashionable person. No one was wearing a bra—women were accepting themselves more. So I tried it for a while. But my husband started making remarks about how "flat-chested" I was, so I started to wear a bra again.

I am a history fanatic and I'd read a lot of classic literature—Greek, Roman, Egyptian. I discovered that Helen of Troy's breast fit into a champagne glass, and in that era this was supposed to be *fantastic!* And mine, being so small, also fit perfectly into a champagne glass and I cried, "Why couldn't I have been born *then?*" More than anything I wanted to find a man who thought *that* was beautiful. I wanted a man who would love my breasts, however they were. I wanted to be *totally* accepted.

My marriage was already on the rocks because my husband was fooling around with countless women. He became a photographer and was suddenly obsessed with nude photography.

That's when it became clear that my husband was literally *obsessed* with women's breasts. He never looked at women's legs, asses—he never looked at *anything* except breasts! So I figured it must be *my* fault, and I discussed it with a psychiatrist. My husband had become impotent, and I thought it was because of my figure. But the psychiatrist said it was my husband who had the sex problem, not me.

The psychiatrist also told me that there are such things as plastic surgery and that it would really help. A year went by and I cried every single day about myself, and finally when I'd put enough money away and I couldn't take it anymore, I went all on my own—still in tears—and consulted a plastic surgeon.

I said to him, "Look, I can't take it anymore! I'm so depressed, I feel so ugly that I don't even want to go out in public. I don't even want to go to work!" Oh, the tears. . . . I spent *hours* with him. He was better as a psychiatrist than any trained one I'd had in my whole life. He was the most understanding, charming man I had ever met, and so kind to me. He said, "I think you're crazy—not mentally—but you're a gorgeous woman." I looked at him and said, "I have to thank you for saying that to me. I hope you're not saying that to patronize me, but I still want to go through with the operation."

He said, "Well, you are very small, and in no way are you ever going to be a busty person. The skin will not stretch enough through mammoplasty, and it's very painful at first. It should become normal with time and if that's what you want to do, fine. But your husband should come in." So he called my husband, and my husband *said* that he was against it. So I said, "It's *my* body

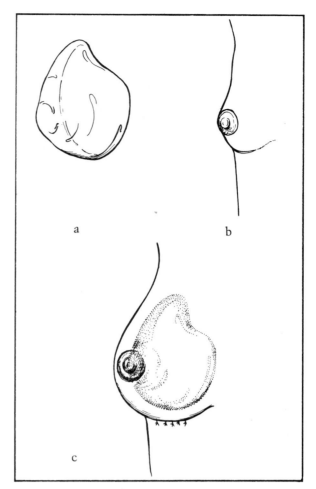

BREAST AUGMENTATION
In breast augmentation, a well-sealed silicone sac that comes in various sizes (a) is implanted in the small breast (b), giving the appearance of a normal-sized breast (c).

and I'm going to do what *I* want!" And I made arrangements to go in for surgery.

I never realized what the pain was going to be like. It was the first operation I ever had in my life. The only reason I kept my sanity in the hospital was because of my doctor—his powers of reassurance were unbelievable.

I went in, had surgery, and never *told* anyone! The only people who knew were my husband and the doctor. Everyone, including my mother, was told I had a flu. The day I came home from the hospital was the day of our anniversary. I was bandaged like a mummy and terribly busty because of all the water retention. Couldn't even move—pain incredible! Couldn't stand or bend over; couldn't use arms. It was probably the same as having a mastectomy. I remember my mother gave me a big hug and a big kiss—"Happy Anni-

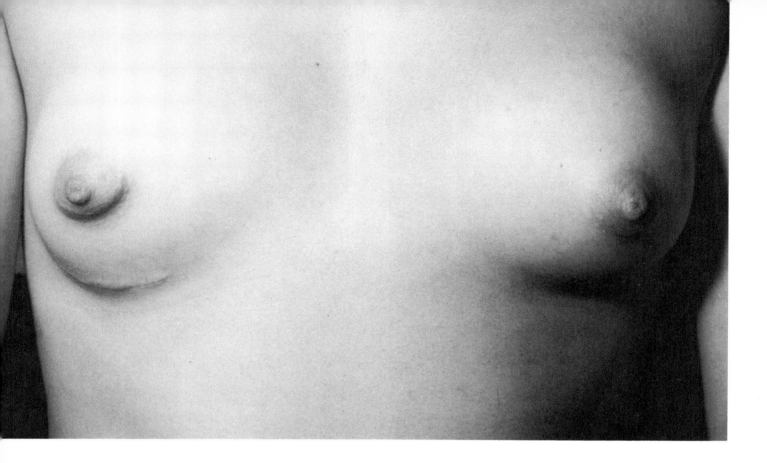

versary!''—and I almost passed out from the pain. I could hardly touch her. I had to tell her I had such a bad flu that my body ached.

And all along I was *dying* to tell someone about the pain I was in but I was ashamed so I didn't. Since I looked the same size as I did when I wore a padded bra before, no one would ever know except my husband. Even after they removed the bandages and put me in a bra, the pain was still incredible. Sex was almost impossible—I couldn't put my body next to anyone else's.

In spite of the pain, I felt more confident. It was unbelievable. I felt like a new person. Before the operation I had lost my sexual desires because of my fetish with my breasts. Now I felt sexy!

It was a *thrill* to go out and buy a stretch bra that didn't have any padding in it. An absolute thrill not to wear bones and corsets and things to make me look busty. An absolute thrill to go out and buy a bathing suit. It was the most *incredible* thing that happened to me! But one breast never healed.

Four months after the operation my husband left me. Two months after that the pain was still incredible and one breast was hard as a *rock!* It was as if they filled the implant with *concrete* instead of silicone. Incredible! If anyone had touched it they would've known it was not real. So I went back to the surgeon. He said I had de-

veloped this kind of scar tissue. It is an inherited thing. He told me I'd have to go in and have the implant removed and another put in.

Okay, great. I was supporting myself as a draftsman. I constantly used my right arm at work and it was the right breast that was affected. When I went in for corrective surgery, I told everyone I had a lump and had to have it removed. The doctor didn't charge any fee—he cried with me.

They removed the implant and scar tissue and said there was an unbelievable amount of it. They wanted to put it in a jar for posterity. In order to remove all the tissue and put in the new implant, they had to make a very big scar. The first implant was done through tiny incisions under the nipples, and you couldn't tell. This time they had to make an incision across the entire bottom of the breast.

That's done, fine. Pain again, worse this time than the first time. Immobility. Can't move my right arm. I am right-handed and couldn't even open a can. I was living alone. Couldn't tell anyone because I was still ashamed. Finally, I told a neighbor that I'd had a cyst removed, so she'd come down once in a while to make sure I had something to eat.

Well, it passed. But I went back to work prematurely because I needed my salary, and fainted. I had a relapse and had to stay in bed for another couple of weeks.

110

When that was over, the breast started to soften and be normal, but I had a terrible scar under my breast. It's been three years since the second operation. My breasts are just getting back to normal touch and feeling. It's like a whole new thing for me—I can actually *feel* again.

Now my breasts aren't bad. I wouldn't say they're gorgeous, but they are probably more beautiful than what I once envied as a young girl. They're firm and always will be. I never have to wear a bra because they are *all* silicone. I have very healthy-shaped breasts and they are very young-looking. I have the nipples of a very young girl—not aged a bit. I suppose as women get older they gain and lose and gain and lose, so they don't have that firmness—they don't have firm skin. Your breasts become aged just like the rest of your skin. *My* breasts are probably the youngest part of my body! (*Laughs.*)

I know a lot of women who cream their breasts every night because they are afraid they're going to sag. I've got news for them—they're going to sag *anyway*. Mine will probably not look too different from the way they look now because they're not real. (*Laughs.*)

Now when I have an affair with someone they'll say, "Oh, when did you have your breast operation?" The first time that happened I was totally flabbergasted! I went through all this to be natural, or rather normal, and then someone says to me, "When did you have your breast operation?" Still, no one in my family knows about the operation. I have *never* undressed for a fitting in front of my mother. I've never even told doctors about it when they've given me a routine examination. No one knows except a very, very few close friends.

I sometimes feel that I went through all that pain for nothing. People still tell me I don't measure up. To this day men still make remarks that I'm flat-chested. I can be out with a group of adult men and they'll still *tease* me about it, even after all that pain and aggravation!

But as I've gotten older I've also discovered how ridiculous men's attitudes about breasts are. A group of people on Madison Avenue and in Hollywood are causing this whole thing—just a particular group of men who are the controlling powers of advertising, films, and the other media. A few men that have a fetish about women's breasts caused this whole damn thing! The only question I'd like to ask men is, "Do you think anything *else* exists besides a woman's breasts?"

I would like to wage a war to wipe out breast fetishes in every American male! I'd kill the man who put the girl on the Chevrolet—nobody does this to *men*. I'd hang him by his toes! You should buy the car because you think it works, not because you think the busty blonde will come with it.

Sex is a great thing, but why do you have to use it to sell your liquor? If it's *that* bad, you shouldn't be in the business. And it's an utter *sin* that most men in this country never read anything else except girlie magazines. If we could only put naked ladies into *The New York Times*, then maybe they'd read, and then go out and vote!

Two months ago, they found three lumps in the breast that was reoperated on, but I refuse to go in for a biopsy. I go through pain every other month—a rare inflammation from the operation; not all women have it. I'm still *paying* for it, still paying my debt.

I refuse to go in for the biopsy because the worst thing that could ever happen to me is to have a mastectomy. If they did that to me, I would feel completely unfemale. I consider breasts part of being a woman. I wouldn't want to look like a man for a million dollars. No matter what amount of liberation, brains, president's wives . . . it doesn't make any difference to me who else had a mastectomy. That's how I'm going to feel. And I swear I would rather have the cancer spread through my body than do *that!*

I've learned a lot from what I went through—being obsessed with my breasts. I'm still learning, believe me, though I relapse constantly. But I think my breasts are becoming less and less important to me. I've learned that the way I felt about my breasts, I also felt about my face, the bump in my nose, my legs, my teeth, my hips, my buttocks, *everything!* . . .

It's been good to tell someone what I've been through. There was a time when I couldn't tell *anyone.* I hope it helps other women realize that some of us have gone through *hell* because of our breasts . . . and it's *not worth it!!*

Rose
Age 32 • Raised in Oklahoma • Ex-Call Girl

My breasts are huge! (Laughs.) Huge! *I'm forever attracting "breast men." Most men I meet pay more attention to my breasts than any other part of me. When I'm with men, I make them feel* proud—*I'm like an* ornament *they can show off!*

Oh, They rave *about my breasts! Of course, I always get these men who at first say, "I love legs, I don't like breasts. Breasts only get in the way"—the same things* I *say about them. And then once the ice is broken and we become friendly, they'll say, "Oh, they're beautiful! I just wish* I *had them. I would touch them all day long!" All these ridiculous things.* (Laughs.) *They swear on a stack of Bibles they're not "breast men"! And, of course,* those *are the ones that are.*

When I was 15 years old, I bought and filled my first 36DD bra. Since then, no man has ever made a serious pass at me without assuring me in the first hour that he was a leg man. Tits!? Why, he hadn't even noticed!

The tacit understanding was that if I did indeed have those giant knockers one hears so much about in locker rooms and sees flopping across magazine covers, why he simply hadn't seen what all the fuss was about! Instead he had been quietly pursuing his birdwatching of ankles, knees, and nicely turned calves.

For years I believed these men, which goes to show how dumb one can be when one puts one's mind to it. And for years I felt sorry for the men who, by some sad twist of fate had gotten stuck with me when they'd have preferred legs. On the other hand, I always knew that if I ever really wanted anything, all I'd have to do was lean forward slightly. Suddenly, the world was waiting to hear what it was I wanted, how fast I wanted it, and whether they could get a better one for me wholesale.

—Eve Babitz, "My Life in a 36DD Bra, or, The All-American Obsession"

I think men would really like to have breasts, at least some men. They must think of breasts as something missing *from them. They say we envy penises, but I don't believe that is true. From my experience, I believe men envy our breasts and they just try to make us* think *that we envy their penises, because really they're jealous of us! So many men I've known have said that they just love them so much, they wished they had them! They probably mean having a pair they could pull out of a drawer and play with at their leisure and then throw in the closet when they're finished! Growing on them? Owning them? I am sure if they had breasts growing on them, they wouldn't like them as much.* (Laughs.)

... men would view my tits and become aflame with desire for them, and they would fantasize about having a pair of their own: "God, if I had tits like those I could fuck my way into a million bucks . . ."

—Eve Babitz

When I first started developing I wasn't at all prepared to have breasts. They came too soon; I didn't want them. I was in the fifth grade, and they were like two doughnuts on my chest.

(*Laughs.*) In the beginning it worried me because the outside part was hard and it hurt.

Boys in my class liked my breasts, but they didn't know what to do about them. Breasts were

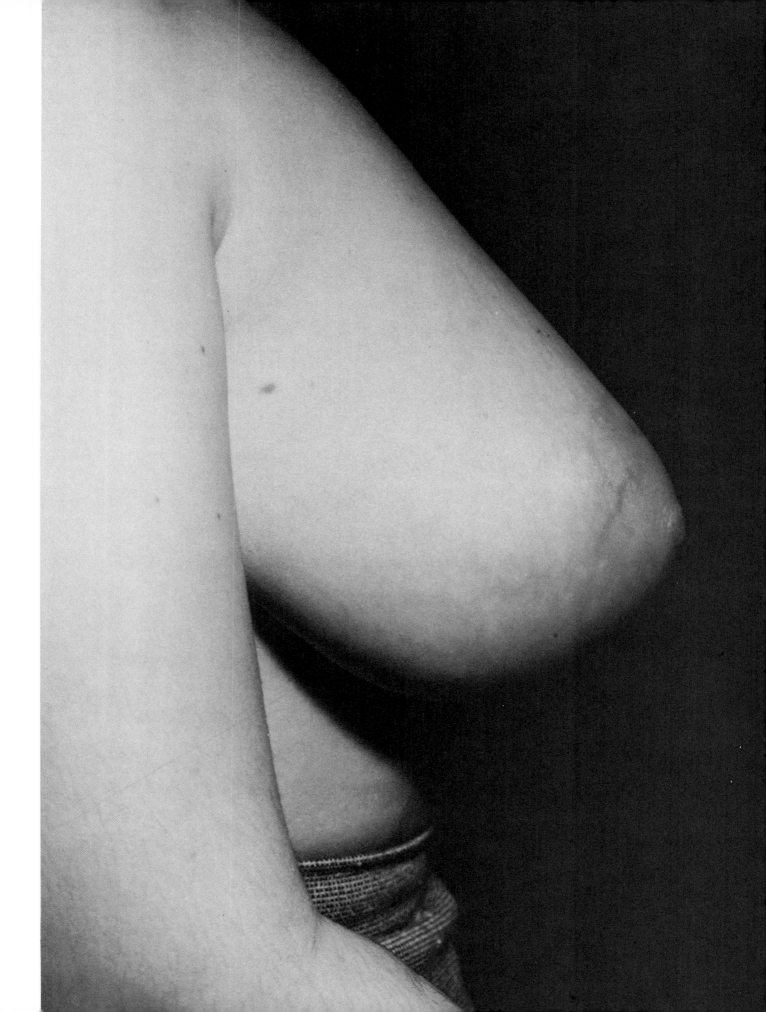

sort of threatening to them. I was also a little taller than they were at that age, so I guess they looked upon me as an older woman . . . in grade five!! (*Laughs.*) I remember being frightfully embarrassed about it. I never had a training bra—I went straight into an A cup and I didn't even want it. My mother told me I had to wear a bra whether I liked it or not! She said I needed support. (*Laughs.*) With an A cup, right?

I remember when I was very young my mother told me what breasts were for and that one day I would have them. *Boy did I!* I had never really looked forward to having breasts. They always looked like they'd get in my way and sure enough they did. *Now* my mother says, "Have you ever considered reduction surgery?" (*Laughs.*) Well, they have gotten kind of ridiculous, you know! I wear a 36DD and sometimes even a 38DD, and I wish I could get a triple D because I *still* have a cleavage with a double D.

I was terribly insecure and never had the slightest idea that I was attractive until I was thirteen or fourteen, after I developed breasts. I was *never* told by my parents . . . *ever* . . . that I was attractive or worthwhile. I can't even remember their telling me that they loved me. So my new appearance made me feel good and worthwhile, and helped me compensate for the love I didn't get.

By age fourteen, I was a 34C and I was getting an awful lot of attention. At first I was a little self-conscious about being looked at so much, but pretty soon I began to notice that boys thought I was pretty, so I didn't mind. I considered it more flattering than anything else. I became proud of my breasts.

It was becoming obvious to me that all this attention was to my advantage and did I take advantage! Oh, you don't know! The *games* I played with those poor little boys. (*Laughs.*) Well, I guess "games" is the wrong word, because I never gave the slightest indication that I'd ever permit them to touch me *anywhere*—not even my *hand.* (*Laughs.*) I was a very hands-off-type kid, but I used to flaunt my breasts a lot. I used to flaunt everything about myself—I became a tease. (*Laughs.*)

Once I had my bra stolen. I lived only a few blocks from the school. Some guy snuck into the house and somehow got into my bedroom, opened the drawer, and took one of my bras. It was all in fun, just like a panty raid, you know. It was because of my large breasts, my reputation. It was a challenge, I guess—male spirit or something. Word got around high school but I wasn't

mad about it. I took it in very good humor and everyone thought I was a good sport.

Around that time, we were on a family trip and my father scribbled some graffiti on a rock. He put my name and my measurements and added a couple of inches to the bust. It was a joke and we all laughed about it. I had a good sense of humor in those days.

Having large breasts helped me think of myself as a sex symbol. Everyone else did! (*Laughs.*) And it certainly didn't encourage me to do anything with myself intellectually. I used to take great *pains* to imitate Marilyn Monroe. And I was even told that I looked like her! I even wore my blond hair like hers.

Although I was always a great reader and still am to this day, I never thought about having a career because I always thought I would grow up to *be* Marilyn! In that way, my breasts harmed me very much. A woman shouldn't think that she *has to be* a sex symbol just because her breasts are large. At the time, I really felt that it was *expected* of me. *Everyone* wanted to look like that . . . and I unfortunately did.

I was popular with boys in a strange way. They liked the way I looked, but I was rather shy and my personality was not very outgoing. How could I compete with *them?* (Laughs.)

I also started getting plenty of, "Shit, she must really be horny." (They get horny so I'm supposed to.)

—Eve Babitz

Being stacked always made it very easy to get dates. You know, in a small town your reputation gets around and a lot of things were said about what I would do, how hot I was, and so on, just because of my large breasts. In fact, it was the farthest thing from the truth. The truth was I was pretty frightened of sexual contact. I noticed that, ironically, after my dates found out that they couldn't touch, only look, my reputation even *grew!*

The very first time I let a boy touch my breasts, I think I was a senior in high school. Touching *over* the clothes only, nothing else. I loved it but I don't know if I thought of it in a sexual way at the time. I mean, I was so totally unawakened sexually at that age. I just knew it felt good.

I still enjoy having my breasts caressed, but it's not really that important. My nipples are very sensitive, but the rest of my breasts are not. I like having my nipples sucked on very much. I usually open my eyes and watch . . . I mean, I love *watching!* My nipples get erect during sex and they stay

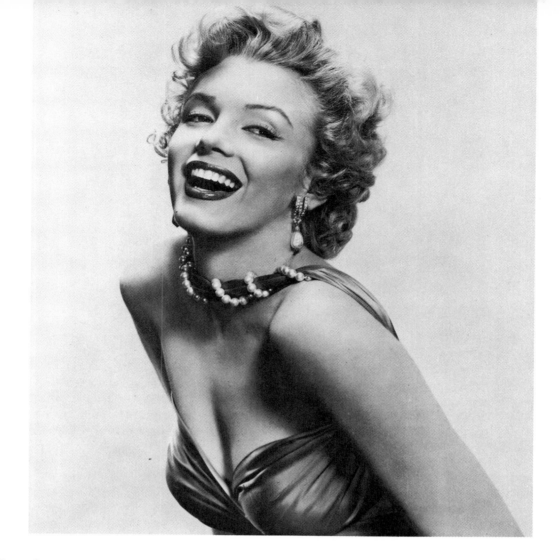

hard for a long time after, but that's normal—I read it in a book. I read all those things.

Somebody tried to rape me when I was about eighteen—I was still a virgin then—but he was too drunk and I was too strong for him. He wasn't violent and he didn't slap me or anything. He was trying to get my clothes off faster than I could get them back on, but I won. I've often wondered if that would have happened if I was built differently. I wasn't bothered much in that way as an adolescent because I lived in a very small town and those things just weren't done. But after I left home at age nineteen and went to the big city—that's when more unpleasant things happened.

●

I always thought of my breasts in terms of using them sexually, or using them to get men, or using them to get men *to do* whatever I want. So I flaunted my breasts all the time. It was very effective, because if you can make a man want you, you can make him do just about whatever you want him to do. It sounds like a sick, terrible

thing to say, but it's true, and I also think it is very unfortunate that it's true. It was easy to become a call girl because of the size of my breasts . . . because men were so *attracted* to them!

It had been a mixed blessing up until then—my breasts or me? That was the question. I got tired of trying to relate on my terms—it was always too painful—so I decided to relate to men on their terms. They were more than eager to foot the bill . . . to pay for my favors. It was so *easy*. Men were constantly propositioning me with dinners and dates and such.

By that time, I'd already learned right from the horses' mouth that men just had this "fatal weakness" for me, and that practically any guy who was *so* attracted to me was willing to pay for his "weakness." The first time money was offered I was twenty-one. So that's how it began. It required very little change in my life-style. I was still being related to as a "pair of tits," but now I was relating to "clients," rather than to so-called "lovers." And my breasts were like my calling card.

I used to have a few guys who would give me

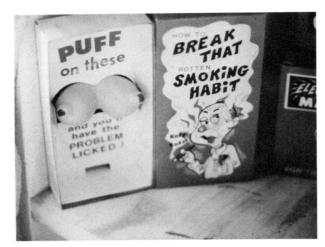

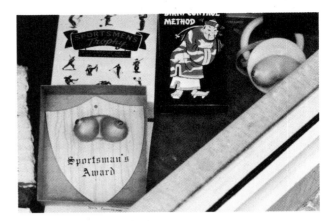

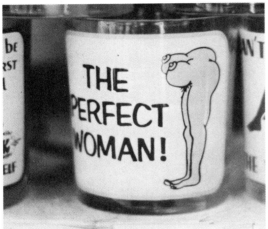

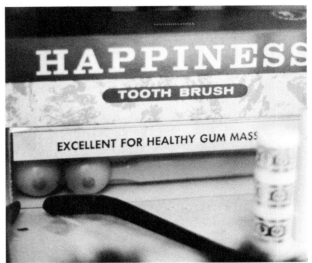

Details from novelty store window

lots of money, but I'm not greedy. I wasn't like those girls that have to make thousands a week. Maybe I wasn't that ambitious, but I preferred having a few regular people. That way, it was more like a relationship, more personal.

Most men really just want company, anyway. But it is still the breasts that attract them. They want me to make them feel like men—the sex is secondary. Men just love to play with my breasts . . . and kiss them . . . and talk about them. Some of them related to me like a "mommy." For some reason I brought out the little boy in them. As soon as they got their clothes off, it was preadolescence! They'd suck and slobber on my nipples like a child.

I used to be able to twirl my breasts in opposite directions and men loved that sort of thing. I'd touch my breasts and that would turn a man on. I'd sit up straight, stick them out, and display them. Oh, men love to look. There were guys who liked to just *look* at my breasts and jerk themselves off!

One man only liked to see me in a brassiere of a certain type—it had to be very satiny and

smooth. He would never actually touch my breasts, but he liked the smooth feeling of the satin. And there were men who loved to come between my breasts. Personally I think it's a waste (*Laughs.*) and very messy, but what can you say—it's their game, right?

●

A few years ago, I went through a period of being a social butterfly. I was escorted to lots of so-called "chic" parties with a lot of boring, stupid people who thought they were so very cool because they had a lot of money or social position. Any man that I went to these parties with would treat me like some ornament. . . . I don't know, maybe like a sports car. It was, "Hey, look at this prize! Hey, look at her tits!" I hated it! Actually, I feel like that *every time* I go out with a man . . . always, always, *always!* It has always been devastating.

My breasts are the first thing that men see and they relate to me *as a* "pair of breasts." A few months ago when I was in an elevator, a guy walked in and when he saw me he didn't even *turn around!* It was fall and unfortunately I wasn't wearing a coat. (*Laughs.*) He just kept staring straight at my bust! Then he started talking to me, still looking at *them,* so I said, "Hey, I'm up here!" He seemed slightly embarrassed, but that didn't stop him.

In an article in *Ms.* magazine that I read the other day—"My Life in a 36DDBra"—the writer said that she was in a supermarket and a guy passed her and muttered "Big tits" . . . just like that. That has happened to me at least a thousand times. I can't even *count* the number of times! (*Laughs.*) And it was so funny the way she compared it to Cary Grant—*recognition!*

Recently, in Ralph's, my local supermarket where anything often goes, there I am trying to decide on some lettuce—lost in thought, idylls of watercress—when I feel a man behind me and quickly, before I can turn around, he says in a low, authoritative purposeful salute: "Big tits." And he's gone.

That's like seeing a movie star. You run up—with all kinds of fantasies beaming through your regular thought processes—you run up to Cary Grant and you say "Cary Grant!"

What's he supposed to do? You've just said his name to him—a tradition, a heritage, a massive plethora of dreams and meanings. It's the same with men and my tits. They cannot imagine my doing anything that isn't somehow connected with how big my tits are. And my tits aren't even *that* big, I mean . . . they're not Cary Grant. They're more . . . John Garfield or Dean Martin. You know, there's that shock of recognition but not the fainting spell Cary Grant would inspire.

—Eve Babitz

●

It's been a long time since I've worn "alluring" clothing . . . two sizes ago. Now, I always wear things that don't emphasize my breasts, like vests or shawls or anything to hide them a little more. I love the winter when I'm all covered up and I hate it when spring comes and I have to take off my coat. If I could stand it, I'd wear a coat in the summer, too! My breasts are much less vulnerable like that, and so am I.

There's also all this having to bundle up. Whenever I go into the street, I have to cover myself with clothes that flow and drape. I cannot wear a tight anything on the street if I hope to have a moment's peace. Suppose, for example, you wanted to go for a nice walk and look at the sunset and breathe in the air at eventide, nice idea, right? No, no, no. Not if you've got big tits and you're not bundled up (Cary Grant can't do it either).

—Eve Babitz

I've learned a lot of lessons about men from my breasts—about how stupid, immature, and child-ish they are—and how cruel they can be. For example, at a party I went to during my social butterfly year, I was introduced to a man who was slightly drunk. He took my hand, but instead of kissing it, he bent down and kissed my breast— right in front of *everybody!* I was so embarrassed! I wanted to die! I wanted to kill him! I wanted to slap his stupid face! I wanted to *scream!*

When a man who I don't love and am not sexually engrossed in talks about my tits, there's something that makes me want to pour cold water into his lap and leave a loose carton of ice cream on his car seat overnight.

—Eve Babitz

My breasts have always made me feel sexy, but it's more than that—my breasts gave me *power!* That's kind of sexy, isn't it? I love using that power against men because basically I really hate them. I loathe them and despise the cocksuckers! I'd love to castrate every fucking one of them! (*Laughs.*)

I hate men for the same reason they *like* me— how I *look,* not what I *am!* They don't even *know* me! The few times I've tried to get through to a man, I was invariably disappointed. In the past few years, I can cope with it much better because I don't feel like much of an "ornament" anymore. I made sure of that.

I started getting heavy in my late twenties. At that time, I had really had it with men. I gained weight deliberately, although I didn't think so at the time, because I wanted to make myself ugly to keep men away from me. I didn't want anything to do with them. I just wanted to be left alone! Unfortunately I still have a pretty face and a big bust, and even though I am heavy there are a lot of men who won't leave me alone. So gaining weight didn't help that much. But the onslaught has let up. I had more time to think things out, to read, to be myself, and I think in the last few years I've come to terms with it. Now I am ready to lose weight and hope I'm ready to handle being thin again.

I don't think I'll ever be a call girl again. I am trying not to be self-destructive anymore and for me that was self-destructive. There was nothing good about it. It desensitized me emotionally and I didn't like that.

Sometimes . . . I would just love to be built like the woman next door. She is totally flat! I've often wondered . . . if I had not had these large breasts, whether my life would have turned out completely differently.

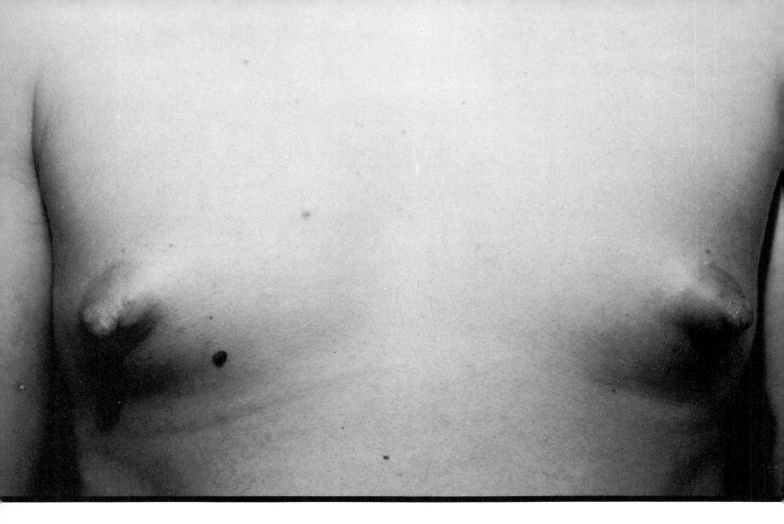

Nancy

Age 32 · Raised in New York City · Unemployed

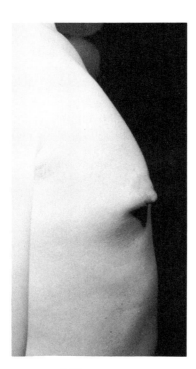

You know that expression, "It's what's up front that counts"? Well, I really lived that. I saw breasts as a "calling card." You know how you give someone your calling card and they see your name and they see where you're at? They "check you out" and then they relate to you. That's the way I saw it. Only as far as I was concerned, I didn't have a calling card.

I always thought that if I had breasts, then they would get the men. You know what I mean? They would be sticking out like this, (motions) and they would be the first thing that would hit the men. First the men would get to them, then they would get to the rest of me, and then sometime after that, to the "person" in me.

When I was growing up, being flat-chested was like a social disease! It not only bothered me, but it also bothered everyone around me. I couldn't even mention being flat-chested to some of my friends. So I usually wouldn't talk about it. But sometimes I couldn't help myself, and if I brought it up, they'd say, "Oh, no, you're not!" They'd deny it! It was like they couldn't believe it was true, that it could really happen to somebody they knew. They reacted as if being flat-chested was something horrible, almost as if I had the curse!

I remember that I always used to ask my mother, "When am I going to develop?" And she would reply, "Well, once you get your period." I didn't get my period until I was fourteen. Then she said, "Once you get into high school." It was always *going* to happen. She put it off like something she took for granted—this *always* happened to everybody, so of course it was going to happen to me. I never felt as though the way I'm built could just be normal and that's that.

I had a friend who lived across the hall from me. We'd been in kindergarten together, and when we were in our early teens I remember her telling me she had nice big breasts—oh, 34D—and how proud she was of that. "Oh, you poor dear," she'd say, and then she told me about some kind of exercise she had done—putting your elbows back or something like that. I did it for a while and gave up when I noticed that it didn't make any difference.

Also, I prayed a lot. I never actually knelt down and prayed, "Dear God, please give me breasts," but I did get very superstitious. I would suddenly get an intuition and then check the mirror to see if there was a change . . . as though magically breasts would materialize. Then I thought that maybe I was doing the wrong thing by looking out for it—after all, a watched pot never boils.

When I was in junior high school, I remember a boy said that he found some other girl more attractive than me. Now this girl was *obese!* She had some kind of physical ailment. Something was wrong with her and she was all blown up like a balloon. So just because I didn't have big breasts, I was so *horrible* that even somebody as grotesque as that girl was better than me! And if that wasn't bad enough, a couple of really nasty girls in my class used to call me "the flat-chested orangutan."

I began trying to create the illusion of having bigger breasts. There was a blouse with ruffles in the front that I wore with a cardigan on top, and I arranged it so that it would sort of *add* to the look. For a long time I tried not to get into wearing padded bras because I just didn't like the idea. It wasn't honest and it felt like cheating. But I finally gave in. It meant not being made fun of anymore.

My mother did all the buying for me because I was ashamed. Right away she got me a bra with *lots* of padding—the damned thing! I even remember the shape of it. Each cup was like half a football. The darn thing was made out of hard rubber and, oh, a *horrible* thing happened in high school with it.

I was walking through the halls, carrying my books in front of my chest, and I *bang* into somebody! Here I am, completely flat, and the goddamned bra is sticking out like this (*indicates with outstretched arms*), and there is *nothing* inside of it, right?—completely *empty!* So the damned hard rubber thing gets dented in, of course, and it *stays* that way! That wasn't so bad because I had my ruffled blouse on, but then the fuckin' thing suddenly snaps back out and makes this incredibly loud "pop," like an explosion, echoing through the halls as I walk to my class. I just *died!*

After a while, I gave up on padded bras and switched to a brassiere with falsies inside. I'd been complaining and complaining, and my mother would say, "Why don't you get some falsies?" and I'd say, "No!" because I didn't want a false thing on me, but I finally gave in. I just couldn't make it into the store to buy something like that, so my mother wound up buying the falsies for me, too. She just gave them to me one day; she thought she was doing me a favor.

Each falsie had a little satin cover over it, and I would put them inside my bra with safety pins. I wore these *same* falsies for a long, long, long time, because I just didn't have the guts to go in and get new ones. Meanwhile, they started to stink and the foam rubber in the falsies got all crumbly and stale with time.

It got so bad that I used to freak out whenever anybody would mention words like "foam rubber." They could have been talking about a *pillow*, but just hearing the word would send shivers up my spine. I was so paranoid that somebody was talking about me. And words like "flat tires" or "pancake," . . . God, I'd *cringe!* Just innocent conversation. They could've been talking about *eating* pancakes, but all those words would make me really paranoid!

I just *hated* it! I just hated the whole thing! I didn't *want* to be wearing falsies! Psychologically, it was a really damaging thing for me to wear falsies *all the time!* Jesus! . . . It sounds so *sick!*

As the years went by, I always used my small breasts as an excuse for all kinds of problems I had. I blamed everything that went wrong in my life on them.

When I was about sixteen, I went to see a doctor, a woman, and I told her this whole sob story about how my life was *ruined.* I went on about how I didn't get asked out because I was flat-chested. Then she told me a story about her son who was going out with a woman who was a cretin. In other words, she was telling me there was still *hope* for me! If he'll go out with a cretin, then maybe some guy would go out with me.

She said ridiculous things and compared me to someone who had a bad case of acne. *That* means that your nutrition is fucked up and besides, it's ugly. It means that you're not healthy. Here she was, a doctor, acting as though there was really something *wrong* with me—like I was unhealthy and deformed, and like it wasn't natural to have small breasts, too. That sure didn't help.

I began to resort to other measures. One time I sent away for a "breast developer" that turned out to be a jump rope . . .

When I was eighteen I went to see a gynecologist. I complained to him about my breasts, so he gave me birth control pills because sometimes they make your breasts swell up. P.S. Mine didn't—no difference!

I was so desperate that at one point in my twenties I went to see a plastic surgeon. First he described the operation, and then he showed me "before and after" pictures. I noticed that in one picture the scars that were supposed to be right under the breasts so that they wouldn't be visible were much further down, a couple of inches below. So I said, "What happened here?" He replied nonchalantly, "Well, that was just a mistake." And I thought to myself, Holy shit! Fifteen hundred dollars he wants for the operation, and here he's cutting somebody up and he makes a *mistake?!!!* So I decided not to do it, and I'm glad. But I was *still* hooked on falsies!

If you wear falsies, the bra is always hiking up whenever you lift your arms because there's nothing to hold it down. The whole fuckin' thing, including the fake breasts, goes! It looks like you suddenly sprouted breasts from your collarbone! It made me crazy to always have that fear in the back of my mind.

Also, if you're wearing all this rubber the air doesn't get through to your breast. In the summer you sweat like anything—it is just incredible. Now I've got little moles or warts on my breasts, and I bet that's from years of being smothered.

I remember that the beach was always a *nightmare.* What do you do when you're getting up and down? You want to lie on your stomach, right, and then the bra top comes down. I was always petrified that someone would look in there and see the *horrible secrets!!*

I could never get a bathing suit to fit right. If it had bones, the darn thing would stick out so far

that it was much too big—bigger than the "falsie image" I had. And the ones that didn't have bones—these little flimsy things—were cut much too low in the middle. I finally got a two-piece with a top that was just a wide piece of fabric that went straight across, without the low-cut part in the middle, so that no one could see that I didn't have anything there. And very important—I would pin my falsies in so they'd never get lost in the water and float away. I made damn sure of that!

●

Can you imagine how it would feel—a guy getting all passionate and turned on, feeling up your *falsies?* They did the whole feeling-me-up number over my bra! They didn't notice the difference! So then I wouldn't let guys feel me up because it seemed ridiculous.

When I got older, I never let a guy watch me undress because I had to take off my breasts! I'd go into another room and take my bra and falsies off, and I'd roll the whole thing into a little ball and hide it under all my clothes. Then I'd come out.

There was one guy I went out with who was particularly sadistic and mean. One night I slept over at his house. I had my bra all scrunched up under my clothes, and when I woke up the next

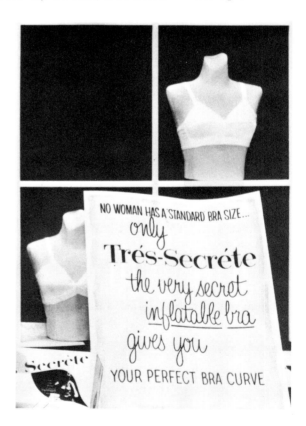

NO WOMAN HAS A STANDARD BRA SIZE...

only

Trés-Secréte

the very secret inflatable bra gives you

YOUR PERFECT BRA CURVE

morning, the fuckin' thing was lying open right in front of my eyes. The bastard stuck it right in my face just to be mean! Just to make sure and let me know that *he* knew.

One man really made a good comment which helped me confront my problem more. He said, "You must feel like you're deformed," trying to understand the way I felt. That really hit me hard and it disturbed me for a long time, but that's *exactly* the way I felt.

By this time, I was *dying* to take the falsies off because I was so uncomfortable. But I was obsessed and worried about what everyone would say if one day I had them on as usual, and the next day I didn't, especially at work. I'd worn them for years at work and I thought I couldn't do without them.

Then I began to notice other flat women around and thought to myself that they were pretty small and nobody was killing them or anything and they were *getting away* with it. So I began to think that maybe, somehow, I might have the guts to do it, too. But how could I walk into work one day without falsies after all these years? There would be such a big *difference!*

So I never got rid of my falsies until I *quit* that job, and then I never went back to visit any of the people I'd worked with. I had to make a complete break. Well, I wore those goddamned falsies right through high school and through this job—about nine years! Can you believe it?

●

I was sexually "straight" for about six years, and ever since I came out as a lesbian, my body has become mine and I am happy with it now. I feel I can do what I want with it, and it's not a matter of how someone else sees it. And I have never gotten shit from other women. It's been four years now, and I've had time to recuperate from the hell I went through before.

Men never took any time to make me enjoy my breasts, to make me feel good about them. I don't think men know what to do with a flat-chested woman, so they ignore her breasts—including the nipple—and make her feel insecure. At least that's what happened to me.

I can't remember how erogenous my breasts

were when I was straight because they were either ignored or abused. Anyway, I was so uptight about them that I hardly felt anything there. Now I always feel at ease with a woman. Lately I have discovered that my breasts are erotically stimulating.

I don't feel bad about my breasts anymore, but whenever I think about them—when I'm conscious of them—I still remember all those horrible experiences and it affects me, you know.

I went to an all-women's dance one summer and it was so hot that some women took their shirts off. I was amazed! I didn't know how to react. Then I saw some others standing around, and you could tell they were thinking about it. Finally, they'd make up their mind and all of a sudden they'd pull off their shirts.

Well, I wanted to do it, too, but the longer I stood there thinking about it the more upset I got, until I finally had to leave the dance. I mean nobody said, "You'd better take your shirt off!" I just left because I didn't want to deal with it, I couldn't confront it.

But I was in such a state of turmoil about it that I almost got hit by a car on my way home. The car actually came so close that it ripped a piece of my jacket off. Isn't that strange?

I've since gone to dances where I was one of the first to take off my shirt and dance. To me, it means I've come a long way. It feels good, anyway. It's ridiculous not to. We'd be dancing and the sweat would be dripping down. Men wouldn't think twice about doing that. So why not?

It always gets me angry when people say I don't have breasts. Even when you are *completely* flat-chested, if you have glands and nipples you still have breasts! I don't like the idea that the way you are identified as a woman is by the size of your breasts. That's obviously a male notion.

Lately, I've been taking karate lessons and doing pushups and my pectoral muscles have developed a bit. Now I am a little bigger than completely flat-chested. So a friend said to me, "Wow, you're getting *big!*" (*Laughs.*) It's funny that it would be happening now, when I don't particularly want to get bigger. Now I am pretty happy with them.

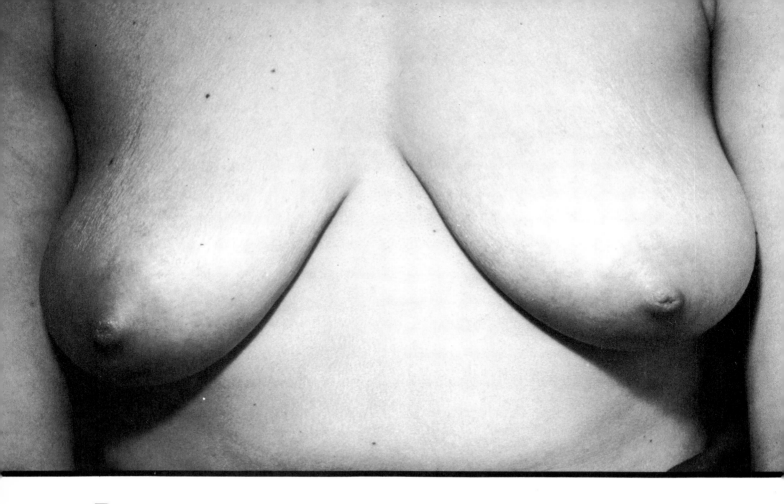

Pat

Age 30 • Raised in "Small Town," Pa. • Social Worker

Now, more than ever, I am extremely proud of myself, of my body, of my breasts. One of my biggest fantasies is just to ride down the highway bare-breasted on my motorcycle. I resent the fact that men do not have to wear shirts and women do, especially in the summer when it's so hot. I see no reason for that, and I see no reason for any woman to be embarrassed by her breasts, no matter what size they are. I just think your breasts are you—they're part of you and they're beautiful.

It took me a long time to understand that, and to understand that maybe I disliked my breasts because of all the outside programming I got. There is a regular kind of conditioning that female children get which says that you have to compete! You have to compete with your body and you're not supposed to compete with your mind. And you have to behave in certain ways and dress in certain ways and wear certain apparatuses to make your body look good. If it's not girdles, it's bras and even padded bras, you know, the whole trip. I hated it all!

When I was little, I wanted to be held, and I enjoyed having my mother hold me so that my head would be on her breast because it was so soft and so comforting. That was always important.

Whenever I hurt emotionally or physically that's where I went—boom—right to Mother, right to the breast. Get in there and get the hug, get the security. Hugs are a big thing with me, especially from Mother, but she won't do that now because she thinks I'm a "big girl" and big girls don't need hugs. She cut that out around puberty. I guess she felt that it was time for me to grow up and she decided that we had to change our relationship. I think the change had some adverse effects on me. I didn't understand what was going on—why she was rejecting me—and why I had to start acting in a different way.

●

Throughout my childhood I was very aware that there was a big difference between male children and female children because I was treated differently. I couldn't do the things that my brothers did and I really hated them for that. I always got messages from my mother and my aunts and the women in the neighborhood. They weren't straightforward but they were messages nevertheless. I remember one time my mother told me to stop playing so rough with the boys or I'd hurt my insides. I said, "What do you mean, I'll hurt my insides?" She said, "Well, you won't be able to have babies," and I said, "Well, I don't want babies anyway. I want to play football!"

I was a real tomboy and I only played with boys—never had any girls around. I remember that we used to say things about "tits," which was dirty, and we'd giggle. We'd hide in trees and look at "tits." As a matter of fact, I remember one lady who had very large breasts. We were fascinated and I don't think it was a negative thing either. It was just that we didn't have them.

One summer before I started getting breasts, a girl I knew was just beginning to develop. One day she had on a sleeveless shirt and her arm was up and I tried to look in the shirt to see her breasts. I was embarrassed 'cause I did that. I said to myself, Christ, you must be a pervert or something. But I was curious and fascinated then, just like all the boys. I *always* was, except when I started getting my own—I wasn't too happy about that. Deep down I knew that meant I had to stop being a tomboy.

I remember it seemed like overnight that I suddenly had these very small breasts, and I *hated* it!

I used to *hit* my chest so that my breasts would go away! It hurt me a lot but I didn't care, I was just furious at my body. It meant so much to me, it took away my freedom . . . it's hard to explain. It seemed very mystical to me that my body was changing and that *they* out there would judge me. I had to start being a girl and I had to be the kind of girl that I didn't want to be. I had to stop playing football and stop playing with the boys, 'cause

that's what they tell you when you are a girl and you have breasts.

I had been in control of my whole neighborhood; I was the biggest one on my block and could beat the boys up. I kept them all in line and they were scared of me; they respected me. What I was afraid of was that when I got breasts and became a so-called "young woman," then I would lose that power. Before they treated me like a boy, too—but now I was different, the "other."

The boys I played with started to comment about my breasts and I got pissed off at 'em all. Everyone treats you differently for some reason and you don't know why, but you're different. Getting breasts changed my status with the boys, which I really resented.

There was a girl in my sixth-grade class who was very well developed for her age. All the boys just loved Lana because she had *big tits*. I remember sitting in class and just thinking that it must mean something if you have big tits, but I didn't know what it meant. It gave you status with the boys but I didn't know why. Meanwhile, I was losing *my* status with the boys. I wasn't one of them anymore. It was very strange and I couldn't understand why breasts meant so much.

There was a rumor going around school that if you took a rubber cup or a soft plastic drinking cup and put it on your breast and squeezed it and held it there for a couple of minutes, it would make your breasts grow larger. I thought that I

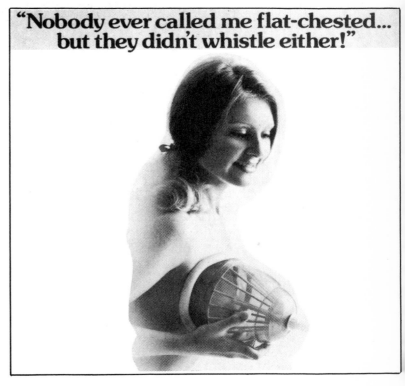

had ruined my chest from beating myself. So I thought, Oh, my God, since I beat them I'd better do that. Well, I tried but it didn't make any difference. I felt embarrassed when I did it; I thought, Oh, Christ, if anybody catches me, they are going to think I'm crazy!

I remember in high school there was always a big stress on breasts which I never could understand. For a while I hated the girls who had large chests and flaunted them because I felt that they were pushing something on me that wasn't my trip. There was one girl I called the "cow" because she had such huge breasts, and I really hated one teacher and used to cut her up because of her big breasts. I was a pretty rebellious kid. I wouldn't do anything I was supposed to do, so if I was supposed to have big tits I wanted to have small ones.

I think that boys go through a similar experience with their penis size, but for girls it's much more obvious and confusing. Everywhere there are cues. On television you could see the bra advertisements hinting that it was an attraction point with boys, that in some way you were rated on how you looked, how you sized up. I thought it was stupid and besides it hurt.

In high school, I wore a 34B bra and I thought of myself as small-breasted. I was afraid I would be rated on that scale of good or bad. In the beginning I worried about it sometimes, and later for most of the time. And what was I worried about? About not being a glamour girl!! I thought of myself as fat and I wasn't. I weighed a hundred and fifteen pounds, but my image of myself was of a fat, flat-chested person. One of the lines that I used when I went out with guys was, "If I turn around, you won't know the difference between my back and my front." It wasn't until much later that I realized that indeed was not true.

Whenever I dated guys in high school, either they got me in the back seat or the front seat or wherever, but the very *first* thing they did was very crudely attack my chest. I hated it and I hated them for doing it because I felt that they just didn't have any understanding of what my body was about. What they thought was turning me on was, in fact, turning me off! I never had the guts to tell them and I just found all my adolescent sexual experiences complete turn-offs.

●

My breasts had a lot of influence on me because indirectly they turned me off to myself—*they* were what I was rated on and I wasn't rated on

me. Men continued to reinforce those negative feelings over and over again.

In my early twenties I began to develop a much more positive image of myself and my body. A lot of it had to do with my own sexual experimentation, and I began to feel that my breasts were very powerful. In my relations with men I had no fear of exposing my breasts. I knew it was an attraction point and I could always flaunt my breasts if I wanted to.

But I didn't become *really* aware of a truly sexual feeling in my breasts until I made love with a woman. I always felt that men were just too rough with me, period, and I resented them for that. I stopped seeing men in 1973.

One of my first positive sexual experiences with a woman was just with our breasts touching, and it was so beautiful. When I danced with a woman—especially one who was the same height as me—and our breasts touched, it was so incredible because we could just feel the softness between us. It's so soft and gentle.

What I like most in making love to a woman is the very softness of the body and especially of the breasts. I like to touch the breasts with my face, with my mouth, with my hands—I feel a warmth and nurturing from them. There's a confidence I feel because I know her body—it's the mirror of mine—and I know how to please her.

My breasts aren't a real turn-on, I would say they're sort of middling. I think it's something that has to be learned—I hope it can be.

●

People have commented that I have large breasts but I don't think I do. To me they're *me*—not large and not small, they're just me. They have a mind of their own. I really can't control them. I mean if I'm walking, for example, I can't stop them from bouncing. If I'm doing anything physical, I can't stop them from moving around. Even if I wear a bra it wouldn't make that big a difference. I'm proud of them now and perhaps that's compensation for the pride I didn't have when I was a teenager. My breasts are a very important part of my personaltity now because I'm a brazen son of a bitch. I'm brazen about my breasts!

I can remember in the summertime, as a teenager, just dying in the heat and wanting to take off my shirt and not being able to. Now I take every opportunity I can to do that outside. Whenever I'm in the mountains with a lot of friends, we run and play ball and dance without our shirts on. It feels so damn good to do that!

I have a couple of dresses that I love to wear that are practically frontless. They're very low-cut and I just love it. It's a sexy, cocky, proud feeling like—"You can't tell me what to do." Nobody can tell me what to do. I always wear my clothing to draw attention to my breasts—I wear my shirts as open and as brazenly as I can, because I think it just demystifies it all.

A couple of Halloweens ago, I painted myself silver and wore a shirt that was open—almost all of my breasts were showing. My whole front was painted silver and my face was silver, too, and I had blue makeup around my eyes. I went into a bar to buy some beer for the party I was going to. I walked in there, natural as could be as though nothing was wrong, and the men didn't know how to handle it at all. They all stood there going "Gaaah . . . ! What's this woman doing in here with her breasts showing?" Some guy said, "Oh, can I touch your breast?" I said, "Yeah, if you don't hurt it," and his mouth just dropped open. That really felt good—that was really memorable.

Once at an art museum, several of my friends were sitting by a fountain and one of the women was going to photograph us. I enticed several of the women to expose their breasts with me. I said, "One, two, three. Pull up your shirts!" And one, two, three, we pulled up our shirts. A male photographer came over and said, "Would you do that again?" We said, "Sure." So one, two, three and the shirts came up and there we were. Then the police came over and began to hassle us.

●

To me, my breasts are a symbol of my womanhood in so many personal ways. My whole involvement with them. I didn't want them at first and now they've helped me feel better about my body. So my breasts have been very important in all the changes I've undergone—in accepting myself and accepting my breasts—it's all tied together.

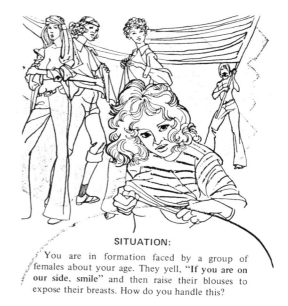

SITUATION:

You are in formation faced by a group of females about your age. They yell, "**If you are on our side, smile**" and then raise their blouses to expose their breasts. How do you handle this?

SOLUTION:

Concentrate on what you're there for. After all, you've seen breasts before. The girls are just teasing and want you to make a mistake so they can ridicule you. *Stay sharp and alert!*

From the U.S. Army Military Police school pamphlet "Keeping Your Cool in a Civil Disturbance"

From my experience, women have a much more open idea of beauty. They haven't been as conditioned as men to treat women's bodies as objects separate from their beings. So I think being with women helped me accept myself and change my attitudes about my body—to know that I don't have to be a Raquel Welch and I don't have to be a sex symbol. I can just *be*, and my body is beautiful no matter what it is.

Breasts are a part of each woman's personal power. In accepting that very important part of your body, you develop a form of power that is not like, say, political power; it's different. It's an acceptance of yourself. That is *real* power!

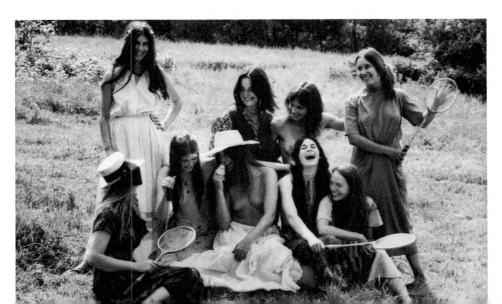

Betty

Age 27 • Raised in Oregon • Science Teacher

I'm participating in this book because now women are going through a time when traditional attitudes toward their bodies are being confronted and are changing. I've never been in a women's consciousness-raising group that focused on the subject of breasts, and yet I think that our attitudes toward our breasts are very important—especially after the incident that I recently experienced with the police. . . .

I love swimming without my top on—it's great. I don't mind showing my breasts at all. I've gone nude sunbathing and I've often shared saunas. At dance class I get dressed in front of people all the time. In more public situations, where strange people are around, I feel fine about exposing my breasts if it's appropriate—sunbathing and so on. If someone is hung up on the fact that my breasts are showing—well, that's their problem!

But if I'm with a man whom I don't know too well, then I certainly feel apprehensive about changing or sunning in front of him, because I don't know what his reaction would be. And my exposed breasts could set up a whole situation that I wouldn't necessarily want to deal with.

Around people I know well, I'm usually a little aggressive about it and maybe it's to compensate for the sense of restriction I sometimes feel. So I might say something like, "Look—it's boiling in here!" or "I don't want to get a tan line," or simply, "I just want to be without my top on. I want to be comfortable, I want to be free. I hope you can handle that."

I really *like* my breasts, and maybe that is because I've gotten nothing but positive feedback about them. Men that I've been with really *like* my breasts and lots of people who've seen me topless have said to me, "You really have beautiful breasts!" So maybe it's easy for me to expose my breasts because they're considered "nice looking." I wonder if I would behave differently if my breasts weren't so nice . . . or if my attitude about them is just a part of my free and easy character.

●

I spent the past summer taking dance classes in a program out in California. We lived in a dormitory on campus that had a swimming pool in the courtyard for the students and faculty.

Some of the women there were like me and had had some previous experiences bathing topless. So after the first few days, some of us began to remove our bathing suit tops at the pool. There was a little tension at first, as different men and women saw us for the first time. Everybody who passed by was confronted by their own attitudes and inhibitions. It seemed almost like a workshop in "practical inhibitions"! The men were very cool about it—there's no doubt that the *type* of people who were in the summer program made this situation possible.

Within a few days, almost *every* woman who came to swim at that pool eventually removed her top, and for many it was a first time. I'm sure social pressure and "taking up the challenge" were part of everyone's decision. But once a woman had struggled with the idea and finally decided to *do it*, it seemed to be almost an automatic, natural thing. It was amazing.

I spent a lot of time down at the pool. I love the sun. I also enjoy looking at other women's bodies and breasts, not out of some sexual attraction, but out of curiosity. Breasts are not something you see normally. In the topless situations I'd been in,

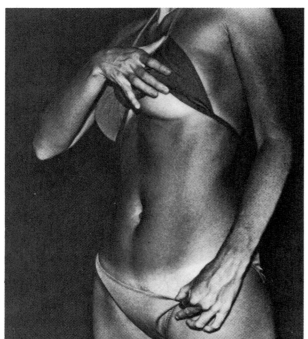

"Some popular desires and/or fantasies (to be tan),"
by Larry Williams

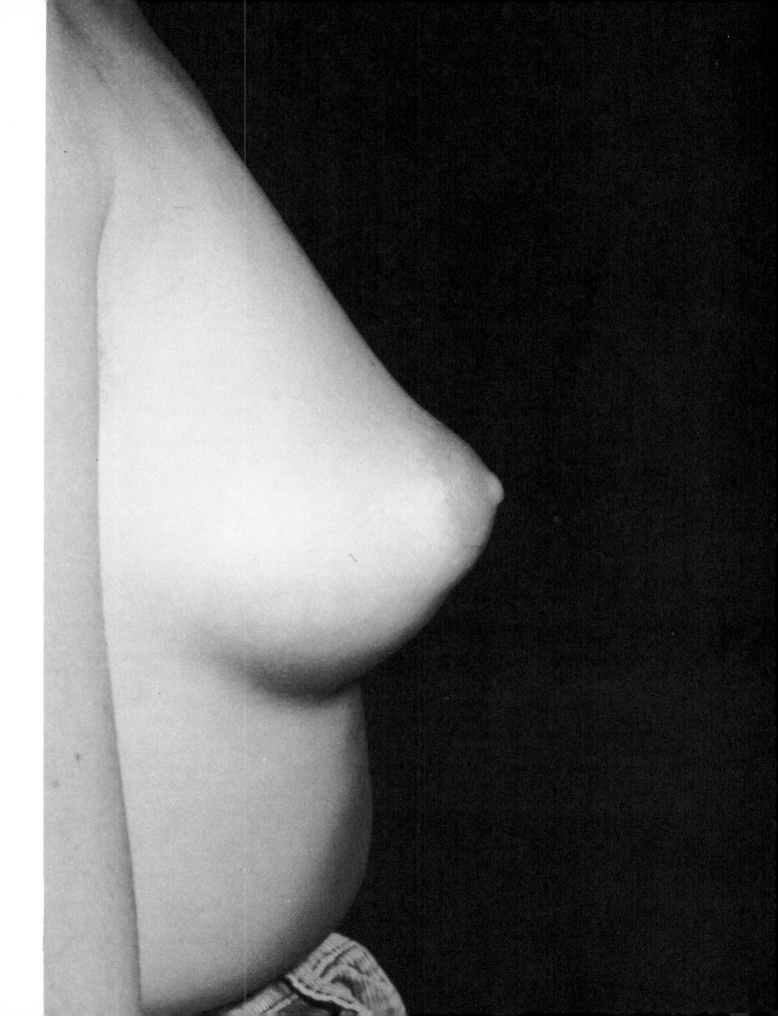

I'd never seen such a wide range of ages and types of women all together. Women all the way up to their forties and fifties were there. There were even some very daring topless twelve-year-olds who obviously had very liberated parents. Many of the people attending the program had young children with them and the kids seemed not to pay any particular attention. It was just a lovely experience and it lasted for nearly two months, until one day the police came.

A friend and I were at the pool, topless as usual, when two young, nice-looking cops showed up. Classes were in session so there weren't too many people around at the time. Anyway, they came over to us kind of apologetically, trying to be really nice, and saying that "personally" *they* didn't care at all. "We're really sorry, but we had a complaint and you will have to put your tops on."

The way they said it made me feel somewhat sympathetic toward them. I thought they were doing the best they could under the circumstances—they came up to us in a particularly friendly way. That is, if someone with guns and sticks hanging off them can indeed come up to you in a friendly way! (*Laughs.*) They were both trying to act very loose, saying how they really didn't think anything of it, but then one of them said, "Well, you know there are *children* around," indicating that he thought there was something *wrong* with children seeing women's breasts. *That* really annoyed me!

To think that children should not see breasts seems really twisted to me. I guess those policemen find the sight of women's breasts a turn-on, probably because when they were children all the

women they knew *always* wore tops. So the *only* time they ever saw breasts was as grown men in sexual situations. Maybe *that's* obscene . . . that they've become conditioned to confuse breasts with sex, rather than as just another part of a woman's body. Of course, sometimes breasts are part of a whole body that is engaged in sex, but then *all* of the body is sexual.

It was probably a good thing for those children at the pool to *see* women's breasts as much as they wanted to and to be done with all the mystique—this hide-and-seek with women's breasts is obviously unnatural and everybody suffers in some way, especially women.

So we put our bathing suit tops back on and the policemen left, having carried out their job of "protecting society and upholding the peace." The police bust (*laughs*) was a big topic of discussion around the pool. For the next few days we all went back into "Western civilization." Everybody grudgingly kept their tops on and felt very *strange* being covered after weeks of being natural.

Some of the women, myself included, were outraged. Some were just annoyed because of the inconvenience of having to tie shoulder straps on the side and rolling tops down without them falling off and, God forbid, indecently exposing our nipples, all in an effort to avoid ruining gorgeous tans. Besides, it was just a *pain* to have to sit around in wet tops.

Although we had been warned of possible arrest if our "indecent exposure" continued, it was very hard for us to keep our tops on. And so slowly, as we began to feel more secure around the pool, and as our run-in with the law was forgotten, one by

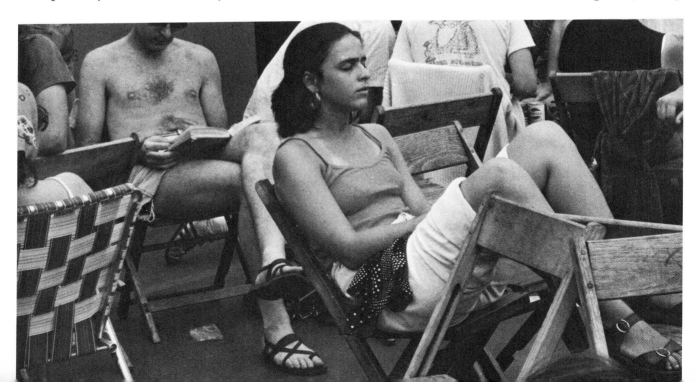

VP aide nude in Hamptons

By **DICK WETTEREAU** and **MEL JUFFE**

A 29-year-old aide to Vice President Mondale has been charged with sunbathing in the nude on a Southampton beach.

Deborah M. Sale, who works on Mondale's staff as an advance person, was arrested nine days ago as part of the resort town's new crackdown on skinnydipping but the arrest came to light in a check of arrest records today.

Miss Sale, an Arkansas native who lives in Washington and summers in the Hamptons, faces a $50 fine if convicted of public nudity. She's to appear in Southampton Town Court tomorrow.

Police say they found her and several others soaking up the sun nude nine days ago when officers swooped out of the dunes of Potato Beach, a remote section of Southampton shoreline between the communities of Wainscott and Sagaponack.

"I was unaware that that law applied to where I was on the beach," Miss Sale, said in Washington today.

Topless bathing sunk

MIAMI BEACH, Fla. (AP) — Bare-breasted bathing is still illegal here.

The city council voted 6-1 yesterday not to change a city ordinance against going topless on the beach.

Councilman Phil Sahl cast the lone vote in favor and said, "God's masterpiece is a well-built woman and, Mayor, you should look into it."

Mayor Harold Rosen was unmoved.

"If we had secluded beaches, like California or some of the islands, it would not bother me," he said.

The change in the ordinance was proposed two weeks ago by the city's Tourist Development Authority, which said it would help draw tourists.

CAROLINE

Baring it

IT USED to be a conservative newspaper, but Britain's Daily Express has fallen on very hard times lately. So on Friday the Express celebrated the engagement of Princess Caroline of Monaco—by publishing a picture of the 20-year-old topless. The sneak shot was one of a set of Caroline and Philippe Junot frolicking on a yacht a few days before their engagement was revealed. The shock the picture has caused in Britain is roughly akin to what would occur if the Christian Science Monitor suddenly displayed bare breasts on Page One.

"In fact, I was unaware of the law and I wasn't really sure of which township I was in.

"Since my job requires I live in Washington now," said Miss Sale, who formerly worked in New York in a city - sponsored educational program, "I haven't been going to the Hamptons much and wasn't aware that South-ampton was applying this statute."

Miss Sale said she was wearing the bottom half of her two-piece black bathing suit and sunbathing far away from the crowded part of the beach when the police approached.

When the police officer said he was arresting her for

Continued on Page 14

Continued from Page 7

"nude bathing," she said she replied: "I was neither nude nor was I bathing."

As Miss Sale recalls, the arresting officer shrugged off the distinction between topless-ness and nudity, saying, "It doesn't matter. It's all the same."

"But the justice of the peace seemed intrigued, she said. Unfortunately, however, he apparently didn't have the town statute for Miss Sale to check. He suggested she write the town clerk and ask for a copy.

NO COURT NOTICE

Miss Sale said that not only hasn't she received the copy in the mail, but she hadn't been notified that she is due in court tomorrow for the trial.

"If they let me see the statute, and if they were right, I would have pleaded guilty. It's one thing to be arrested for something you really believe in—like a civil rights issue you're really concerned about—but this is

really not my issue," she said with a laugh.

Miss Sale, speaking with a marked southern accent in the telephone interview, said she wasn't sure that the case was important enough for her to get a lawyer. She said she felt inclined simply to plead guilty if the law, as she reads it, does indeed prohibit topless sunbathing.

NOBODY AROUND

"But I'm afraid I was a rather innocent victim," she said.

"I was in a secluded area of the beach and far away from the other people when the police started patrolling the beach. I guess they just came upon me first because I was farther down the beach than anyone else. Ironically, I had walked way down the beach in order not to be surrounded by people."

Miss Sale, who rents a summer house in Bridge-

hampton, recalled that the arresting officer suddenly appeared and said: "Get your identification and come with me."

'PERSONAL CHOICES'

"I was surprised that they instantly arrested me, instead of giving me a warning, considering the type of law it is.

"I thought I was in a secluded area where for a number of years people basically have made personal choices as to whether they wore the tops of their bathing suits."

Maxine Burns, Mondale's deputy press secretary, confirmed Miss Sale's arrest and pointed out it wasn't connected with efforts by "free beach" advocates, who had threatened to stage a mass nude-in Saturday at Gibson Beach, just west of Potato Beach.

Although the demonstration never materialized, Southampton police had another busy weekend as they arrested a dozen nude sunbathers at various town beaches.

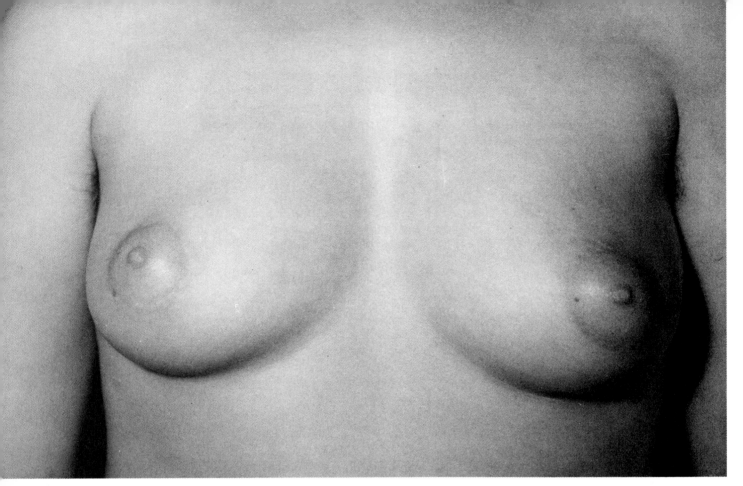

one we took our tops off again—though not everybody this time. Regretfully it wasn't the same. We were all much more cautious and tense. It was no longer the free and easy and relaxed thing it had been. We were breaking the law—*criminals!* Now, taking your top off at the pool was a statement rather than the most comfortable and natural way to be. Luckily the summer was almost over anyway.

●

A wonderful thing happened in California about a year ago. They had a topless march which was publicized on the radio and in the papers. Women marched through the downtown area, because on some beaches toplessness had become a legal issue. Now, I think they allow it in certain areas. So maybe things are changing, as far as sunbathing and swimming go. . . .

But on hot summer days when men take off their shirts and there I am with my lousy tank top . . . I hate it! Traveling in Norway and Denmark it was wonderful. In Denmark all the women go topless down at the beach. When I was hiking in Norway, I came upon a woman who just had her bra on and her shirt wrapped around her waist. She obviously wore her bra because it is simply more comfortable to wear one when you're hiking up and down hills. And the men that passed her on the trail didn't even bat an

eyelash. I thought that was great . . . so reasonable!

She wasn't the only woman I saw like that while I was traveling, and it just made me so happy. If a woman can wear just a bra outdoors in these countries, then I'm sure from there it is no big step to taking the bra off. In this country a woman can walk around with the skimpiest bikini or halter top, but *never* a bra. That would be indecent.

Although I usually don't wear a bra, I do wear one for teaching. I have to because I teach older high-school kids. It would just be stupid not to wear one then. It's too hard for the boys and they have it tough enough as it is. I mean a lot of them would relate to me as a sexual person instead of as a teacher, so . . .

I've often thought of not wearing a bra, ever. That would be great, but I can't do it because of my work. I mean if my business is to teach, it is up to me to make communication as open as possible between me and the kids, so I don't want to set up circumstances that will get in the way. When I wear a bra, I wear the most minimal, least structured one I can find—kind of a token bra.

How would you describe your breasts?
Firm . . . conical, I guess. They're really soft—the nipple is the softest part of my skin.

130

My breasts hang at different angles—they are different from each other. It doesn't really bother me, although it's interesting. I've gone through the whole rolfing process [a system of body realignment designed by Dr. Ida Rolfe] and my breasts have changed a little since then.

Breasts alone cannot actually be rolfed since they are not muscle tissues, but the therapist did work on opening up places between my ribs. She went all around and underneath into the chest muscles. Before that, my whole left side was caved down a little bit more, probably because I had a bad postural habit as my breasts were developing so that this breast just sagged with the development of the muscles underneath. After I was completely rolfed, my breasts became more evened out.

I guess I think my breasts are beautiful. I don't like to waste a lot of energy in self-pride, but people like them so they *must* be beautiful. Maybe the reason men like my breasts so much is because they're really firm—my muscles are very developed from a lot of swimming. And probably the most important reason is because *I* really like them.

There's one man I take dance lessons with who's a very good friend, not a lover, and every time we see each other he goes, "Tsk, just gotta squeeze your titties, Betty," and he does. That's become his way of greeting me, 'cause he really appreciates that part of me. If he *didn't* do it, I would think something is the matter with him. I really dig it that he appreciates my breasts in a nonsexual way, so it's a good relationship.

How do you like your breasts touched during sex?
I like all kinds of things. I like being touched really firmly because I have very strong pectoral muscles, so that feels real good. Soft and almost teasing feels nice, too. I like anything, as long as it's done right.

If there's one thing I *hate* in lovemaking, it's when somebody thinks he knows what turns me on, and then he just keeps doing it over and over again. I can't stand that! I'd much rather have somebody explore my breasts like they're a new world—that really turns me on. It's more the *attitude* of the person that turns me on, rather than specifically *what* they're doing.

Have your breasts taught you anything?
I suppose they stand for how I feel about myself. I'm not hung up about them compared to most people. They reflect my own unselfconscious attitude—I feel loose and easy with them, which is the way I feel about myself.

When I was growing up my mother was pretty relaxed about any of us kids seeing her nurse or coming into the bathroom while she was taking a bath, and I think that affected the way I now feel about myself.

Also, after high school I had a long, beautiful relationship with one person so I didn't feel that I had to go out and lose my virginity or do weird numbers with men. My sexual development was a gentle, slow process with someone who cared for me, and I think that has a lot to do with how I have come to feel about my breasts.

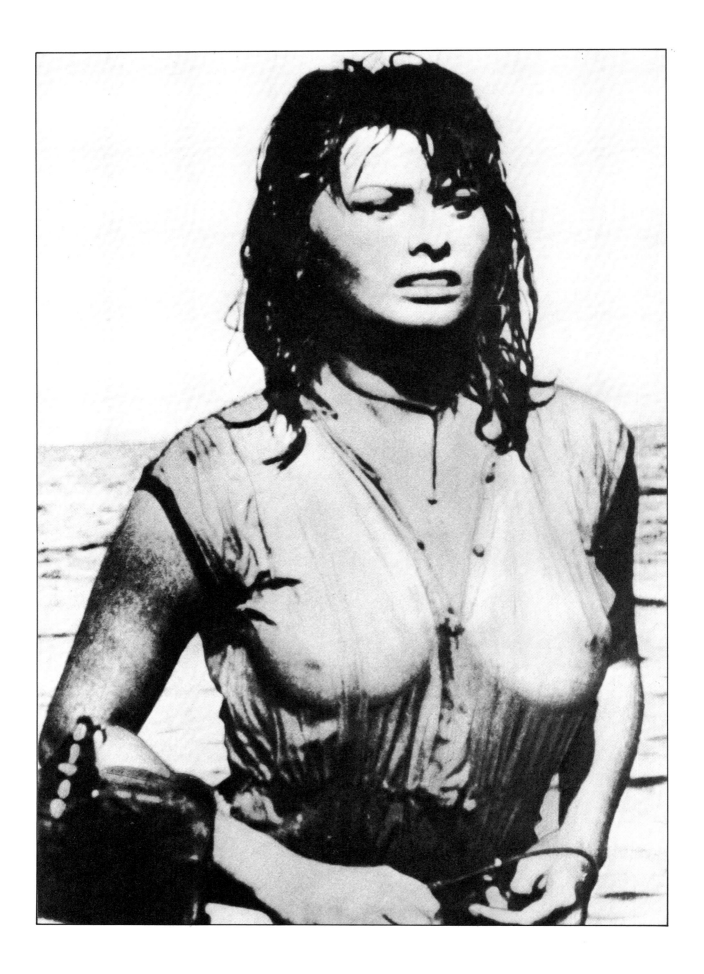

Sandra

Age 33 • Raised in New York City • Feminist Activist

When I was leading consciousness-raising groups a few years ago, I got women to talk and it was all very vital and important at that time. But now, when I think back on it, God! What did we say? So much complaining and refusal to take responsibility for ourselves. But then again, it's also true that women are oppressed, so it's tough.

Now in my life I tend to think that things are much more complicated—there is more than meets the eye going on concerning breasts and sexuality and men hooting on the streets and what not. So I am slightly suspect of the value of a sociology of people's impressions of their own experience, something that isn't more historically or scientifically based. I'm just not sure what you get out of talking to a lot of people.

In the C.R. groups, we used to have discussions about "How I feel about my body." I remember that I never got involved in dealing with my breasts very much. Somehow, it's an area of my body that doesn't have a whole lot of meaning for me.

Of course, that's not true for other things about me. There are some things about my body which I have had such a severe prejudice about that nobody could change my mind. My breasts, though, are a subject about which I have had very little conflict.

◄ *Note: Sandra excused herself from having her breasts photographed, giving a number of explanations—"busyness", etc. When told it could be done at her convenience, she replied: "Why don't you just use a picture of Sophia Loren's breasts and say they're mine!"*

I was quite surprised when my breasts began to develop. One day I looked down in the bathtub and I had breasts. They grew so fast I didn't really have any expectations but I did want them to be "beautiful."

At that time, breasts seemed to be very important sexually for a woman. You know, the fifties, seeing actresses in low-cut gowns and the whole sweater craze. I wanted to wear a tight sweater with a belt just like in the movies.

My breasts made me feel womanly, and I was very thrilled at becoming a woman. I was very thrilled when I menstruated. I was very thrilled when I got hair under my arms. I was thrilled that I was going to have sex and going to have children. Sexuality wasn't frightening to me. I was very "into" growing up and positively disposed to becoming a woman in general.

It seems to me that when I first had sexual experiences I was more shy about my breasts than about other parts of my body. I guess it was be-

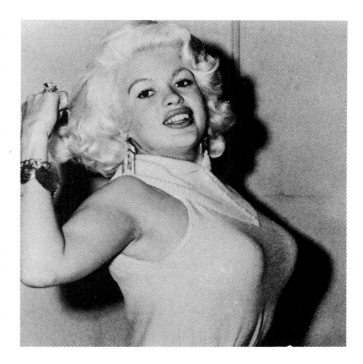

cause there was such an emphasis on breasts in the culture. The images that you see are so unnatural when you compare them to your natural breasts, which aren't as perfect or as spherical or whatever. Also, I just imagined that everyone's pubic area looked the same, so there wasn't as much identity crisis around it as there was around breasts.

I remember when I was a teenager, pressing my breasts against somebody was very exciting—that *alone* would be exciting. That might have been because for a time that's *all* there was to do. But I also think that as adolescents we are not very developed vaginally, so breast stimulation is more important than other kinds. Everything comes together then—the sexual energy and the permission to go with boys, as well as getting breasts—so the excitement is much more mental. After a while there's a limit to how exciting or satisfying the breasts can be.

There were all those games about whether somebody could touch my breasts. But after all the fuss, I ended up thinking, What is this? This isn't what it's cracked up to be! So very early, I began the odyssey that you make through your sexual experiences. I began having sex, so my sexual experiences didn't revolve around my breasts for as long a time as they did for most girls. Though your sexuality begins with your breasts, the sexuality of your breasts becomes less and less important as you grow older.

When I was growing up, there was so much torture associated with bras and clothing in general. There were different levels of dress for *everything*. Being a young girl was so formal and time-consuming. There was Friday dress and Saturday dress and, you know, Sunday afternoon. There was school dress and after-school dress . . . oh, all kinds of dressing, and there was a lot of peer pressure about it.

Different dresses required different bras, and finding a suitable strapless bra was always a big deal. All this nonsense, spending an inordinate amount of time being concerned about them and shopping for them—pink bras and blue bras. For me the pain of adolescence had less to do with my *body*, and more to do with the social craziness. When I was fourteen and fifteen, it was just like a torture rack of adjustments. It was all socially imposed, and all such an unnecessary *waste!* I'm very resentful.

So ten years ago, when bralessness became popular among feminists, I stopped wearing a bra. By that time anyway we were wearing "no-bra" bras,

right? So what was the point? It was just another expense.

Since then I've dispensed with all unnecessary trouble—laundering and other stuff, and things that rip. You really have to wash bras by hand so they don't get all wrinkly and frayed. Slowly, I started wearing leotards which pressed me flat. I liked it because it looked "tough."

●

I don't think I ever saw my mother's breasts. She is a person who gets dressed as soon as she gets up in the morning, so I always remember her covered up. I am sure she had a special bra when she breast-fed me or my brothers, so she could just open her dress without exposing her breasts.

My mother isn't puritanical; she's just a very, very decorous person. In some way, though, she drew attention to her breasts by *covering* them up a lot. My mother also had a habit of talking with her arms crossed over her breasts which hid them, but on the other hand could be interpreted as saying, "Look at me—look at my breasts."

When I was a teenager, my family doctor told me that when his wife was a young girl in the flapper era, they wrapped their breasts so that they would look flat. He obviously said that to make me feel guilty because my generation was so different—into bras and tight sweaters and display. So he was warning me—it was one of his obsessions—that because women were displaying their breasts, the world was going to hell!! The guilt he evoked in me is something I haven't forgotten.

I spend my summers out in the country and many people go swimming there without any tops or even bathing suits for that matter. Most people think that's so terrific, but you know, it has no attraction for me. I would rather keep my top on.

I'm not interested in having people look at me in *that* way. I have a sense of privacy about myself that I only reveal when I want to. My breasts are generally covered up, so that to uncover them is an *event*. In a way, exposing women's breasts probably defuses and desexualizes things ultimately, but I'm not sure whether that's good or bad.

I think I will always cover my breasts—going bare-breasted scares me. Since breasts have particular sexual significance, people are drawn to look at them, and I guess that makes me feel vulnerable.

I feel more in control if I have a little something

between me and other eyeballs—a little protection. Perhaps it's like wanting my own space or something. Even in my own house I never go naked, and when I sleep I always wear a nightgown.

How would you describe your breasts? Do you think they are beautiful?

You know, it's hard to talk about myself that way, but, yeah, I'd say they're beautiful. My breasts are very round, not conical like other people's. They don't stand up as much as they did when I was younger; I guess it's gravity. They have some stretch marks, but that's all.

The things that happen to my body with aging don't disappoint me really. I don't wish I had a younger body, and I don't feel competitive about it. I see my stretch marks as distinguishing characteristics, like a few gray hairs for a man, I guess. I attribute them to . . . maybe not wearing a bra. Maybe I'm just getting older. My body has changed a lot, even in the last few years. It has sort of settled.

I look at myself and I see that I'm older. I see that being very pretty is not going to be the same factor it was in the past. I see that my life is passing, that it's gonna end—that it's *actually* gonna end at some point—and I'm not going to be on this earth forever.

●

A year and a half after the initial interview, Sandra was contacted for a follow-up statement about why she refused to have her breasts photographed.

I just feel very private about my body. Also, the kind of work I do involves publicly expressing ideas, and this other part of myself, my breasts, I just consider private.

Whatever photographs of me that have appeared in connection with my work are of my *face*. My face expresses my personality, but I don't think my breasts do that at all. Just looking at your face, you see your own mortality. But I don't particularly see *that* in my breasts. I very much doubt that breasts take on a shape according to personality. So they don't really express *anything* about me. I mean my breasts are just part of the body I was born with. They're just an accident in a way.

I don't feel any more positive about being photographed now than I did at the time of the interview. I've often thought of it. I remember we had a joke that passed between us. I said, "You can use photographs of Sophia Loren," and you said to me, "Well, that's just the problem." But I thought I understood perfectly why I said that; if you're going to have a photograph of me in the book, use one that is beautiful. I was joking about the whole theme that you're raising in the book—about there being an "ideal" breast that women measure theirs against.

It seemed particularly ironic for you to be saying that. You made that "joke," but I wondered if there was some truth in it.

Sure, sure, sure. . . . But generally I feel positive about my body and I don't . . . ummm, you know, my not wanting to be photographed is just a question of privacy. Didn't any *other* women say they didn't want to be photographed?

Very few.

Then I'm really surprised that more women didn't feel that way about the issue of privacy. Most women don't expose themselves so easily . . . but who knows?

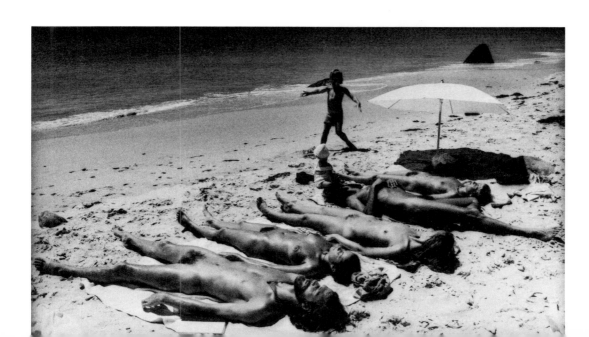

Fran
Age 34 · Raised on the East Coast · Anthropologist

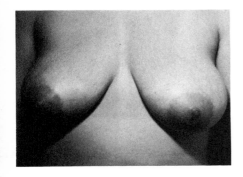

I don't particularly like my breasts right now. They're just too saggy and large according to the ideal of body proportions. The largeness of my breasts is one of the reasons that they sagged, but that's not the only reason. I think my whole body is too . . . lush! I'm afraid it's going to run to fat when I get old. I'm always fighting my body—it's always expanding and I'm always trying to contract it. The fact that I gain and lose weight so often must have affected the elasticity of my skin, and that includes my breasts. My sagging is a great source of self-consciousness for me, and I think that is totally cultural—one hundred percent!

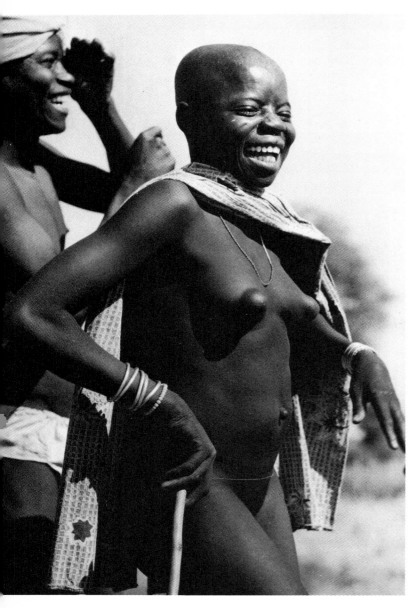

The Sherpas—a mountain people of Nepal and Tibet with whom I lived while I was doing fieldwork—have a very matter-of-fact attitude about the body. Breasts are not erotic at all. They're purely functional.

In many cultures sagging breasts are a sign of *beauty* and are sought after. Because sagging usually accompanies pregnancy and childbirth, it means that a woman is grown up and has achieved stature. In most tribal societies a young girl isn't fully considered a woman *until* she's had a baby and fulfilled her biological role. And when her breasts sag it is a sign of that maturity. So long as she has these silly-looking adolescent breasts that are pointed up in the air, she's still considered an immature person—a girl—and she hasn't reached full status as a "woman." There are even some tribal cultures where that idea is so fetishized that women tie *rocks* to their breasts to cause them to hang—the more they hang the better!

Most tribal societies don't favor upright breasts. That is mostly a Western cultural ideal. From a tribal society's point of view, we always want to look *immature* (*laughs*) and there's a lot of truth in that. We have such a youth fetishizing culture and the cult of the upright breast just goes along with it.

You'd think that with all the information I've been exposed to I'd feel better about myself. But when your whole upbringing and your culture have made you internalize these fetishes as ideals, there are just too many pressures working on you. I am a product of my culture.

●

I went through puberty and adolescence in the fifties—those were the days when women wore

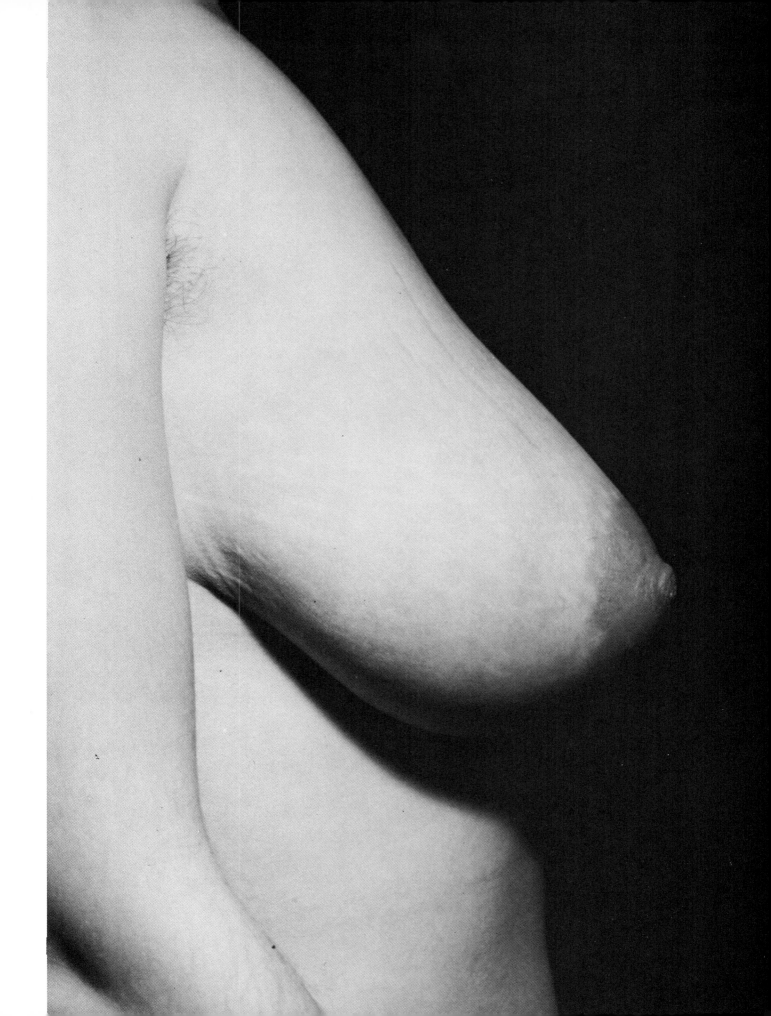

pointy bras and tight sweaters. Then, the cashmere sweater was the *ultimate* thing, not only because it was expensive, but also because it molded itself to your body. And the *bras!* They were like twin machine guns, such pointed things! Everybody would hike them all the way up to their shoulders and wear them sticking straight out like a war weapon! I don't think they still make those bras—they're probably collectors' items now! (*Laughs.*)

I got pregnant when I was sixteen—it was my first lover and probably on the second fuck! It was just a *horror!* I was petrified! So I went five months without telling *anybody* and finally had an illegal abortion. That's when my breasts started sagging.

I've always thought of that event as some mythic "before and after" turning point. "Once upon a time" I had terrific breasts, like the ones in the magazines—the "great American dream"—and then I committed this sin and God punished me. It was like the Garden of Eden. Now I've been cast out and I am eternally damned with these unacceptable breasts!

The sad part is that it happened at the *bloom* of adolescence, sweet sixteen going on seventeen, so I didn't even have my *terrific* breasts very long. Now I try to remember what they were like and I can't even conjure up the vision. I think to myself what a schmuck I was that I didn't appreciate them then! At the time I was ashamed in a diffuse, adolescent, what-is-my-weird-body-doing way, so that I didn't pay much attention to my breasts directly. And now I regret it.

●

Since I'm very self-conscious about the way my breasts look, I *always* wear a bra. It would be very hard for me not to wear one in public, but I even wear a bra in the house most of the time. I get very turned on by a new bra or a new bathing suit—anything that makes me feel good about my breasts and makes me look sexy to myself. Uh . . . I . . . uh . . . (*pause*) I often masturbate when I get a new bra in response to the way I look in the mirror.

I can't help it but I really have to fight my self-consciousness in sexual situations, when I'm undressing myself in front of somebody. I have to psyche myself up to overcome it. My bra would be the last thing to go, except that it's unaesthetic to have your bra on with your panties off (*laughs*), like a naked man with only his socks on. It's pretty tacky! So I don't do that, but I *would* if it didn't look so weird.

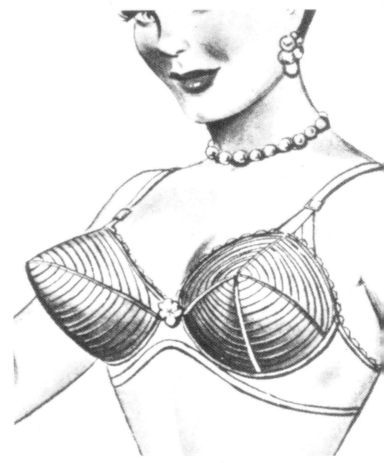

Men have accepted my breasts . . . nobody has ever said, "Get out of bed, I can't stand them!" (*Laughs.*) Yet I'm sure that they're not terribly excited by them either. I think my breasts get less attention from men during sex now compared to when I was younger, and at times I feel cheated. I like to have men play with my breasts and they just don't do it enough, and yet I've never asked a man to pay more attention to them. I wonder how a guy would respond if I said, "Hey, listen, up *here,* too!" (*Laughs.*) Except I don't want to call attention to them so at the same time I'm very ambivalent.

I assume aging is going to bring more of the same self-consciousness that I've already got. In our youth-worshiping culture it's going to be more of a problem to take off my bra with every year (*sighs*) . . . unless, of course, I make up my mind to overcome it.

Have you ever thought about changing your breasts?
    Yep. . . .

How far did it get?
    Well, I wrote a letter to a plastic surgeon. (*Laughs.*)

Oh, really?

Really! Funny you should ask. That's really *embarrassing! No one* knows that! I don't think there's a human being on earth who knows I wrote that letter.

I read an article in a magazine in a doctor's office about the booming trade in breast plastic surgery. It mentioned four big plastic surgeons who were all outside the United States. The point is that they're not just technicians, it's a whole high-society trip. It's *the* thing to do in the jet set to fly to Rio and go to a plastic surgeon's clinic for a month. These places are half clinic and half spa. You get *everything* all patched up. You get your ass lifted and your breasts made bigger or smaller and your creases "ironed out"—a complete overhaul! It's a very elite and expensive thing to do.

One of the surgeons mentioned in the article was in Sweden, and since I was going to be in Europe that summer anyway . . . *(laughs)* I wrote him a letter and asked how to go about making an appointment. I told him I wanted to have my breasts lifted. He answered the letter with a cordial reply and you know, I never did anything more about it. Theoretically, it's really creepy and obviously I just couldn't go through with it—I don't know if I ever really would. But definitely, I've gone beyond just thinking about it.

●

I don't know if anybody has any good explanations why breasts have become *the* fetish about the female body in our culture. I mean it's obviously not universal. Different countries seem to fetishize different parts of the body, and I don't know why Americans are particularly into breasts.

You'll find breast symbolism in some primitive tribal cultures, though not very highly fetishized. Breast symbolism seems to originate in early agricultural societies with fertility imagery like the Mother Goddesses. Then the breasts start to get much bigger . . . *(laughs)* metaphorically speak-

Venus of Willendorf (left) and breast idol from Dolni Vestonice (center), about twenty-five thousand years old; Great Mother from Senorbi (right) somewhat more recent.

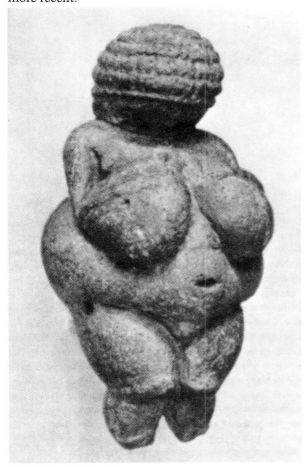
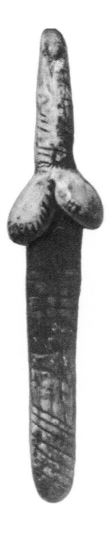
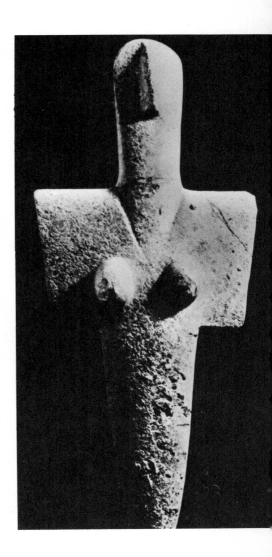

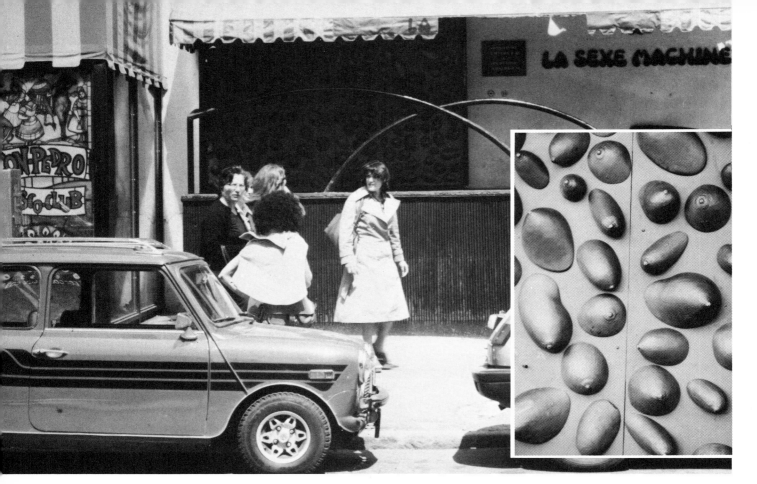

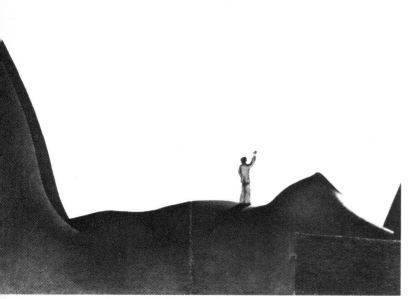

Cover of airline brochure

ing. But no society has the *degree* of preoccupation with breasts that Western culture has today. It's just not found elsewhere.

Somehow I think this entire issue is related to nursing. As long as a culture keeps the tradition of nursing, the breast remains part of the func-

tional aspect of life. Except that they represent fertility, they are not such *symbolic* objects. And then there's no hang-up about breasts—either about exposure or as a sexual object—though of course that's variable from culture to culture. In premodern cultures, for example, the exposure of women's breasts is a nonissue, yet there are also some cultures that have developed a thing about covering the breasts even though breast-feeding is the norm.

If a culture becomes clothed because it has been missionized, that is a whole different thing. Interestingly, the *first* thing missionaries do when they come to tribal cultures is put blouses on the women—immediately the women have to start covering their breasts! It's always interesting to see what happens to people's ideas about modesty after they're clothed. Being clothed usually tends to affect a culture's notions of modesty and sexuality so that women, for example, become embarrassed about exposing their breasts.

The Sherpas, however, who are fully clothed from their neck down because the Himalayan climate is so cold, still have no compunctions about nursing in public or about a woman taking off her top to wash her hair out in the sun. And of course they have a very strong breast-feeding tradition.

So I have an idea that our culture's fascination with breasts might in some way be related to its rejection of nursing. Since our cultural ideal is the "immature" adolescent breast, we must *not* nurse in order to stay youthful, that is, beautiful. There seems to be a vicious cycle there—the more of a youth fetish there is, the less nursing there is, the more fascination there is with women's breasts, and on and on. . . . I can't prove that this is true but it's a strong feeling I have.

That's the anthropologist in me speaking. But personally, as a product of my culture, whenever I see breast-feeding going on in public in *this* country, even though I think it's fine, it always jolts me a little. I can't help myself because it's just not that common. Given the cultural context, I have a fleeting thought about whether the woman is being exhibitionistic. I can't help it.

How did you feel about being interviewed?
You know, when I remembered that thing about bras and masturbation . . . For a moment I almost wasn't going to tell you. I was embarrassed. But I decided that I'd done all the rest of the interview and I might as well. And, you know, I'm glad I did.

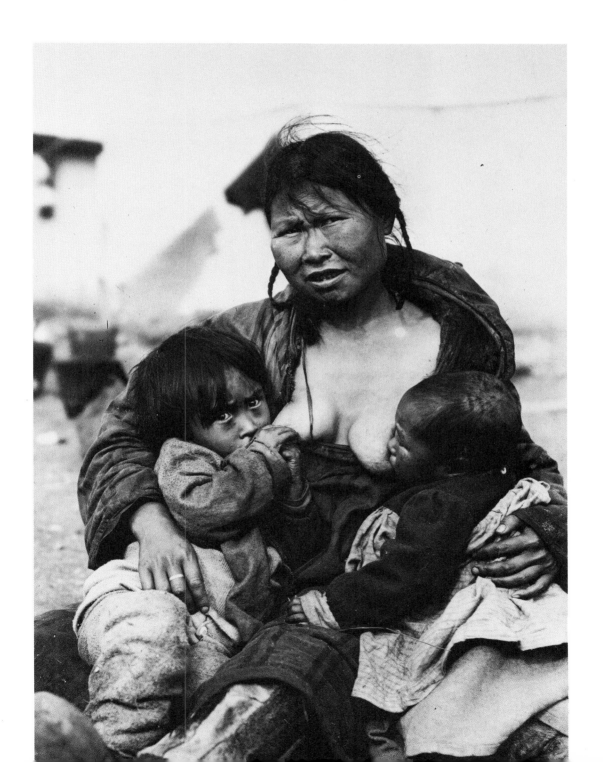

Pregnancy and Breast-feeding

• I think that my breasts will become uglier during pregnancy. I will probably be repulsed by them.

• When I become pregnant, my breasts will really take on functional meaning. They won't just be there as decorative objects and I'm sure they'll feel different, too. I'm hoping to feel that my body's like a sacred temple housing life.

How did your breasts change during pregnancy? How did you feel about the changes?

• The first time I really thought about the possibility that I might be pregnant was when I noticed my breasts changing.

• As soon as I was pregnant I was amazed that I could squeeze my nipple and a drop of fluid would come out.

• After about six weeks the Montgomery's glands—the little bumps on the aureole—began to get very prominent. Then the nipples and the aureole became very dark. I remember looking at the changes in wonderment. It's amazing what happens!

• Physically my breasts were much more tender and sensitive to the touch. I couldn't squeeze them or anything like that, so all during pregnancy I had a new feeling in my breasts. I became aware of them in a completely different way. It was through my breasts that I first began to really *feel* pregnant because they were sensitive months before my stomach showed.

• Right away my breasts got bigger. The nipples stood out more and *everything* was harder. My breasts really looked beautiful, but I think that's true about every pregnant woman.

• I was once pregnant for seven weeks and my breasts got huge and hurt like a son of a bitch! The nipples got really dark and there were purple lines running through them. It really scared me! After my abortion I got really pissed off because my breasts didn't shrink much.

• During the first month of pregnancy my titties got two sizes bigger and fluid just poured out. I couldn't believe it! They were so big and so wonderful . . . Oh, I was thrilled to death! I thought, This is the way to be. I'm going to stay pregnant *forever*. But the pregnancy was ectopic—the fetus was growing in one of my fallopian tubes—so I had to have an abortion. The doctor gave me some pills and the next thing I knew my titties were right back to nothing again. What a disappointment.

• When I was pregnant I was very glad that my breasts were getting bigger, and that was a big factor in my keeping the baby. I knew that my breasts would get even bigger and I was hoping they would stay that way. But after a while, I remember feeling very panicky that they were going to get *too big!*

• Naturally my breasts got bigger when I was pregnant and people noticed that. I must say I enjoyed the attention, but I worried about getting stretch marks. Before, I had been concerned about being flat-chested. There's always something to worry about, *always!*

• So far I've gone from a 34B to a 36D, which is quite a way to go. I keep thinking to myself, Wow! And this is only the *beginning!*

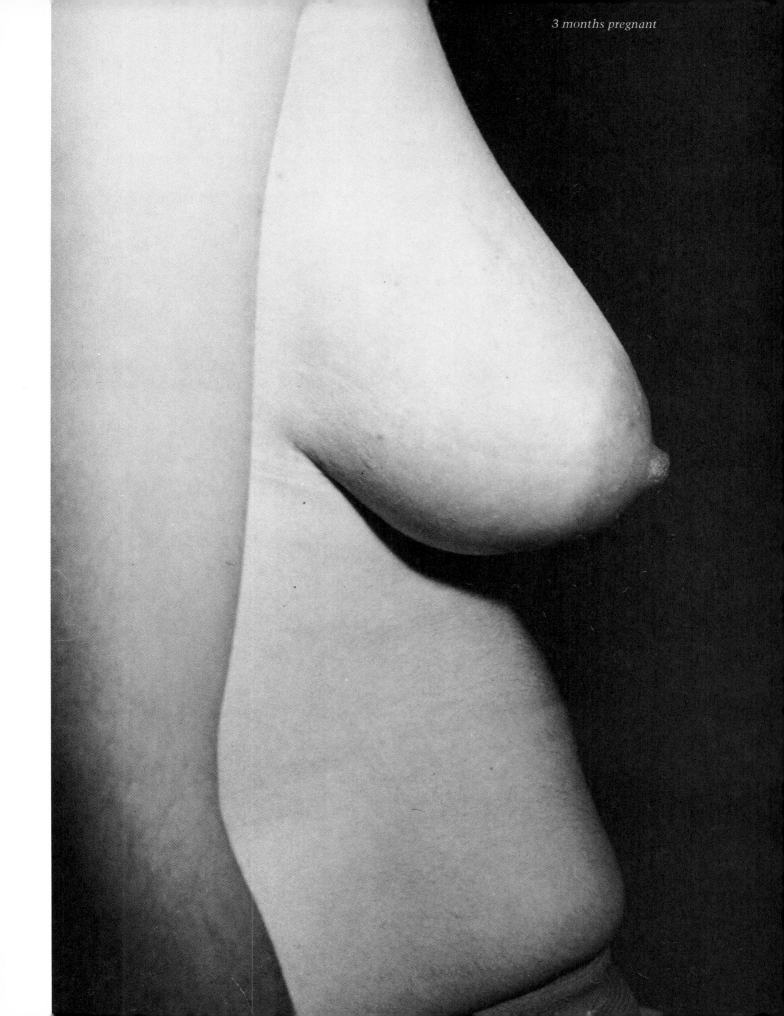

Beverly • 6 months pregnant • Part I

I really like my breasts right now. Since I was never particularly large-breasted, it's fun being pregnant and having my breasts inflate a little bit! (Laughs.) I'm also a lot more conscious of the real *function of my body—pregnancy has done that. And it's helped me get away from all those myths we're taught when we're growing up—you know, about how a woman's body* is *supposed to be. I really feel good about my body now.*

When I was in my teens, my mother laid the same cultural rap on me that everybody else got, and she *still* does even now. A couple of weeks ago, I sent her a picture of myself because she wanted to see how I look pregnant. She wrote back, "Oh, you've got breasts now," (*laughs*) as if I didn't have *any* before. I was wearing clothing in the picture, but you could tell that I was bigger. My mother always accentuated that part and subtly made me feel lacking.

How would you describe your breasts now?

Rounder on the outside and flatter on the inside—it's all out and underneath, with no cleavage. I think they're friendly. (*Laughs.*) Hello! I guess now that I'm pregnant they're more beautiful to me than they were before. I'm finally becoming friends with my breasts.

When I first got pregnant . . . (*sighs*) . . . I looked at myself in the mirror in fascination. You know, I hadn't *really* looked since puberty. Every day I'd look to see what changes there were in my breasts and in my pelvis. My nipples have gotten darker and larger. Just watching and feeling my body change is an incredible experience—I love it.

My breasts are more uncomfortable sometimes, just because they're harder and fuller than before. When I lie on my stomach it all pushes up and feels very funny. I'm not used to having it there. And I've actually thought (*pause*) . . . Well, now I'm not sure I'd want all *that* there all the time. But otherwise my breasts are pretty comfortable.

I *hate* wearing a bra! I don't usually, but it's really necessary right now. Even though I'm not particularly big, I'm starting to feel some strain on my breasts. For a while I had to force myself to wear a bra, but by now I'm used to it.

I don't know if I'll wear a bra afterward. I'll see what state I'm in. I hope I don't have to. If I get a lot of stretch marks and sagging I might wear one. I'll let my breasts tell me. If they want it, they can have it. (*Laughs.*)

I don't know if my breasts will change from breast-feeding. A lot of people say they get smaller and smaller. I don't relish that, but what can I do?

Have you thought about whether or not you will breast-feed your child?

Yes, I can't imagine having a baby and not breast-feeding if you can. It's got to be the most wonderful experience. It's just part of having a baby, really.

Do you think your feelings about your breasts will change after you breast-feed?

I'm enjoying being pregnant and seeing my body work, so I think I'll enjoy myself even more after experiencing the complete cycle to its fullest. I know that will affect how I feel about my breasts afterward, but I don't know what that effect will be. . . .

144

(Part II on page 154)

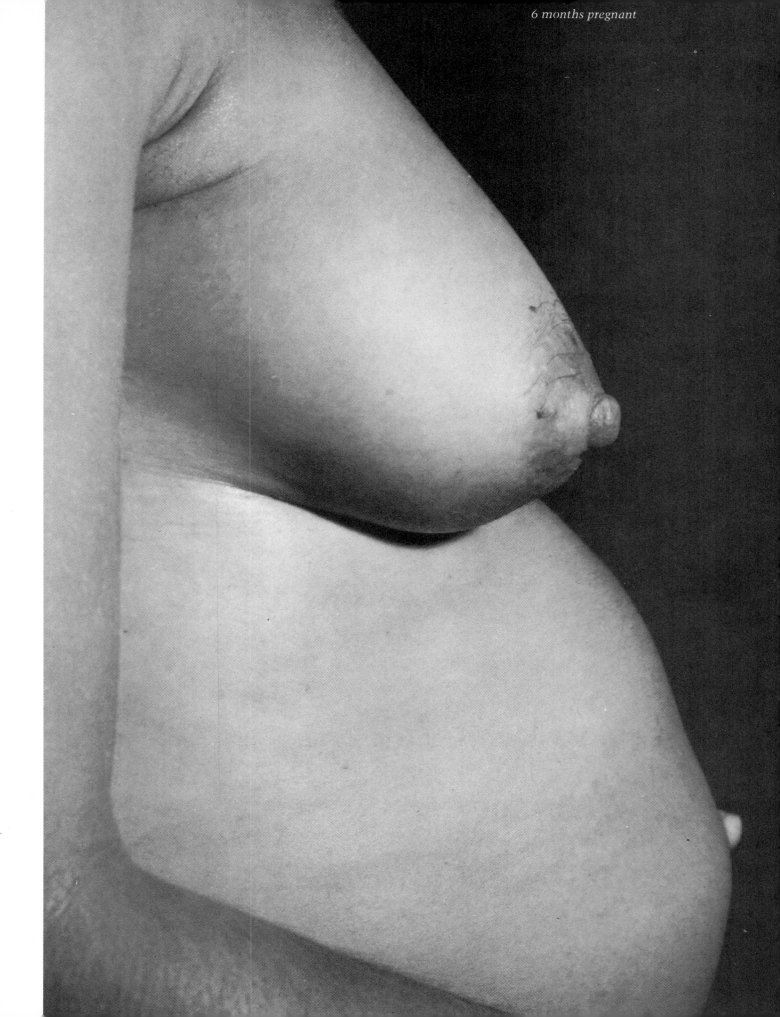

• *I've seen my sisters and other pregnant women and I noticed that automatically the breasts get very full and healthy looking* (laughs), *almost ripe, ready to be picked and eaten. I think the dark nipples are really very beautiful —they're so striking.*

Daphna: Your reaction is interesting because I've shown pictures of nursing and pregnant women to other women and some have said, "Ooh, the dark nipples are so *ugly!*"

That's probably because they've never seen nipples like that before. They're used to seeing pink nipples in the magazines and they don't realize that women actually get brown nipples when they are pregnant. I've seen them change from pink to orange or dark brown and I find it beautiful. The contrast is so strong—the nipples look like chocolate.

• Being blind, I couldn't see the actual changes in my body, but I liked the feeling of being pregnant. My front was a very funny shape. My breasts loomed larger, sort of doubling over my body, and there seemed to be a little recess under them and then a great big belly. I could also feel my nipples protruding a lot more than they had.

• I loved the way I looked when I was pregnant. I felt fertile. For the first time I felt I knew what it truly meant to be a woman. And also for the first time in my life I could actually fill a bra! (*Laughs.*) I *loved* it! I stood in front of the mirror all the time and just *stared* at my breasts—forget about the stomach.

• My breasts didn't grow much in either of my pregnancies. That's what upset me. I figured that now I'd have a real big pair. Forget it!

• Oh, my breasts were gorgeous! Well, gorgeous to most people, *horrible* to me! They were hard as rocks and monstrously big. *Huge!* To men they must have been *unbelievable*—a man would have died! (*Laughs.*) I just sort of gritted my teeth and got the biggest bra that I could find.

• While I was pregnant I had enormous breasts that stayed up. They looked like they did when I was eighteen and were very attractive, but ironically I wasn't at all interested in sex during pregnancy, so it was very conflicting. I didn't want my husband to bother me, but he was very turned on by my breasts, so it was hard.

• One day in the last stages of my pregnancy, I was on top of my husband making love. I was so big there was no other position I could take! In the middle of my orgasm, my nipples started squirting milk. It dripped all over him. (*Laughs.*) I was delighted and thought it was very funny, but he was absolutely horrified and repulsed by it. Many men are revolted by breast milk, for all kinds of reasons.

• My breasts are really fun now—just the fact that they're going to start making milk. They're like a toy. (*Laughs.*) I started having colostrum pretty early in pregnancy, in about the sixth month, but I didn't start expressing it until the eighth. I enjoy seeing the colostrum come out, so I'm sure that when I'm nursing I'll get a big charge out of it. (*Note the drop of colostrum in the photograph.*)

I didn't enjoy having my breasts fondled much before I was pregnant, but now I do. Sometimes when I have an orgasm, colostrum squirts out. Imagine what it'll be like when I have milk—I'll be squirting the walls! Oh, it will be great! (*Laughs.*) I'm really looking forward to nursing.

I love my breasts now. I wonder if the pleasure I take in them now will diminish when they've done their job and I stop nursing? Will I go back to

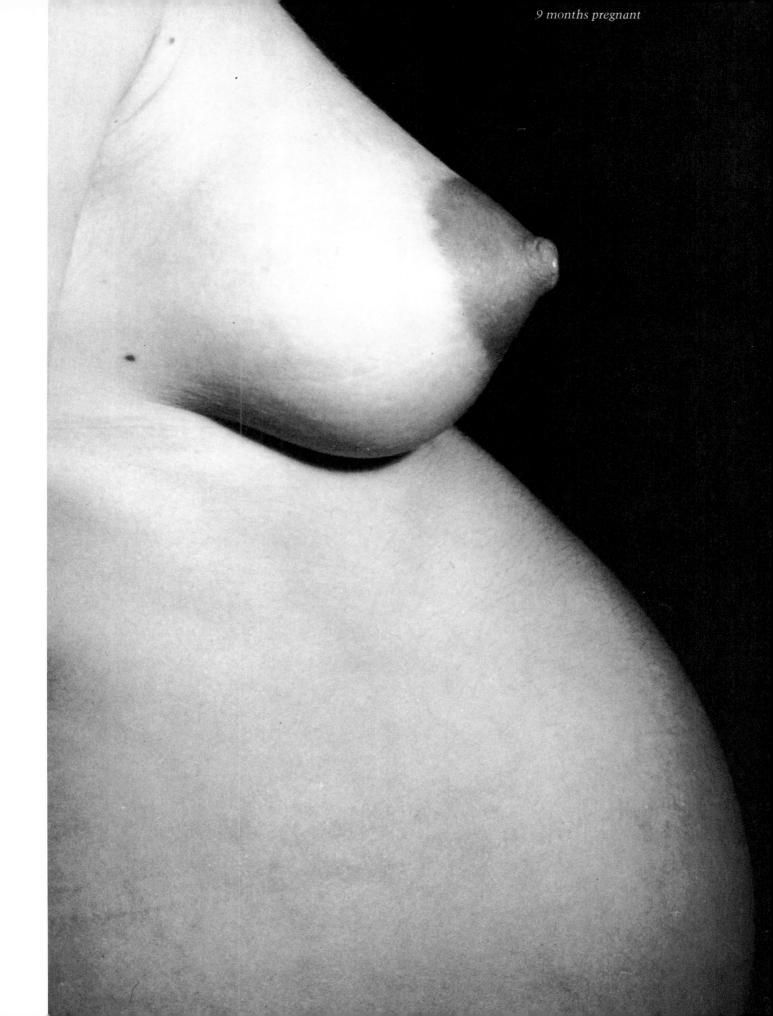

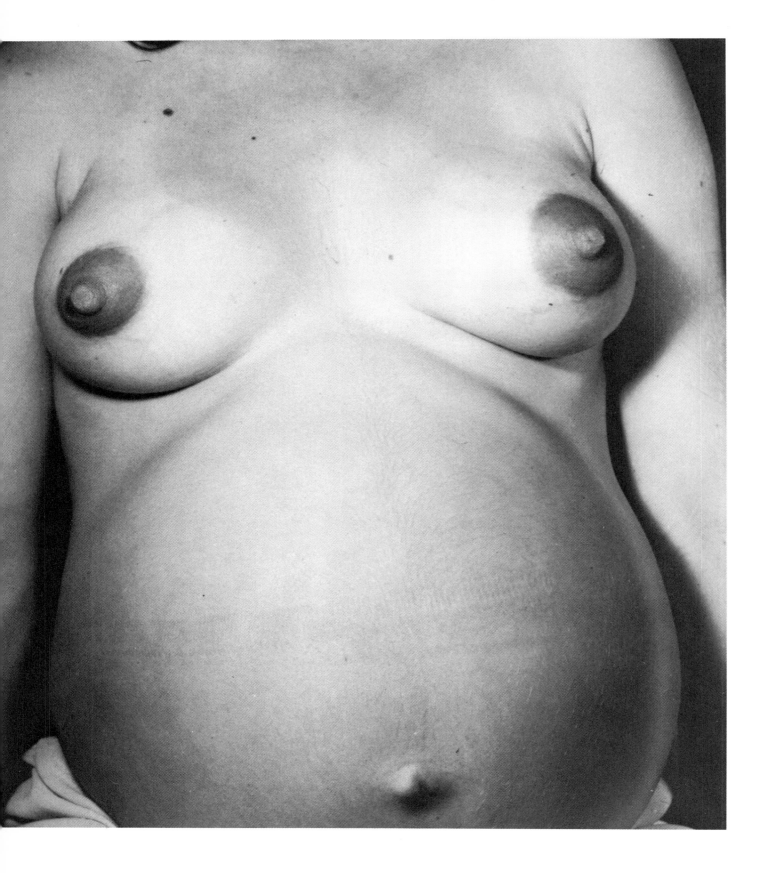

being indifferent to them? I just wonder how I'll feel about them when it's all over.

• During my pregnancy I got to love my breasts and I cared for them in a way that I couldn't have imagined before. Toward the end I began to lubricate my nipples with special cream to prevent them from cracking. I stimulated them and did what I had to so that they will be tough enough to breast-feed the baby. My breasts have done wonderfully up till now and I'm pretty confident that they'll do just beautifully when the time comes to nurse. It's the most natural thing in the world, so why shouldn't they?

Would you breast-feed if you had children?

• I don't know if I would breast-feed or not. I've never seen women breast-feeding, except in documentaries or in *National Geographic* magazines.

• I think the idea of breast-feeding is neat. I would definitely do it. I can imagine it being very nice to snuggle a little thing right here and have him suck on your breast. It might be a real turn-on.

• I don't know if I will breast-feed. It'll depend on how my husband feels about it and if he's supportive.

• It is incomprehensible to me not to want to breast-feed. When I was much younger, I once bought a *True Secrets* magazine—you can imagine what *dreck* [garbage] it was—and put it inside a *Newsweek* so I could read it. There was a story about a retarded girl who got raped and blah, blah, blah, but she had a baby. The article constantly talked about how she was missing things "upstairs," but there was one moment of clarity in this retarded woman's existence when she fully understood the milk coming through her breast into the baby's mouth. At that moment she was whole and connected, and she wasn't missing *anything*. It had such an impact on me, I never forgot it.

• I'm very mixed up about whether I would nurse. On one hand I feel that I should, but on the other I wouldn't want to because I'm afraid my breasts will get wrinkled and become ugly and that's what scares me.

• If I ever have a child I don't know if I would breast-feed it or not. I'd try to talk to people whom I really had confidence in to find out if it's good for the baby or not.

Did you breast-feed or bottle-feed your child? Why?

• I didn't make a conscious decision. When I accepted the fact that I was going to have a child, breast-feeding was just something that I assumed also.

• I didn't breast-feed my child. I didn't even *think* about it. There was no special decision *not* to because at that time it was normal to bottle-feed. They taught me how to prepare formula in the hospital, and I made it and she just drank it. It would have been abnormal to breast-feed—they would have thought I was *nuts! Nobody* did it.

• I always knew I would breast-feed. I come from an old breast-feeding family. (*Laughs.*) My grandmother had fourteen children and nursed them all. I grew up wanting and even dreaming of being able to when I had children.

• I breast-fed because my mother would have been outraged if I didn't. All the women I knew breast-fed, so I never considered any other way.

• My mother thought feeding a child from your breasts was disgusting. "Only animals do it," she'd say, so I never even *considered* it.

• I was informed by my mother that breast-feeding was what I should do. And since I was still rebelling against her, I didn't want to *because* she told me I should. I ignored her and didn't nurse.

• My mother was upset that I wanted to nurse because then *she* wouldn't be able to feed the baby, but despite her protests I decided to nurse my children.

• I didn't breast-feed my daughter. I had some preconceived ideas that it might not be so pleasant, that it might hurt or something. And what if you're tired and the child's still hungry?

• I never considered breast-feeding. Absolutely not! Oh, I could not imagine a child sucking on me—that pulling, that constant irritation. I don't like being sucked on anyway. The whole idea of breast-feeding completely turned me off.

• All of my children were breast-fed. In those days [1920s] everybody thought that if you nursed your children until they were two, you didn't become pregnant. I don't know whether it works or not, but that was the reason a lot of women nursed.

• One of the reasons I breast-fed my son was because of breast cancer. I used to be a nurse and I also worked in obstetrics so I knew that breast-feeding could possibly help prevent breast cancer.

• I grew up with the idea that you should raise your children with total devotion. You breast-feed them and love them, and in turn they suck your milk and take your blood and your strength and your teeth and your hair and your tits. So I didn't even *try* to nurse because I was scared to death of it!

• My husband was very concerned that I would "ruin" my breasts if I breast-fed. I was so upset that he felt that way, that I decided not to.

• I nursed all my kids, but I think fear of ruining the breasts plays a large role in a woman's decision about whether to nurse these days. Several women I've known didn't nurse for that reason. I object to magazines and all blaming drooping and stretch marks on nursing. It just isn't true. It's more a result of pregnancy than anything else.

• Within the past year *Glamour* magazine had an article that blamed droopy breasts on nursing. I wrote a letter to them objecting to it and got a nice apologetic reply saying that they would retract the statement and perhaps do a follow-up article. But I doubt if they were aware of the damage they were responsible for.

• I read in a book that you get stretch marks just from being pregnant even if you don't nurse. So I figured, what the hell . . . I might as well nurse!

• I didn't nurse because of what happened to my mother. She breast-fed us and her breasts looked like two rocks in a sock. They were long, pendulous things that hung down over her belly—she could sling them over her shoulder. I always thought they were ugly. So when I had my child, I thought about the disastrous things that had happened to her breasts and I decided I wouldn't nurse. I didn't want my breasts to look like *that!* I slept in a brassiere for two months until the milk dried up. But even then my breasts didn't look the way they used to.

• A lot of women in my family were afraid to nurse because of ruining their breasts—you know, stretch marks and stuff. All my aunts said, "Oooh, I wouldn't nurse because your breasts will sag and get stretched out and it will *ruin* your figure!" But I ignored that advice because all my friends who had breast-fed had good experiences—it hadn't destroyed *their* breasts.

• In the beginning I didn't want to nurse. Thank heavens for the doctor. He said, "I don't care about the baby, but if you nurse, your uterus will be in good shape and you won't get troubles later on. Every suck on that breast is like a suck on the uterus. Out comes the stuff—the afterbirth. And the contractions are like exercise—it'll make you strong and give you a flat stomach. You like a good body? Then the baby's got to suck!" So that's how he talked me into it.

• I didn't breast-feed because you have to be a certain type of person to do that. My friend would sit casually and breast-feed her child in front of three or four girlfriends, but I would never, *never* do that. Not even in front of my own family! I don't like the idea of whipping it out in a restaurant, where I have seen it done, but even in the most intimate of situations I would never do it.

• You know, the idea of having to breast-feed in front of other people never occurred to me when I was trying to make up my mind if I was going to nurse. It would have been terribly inconvenient if I would have had to stay at home all the time. I wouldn't have been able to take it.

• I breast-fed because it's healthier. Immunities to various diseases are passed on in the milk. I'm allergic to cow's milk and that has caused many problems for me, so I would never put *my* child in the position of having to cope with anything other than human milk. I don't see how you can take a newborn baby and put it on synthetic food—it seems weird to me.

• I didn't breast-feed because I didn't want to get tied down. I wanted my husband to take care of half the feeding, without my baby having total reliance on *me*.

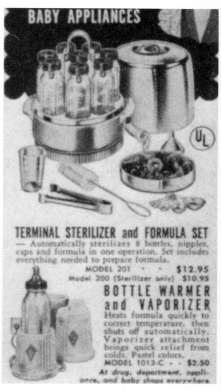

"*The easy, safe method of scientific feeding*"

• I nursed because the equipment was there. It was the most practical and convenient way of feeding a baby. The milk never goes bad, it's always the right temperature. Wherever you are it's always handy. And I didn't feel like washing out bottles and making formula day and night, and shlepping it all around with me wherever I went. It was easier just to take off my blouse and say, "Here it is, kid." I nursed just for convenience sake, really.

• I didn't breast-feed my children because I couldn't give them *all* my attention and keep my husband, too. If I had given up my life with him for my children, someone else would have taken my place. I am sure of that.

• First of all, I decided to have a home delivery—that came first—and breast-feeding just went right along with it. I was a little concerned if I'd be able to nurse, but the midwife said, "Oh, sure, you'll have enough milk. Many small-breasted women have more than enough milk and even donate some to milk banks."

• I had a subconscious reason for breast-feeding that I only realized recently. When I was in high school, I couldn't save money by sneaking through the subway turnstile like my small-breasted friends could, and I was always getting teased about it. So now I could get back at them—I'd save money *this* way! (*Laughs.*)

• I breast-fed because there was no other way sixty years ago. Who had the money for bottles and formulas? Especially if you had your own!

• Since she's my one and only, I wanted to experience the whole thing as maximally as I could. It was also the best thing I could do for her.

●

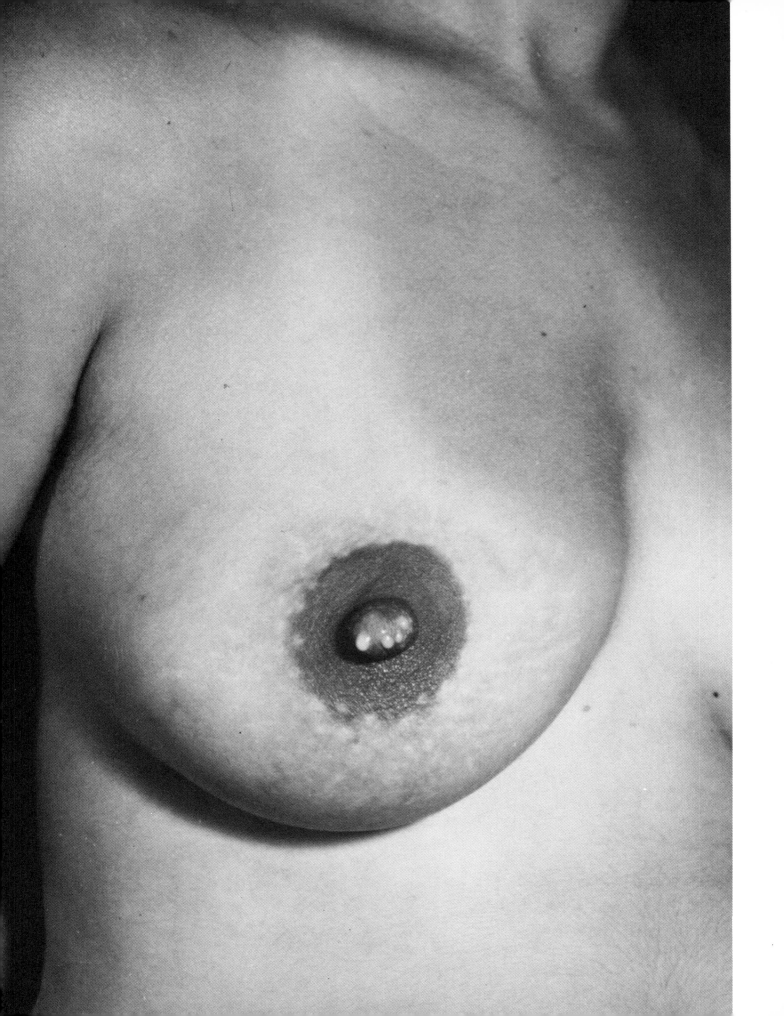

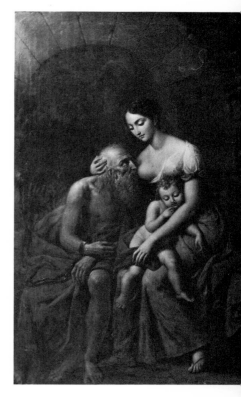

• When I was a child, I wondered how milk came out of the nipples. I thought you had to have holes *pierced* in order to breast-feed (*laughs*) and that frightened me. A few years later, when my breasts began to develop, I examined my nipples to see if any holes had appeared. I was worried, because if they did, they were microscopic.

• I think it's fascinating that breasts can hold milk—it's something magical. I didn't realize there are so many holes—I always thought there was just one hole.

• The milk that comes from your breasts contains almost everything one needs to live, so it is life-giving for the child that comes out of your body, and can be for others, too.

There is a series of paintings done by artists throughout the ages, known as *Roman Charity.* They depict an old man with a beard whose ankles and hands are tied. A young, very plump woman with bursting breasts is suckling him. This image has stunned everyone! What is this tied-up old man doing sucking this young woman's breasts?

This theme goes back to Roman times and is based on a true story about an old man who was imprisoned and left to die of hunger. The only person he had in the world was his daughter who was allowed to visit him. The jailers were absolutely *amazed* that after weeks and weeks passed, the old man still didn't die. But then they discovered that his daughter, who had just had a child, was breast-feeding her father and keeping him alive!

• It occurs to me that when you breast-feed, food is coming out of you and going into another human being, so through the nipple flows life and creativity. And the "life-giving" character of the female of the species should be symbolized by the nipple because it is not just the fact that a child is born out of a hole in a woman's body that makes her a "life-giver." Giving birth is not enough! Children can come out of our bodies and be left to die if they are not wanted, and then what? But the nipple is truly a transmitter of love and life.

So help me God, I've never thought of it in this way before!

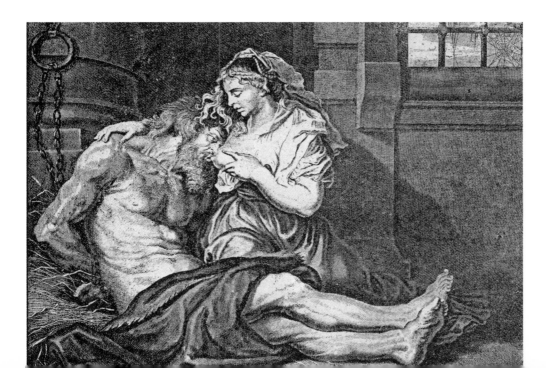

Beverly, Part II

. . . As nature would have it, our baby chose to come eight weeks early. The event was filled with considerable anxiety and I've been the full gamut with my breasts. I've had more contraptions on them than I ever dreamed possible.

During the six weeks that the baby was in the hospital, I worked desperately to maintain my milk supply. She was too tiny to suck, so I had to use a breast pump—a most unaesthetic experience. When the milk first came in, all was great. It was wonderful to feel my breasts function, and it was fun if somewhat painful to squirt milk into a jar. My milk supply diminished rapidly after ten days, but I worked hard to keep what little milk there was going.

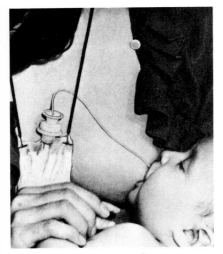

Lact-Aid® nursing supplementer

In addition to hand and electric pumps, I used a Lact-Aid when she came home from the hospital. It's a gadget that supplements formula through a small tube on your breast which the baby sucks on while sucking on you, thus encouraging your own milk supply and feeding the baby formula at the same time. However, it requires tremendous patience and effort.

As my anxiety increased, I realized that those vibes were being passed on to the baby and that it would be healthier for her if I were more relaxed and happy. I gave the Lact-Aid one month and then realized I had to quit or go crazy. That was a difficult and traumatic decision for me, because I'd been very attached to the idea of breast-feeding.

The emotional pain of that time has diminished somewhat now. It was very intense then because I wanted desperately to give milk to my baby, but without her stimulation my body didn't want to cooperate. I felt a sense of failure and at moments like "less of a woman," although I knew intellectually that wasn't so. I felt that my inability to feed her from my breasts was adding to her already traumatic beginning of life.

I'm just beginning to realize that there are things about the whole premature birth experience that are buried deep within me and sometimes I even find myself blaming her. But those moments are short-lived compared to the fullness of having a new baby in the house. When I see her smile now, and recall that exactly a year ago she was just starting to put her cells together, it blows my mind. That's a real birthday.

Slowly, I'm coming to accept the fact that I can't control her life. She's started off in the world in her own special way, as we all do. But a mother's instinct to protect is strong, so it's a slow and painful learning process. I still hope that someday I'll have the experience of breast-feeding, but for now I've put that aside.

What were your first experiences breast-feeding?

• With my first child, I had no problems breast-feeding whatsoever. Everybody was shocked because I should have! Both my children were cesareans, and I didn't know that if you have a cesarean you're *supposed* to have problems with breast-feeding. Cesarean mothers are often made to believe that they can't breast-feed because the whole hormonal cycle hasn't really occurred, but I had more than adequate milk the first time. The second time, though, I *knew* that I was *supposed* to have a problem. I tried to force the baby to nurse a lot the first couple of days and he wouldn't. But the problem was all in my mind. I still have milk in my breasts—I've had milk in them for four and a half years straight!

• I tried to nurse my baby but I was not successful because I had a cesarean delivery, which meant I couldn't breast-feed right away. I was really sick, sick, sick, so I didn't even *see* her for four days. I developed an infection and when the time came, I finally put the baby to my breast. The mouth was moving but nothing was happening—no milk was coming out! After a while the baby literally looked up at me with an expression on her face as if to say, "Are you for *real?*" It was too late. She had already been bottle-fed.

• I had a home delivery, and immediately after the baby was born, before the cord was even cut, I put her to my breast. She was slippery all over and I didn't think I could really hang onto her. I tried to get my breast in her mouth while she was still wiggling around, and after a bit of fumbling she finally caught on. She sucked right away—they have such a strong instinct to suck. It was an incredible feeling.

• I was very scared the first time I nursed. When they brought her to me—this little thing—I didn't know what to do with her! (*Laughs.*)

• There was a special nurse who came in and explained everything about breast-feeding. She was there to help, which was something new in that hospital. She explained how to press the top of the breast to keep it out of the way of the baby's nose so it wouldn't stop him from breathing.

• My doctor had to *show* me how to nurse—yes, a man! If he hadn't, I wouldn't have known how.

• The baby took the breast right away and there wasn't any problem. He knew what to do. They told me in Lamaze classes to take the nipple and rub it on the side of the baby's face that was closest to my body and the baby would automatically turn its head, and he did right away. Even when his father held him he'd turn his head toward his daddy's chest, looking for the breast.

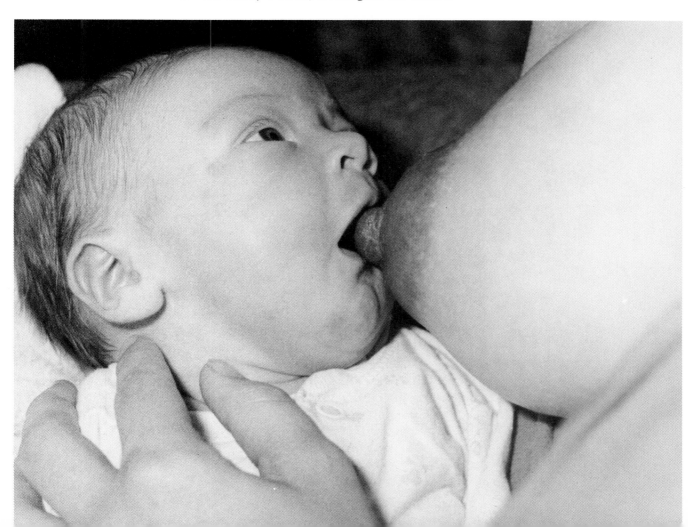

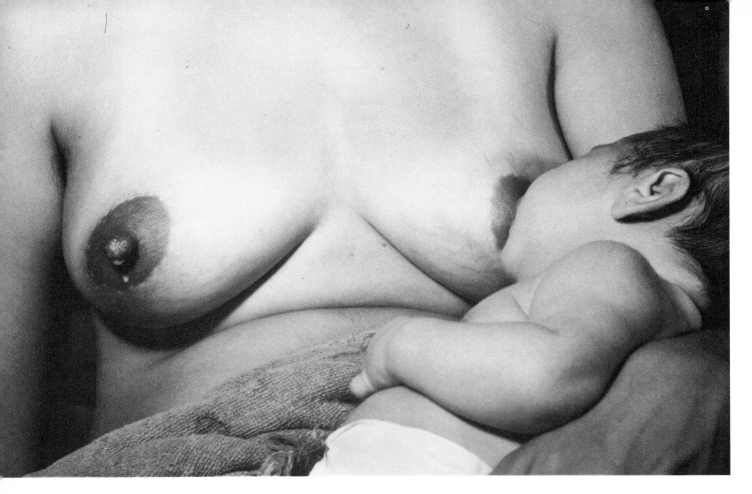

• The first time I nursed was really shocking—it was amazing and horrible at the same time. I was in a hospital with a nurse shoving my breast in the baby's mouth, telling me, "Only give him two minutes on each breast and then get him off," and making remarks like, "You're going to spoil him!" They have a thousand weird ideas. If you don't fight them they keep you on a very rigid schedule which *ruins* your breast-feeding. Hospitals and routines really discourage the easy flow of time and space in which mothers and infants get to know each other.

• The whole thing seemed a little ridiculous at first because the baby doesn't *know* how to nurse. He knows how to suck, but he'll suck anything that he can get into his mouth. It was very frightening in the beginning.

• First time nursing? A laugh. She missed the nipple and gave me a hickey. It took a tough old Polish nurse to show me how. I had to lie down and hold her to my side and *work* at it. After about three days we finally got it right.

• After I gave birth, I couldn't imagine milk coming out of my breast any more than I could imagine milk coming out of my elbow or my feet, so I didn't think it was going to. I think that's why a lot of breast-feeding fails. You don't believe that milk will come out of you, so you just unconsciously stop it.

• When I was born my mother had wanted to breast-feed me, but a nurse told her, "It doesn't look like you can make any milk," so she lost her confidence. Her heart was in the right place, but she was discouraged. At that time [late 1940s] the formula industry was very influential.

Without guidance and support it's practically impossible to succeed at breast-feeding. Pioneer women and tribal women still lived with their relatives and got a lot of encouragement to breast-feed and saw it happening naturally all around them, so instead of being something strange, it was the inevitable natural flow of events after childbirth.

156

• My first two children were born in the twenties and they were brought to me to nurse as soon as they were born. With my second two, who were born in the forties, I had to *fight* to nurse. I was an M.D., so I had a little more latitude to say what I wanted or didn't want. Yet even my obstetrician made remarks like, "Oh, you'll get tired of it." Of course, I didn't.

• I didn't get enough encouragement to breast-feed and I'm sure that had a lot to do with why I didn't last longer. I'd had natural childbirth and I wanted the experience of breast-feeding. I didn't know if I would have another child, so I wanted to try it all. But I was very discouraged by the nurses. That was in 1967, and I was the *only* woman in the ward that had natural childbirth.

The nurses were hostile about me breast-feeding. They would wake me up in the middle of the night to breast-feed and it was awful! They gave her sugar water or milk before they brought her to me and so she wouldn't take enough milk. And then there wouldn't be enough milk in my breasts for her the next time. On top of it all, because she didn't take enough milk from me, it would squirt all over after they took her away and it was a mess.

I felt angry about the way I was treated—I fought my way through that whole clinic. They injected a lot of women with stuff to dry up their milk, whether they wanted to breast-feed or not. Then the women would wake up from the anesthesia and want to breast-feed their babies and there would be no milk. So the nurses put the babies on formula without explaining what they had done.

• I announced to the doctor that I didn't want to breast-feed and then after my daughter was born, they forgot to give me the special pills. My breasts got big and very sore, but because I used to feel, "I'm in your hands," when faced with doctors and hospitals, I let it get very bad before I said anything. By the time they realized what happened, they had to put *ice packs* on my breasts. I thought I'd die—the mortification of it all!!

• The nurses didn't like the fact that I was nursing, and I think a lot of it was because I am blind. They felt that it would be easier to bottle-feed. But that doesn't make any sense to me—obviously it's easier to breast-feed, particularly for someone like me.

• The nurses didn't bring my daughter to me often enough. She must have been screaming a lot in the nursery, because when they finally did bring her in she was too tired to nurse. She would just fall asleep in my arms. The nurses would say, "Wake her up! She has to eat!" And they would pinch the bottoms of her feet or slap her.

• It is very hard for a baby to nurse on a rigid schedule because they want to nurse very often in the beginning. But luckily you could go in and get your baby any time you wanted. You could even have the baby in the room twenty-four hours if you wanted to.

• They allowed me to go into the anteroom of the nursery—a very sterile-looking room—every three hours, and I had to put on a sterile gown in order to nurse the baby. They even made me *wash* my nipples! I had studiously avoided using soap on my nipples for many weeks before so that they wouldn't be brittle and crack, and then they insisted that I *wash* all the natural oils off, which the Montgomery's glands secrete. I couldn't wait to get out of there.

• In the hospital they tell you, "Wash yourself every time you breast-feed your child. Make sure you are *clean!*" What kind of dirt do they think we have? They want us to wash ourselves inside and out. I wash myself when I take a shower, but I don't go into orgies of cleanliness just because I'm nursing.

• I was in a Catholic hospital and they really put me through the mill about breast-feeding. The nurses told my husband that he should *leave* the room. They said, "Don't you respect your wife's *privacy!*" And every time I nursed—I was the only person who did—they drew the curtains around the bed, as if I was doing something *obscene!*

• When I had my baby, I was put in a room with five other women, all of whom were going to bottle-feed. Then the nurses brought in all the little babies and gave them to all the mothers for the first time, and each mother pulled out her bottle and fed her baby.

When they gave me my baby, I wanted to breast-feed, but I just couldn't! Seeing all those efficient mothers bottle-feeding their babies, I sat there for a long time feeling awkward and totally perplexed. I didn't know what to do. It was so strange being completely dressed with my new baby all bundled up, just after we had been through the whole birth experience and been completely naked.

All of a sudden I had an inspiration. I jumped out of bed, took off all my clothes and all the baby's clothes, jumped back into bed, and put the baby to my breast. I just didn't know what else to do. Then I nursed and was perfectly happy. The women were all shocked so I blurted out some apology but I don't think they really understood.

• After my baby was born I wanted to nurse as soon as possible. But the hospital had an official twelve-hour waiting period before mothers could bottle-feed their babies and they wouldn't let me nurse! Before a baby gets a bottle they must make sure that its digestive tract is okay, because if the baby aspirates formula it can damage the lungs. This is *not* the case with colostrum, which is what you have in your breasts until seventy-two hours after birth. But hospitals are geared to bottle-feeding, so they work on schedules and do testing and all sorts of unnatural stuff.

I was furious that they insisted I wait because all the good stuff in the colostrum, which the baby is supposed to get, was going to waste. What's more, I *needed* to nurse and I knew my baby needed to nurse, too, and they weren't *allowing* it. I pleaded and argued with them and finally, after tremendous aggravation and heartache, they allowed me to breast-feed before the official waiting period was up.

What gets me is that I had to *fight* for it. The whole institution was against me! It's such a frustrating and desperate feeling because I was fighting for the good of my child, and all they talked about was "rules." The organic one-to-one relationship of breast-feeding disrupts the hospital's assembly-line routine.

It's so screwed up—they've made everything so complicated when in fact it's all very simple. The nurses feel that it's necessary to watch the baby to make sure it's healthy. Of course, they've got thirty babies in the nursery and they must watch all of them, whereas if they gave babies to their mothers, the mother would have only one to watch, and being more personally involved would obviously do a better job.

The hospital's attitude is that you're sick and the baby's sick, so they treat the whole process of childbirth and breast-feeding like an illness. I tried to convince the nurses to bring my daughter to me for her night feedings, and they tried to convince me that I needed my sleep to regain my "health." So I told them that it is natural to nurse around the clock and that breast-feeding has been around a lot longer than hospitals. But they still refused—"We can't run a hospital without rules." Realizing that it would affect my milk production, I tried to avoid getting too upset because I knew I would be going home within a day or two, thank God, and then everything would be okay.

• When I brought the baby home, I had a practical nurse who had never been with a nursing mother before, so she really steered me wrong. Her major concern was that I should rest, so she wouldn't bring the baby to me on demand. Meanwhile the baby was crying endlessly, so she tried to give her sugar water in a bottle, but I wouldn't permit it because *I* don't even use sugar.

The nurse would bring two or three glasses of milk each time before I nursed, until she almost drove me *crazy.* I called my pediatrician and he said, "Does she actually think that if you drink milk, ten minutes later it's going to come out of your breasts? That's the silliest thing I ever heard!" I didn't calm down until the nurse left and I started breast-feeding my baby on demand.

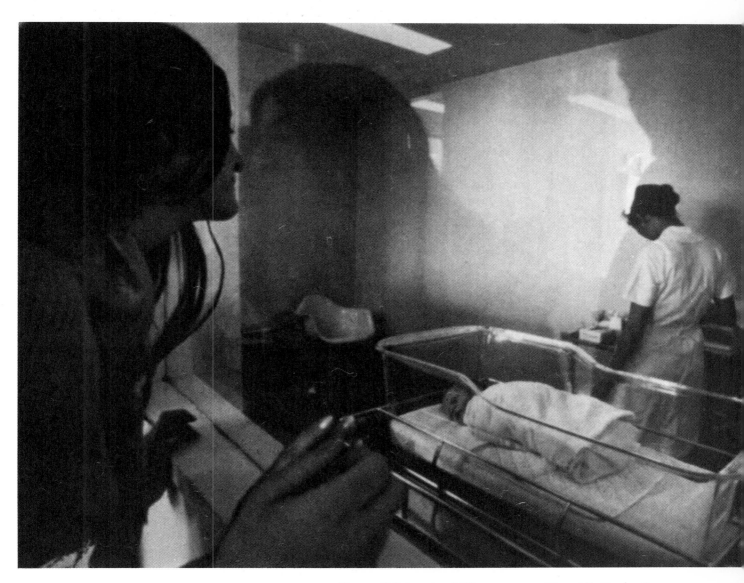

Photo: © Sebastian Milito, courtesy Time-Life Books, Inc.

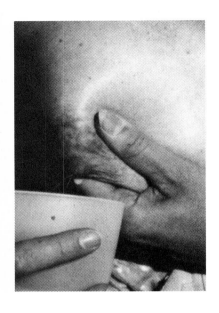

How did it feel when the milk came in?

• There's only colostrum, a clear liquid, in the breasts right after giving birth. The milk production doesn't start until a few days later and it all happens at once. You can feel the milk coming in, and if you're asleep you wake up with enormous breasts just full of milk. It's a very dramatic experience.

When my milk came in I leaked all over the place. My breasts became extremely hard and engorged. It was painful for the first few days, so breast-feeding was actually a relief.

• I practiced expressing colostrum while I was pregnant, so I was physically ready and didn't get engorged—ouch, swollen tits!—when my milk came in.

• For three days I had colostrum. The milk came in the day I left the hospital. Oh, that was exciting! When the milk let down there was a stinging feeling. Then it started to flow, and if I hadn't had a bra on it would have leaked through my clothing. After a month or so it got under control. My milk became regulated to the baby's needs and didn't let down as much while he was asleep. At first I only had to *think* about him and my milk would start dripping!

• When my milk came in I was really excited and happy, but then I was faced with the problem of too much milk. It seemed that every minute I was soaking wet. I went through tons and tons of nursing pads, one right after the other, and the milk kept pouring out. I used to sleep with heavy towels all around me and I would still wake up sopping wet in no time. I walked around my apartment virtually topless the whole time.

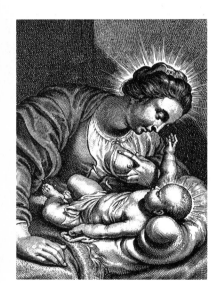

• At first I had so much milk that the baby couldn't empty my breasts. There was no way I could express the milk myself, so my husband had to. He gently sucked the milk out and he actually swallowed it. He was delighted to do it.

• When my daughter didn't nurse enough, I would wake up at night lying on my back with the milk squirting out like two fountains. I could just touch my breasts and milk would go shooting across the room. I could've been a wet nurse! Sometimes I even nursed my friend's baby and mine at the same time.

I also contributed to the mothers' milk bank. All over the country there are milk banks that buy it and freeze it. They use the milk for sick or allergic babies, or with mothers who can't or won't nurse. Mother's milk goes for *a lot* of money.

Did you have any complications while breast-feeding?

• Nursing was terribly painful the first few times with this *thing* chewing on my nipple! I had no idea—I thought it would be easy. I remember thinking, My God, why did I ever want to do this? And I kept wanting to tear him off and send him away. Ouch! The baby was very hungry, so he really worked away at me, and my breasts just weren't used to all that attention so it hurt. I knew that I just had to get through it, that the pain was going to pass. It took a few days for my breasts to toughen up and accept the gnawing and pulling. Then nursing became nice.

• When I was pregnant, my obstetrician told me to rub cocoa butter on my nipples to toughen them and prepare them for nursing. I ignored him—never did *anything* to prepare my nipples—and I never had any problems. I just figured that peasant women didn't do that, so why should I? Who has time to rub cocoa butter on their nipples?

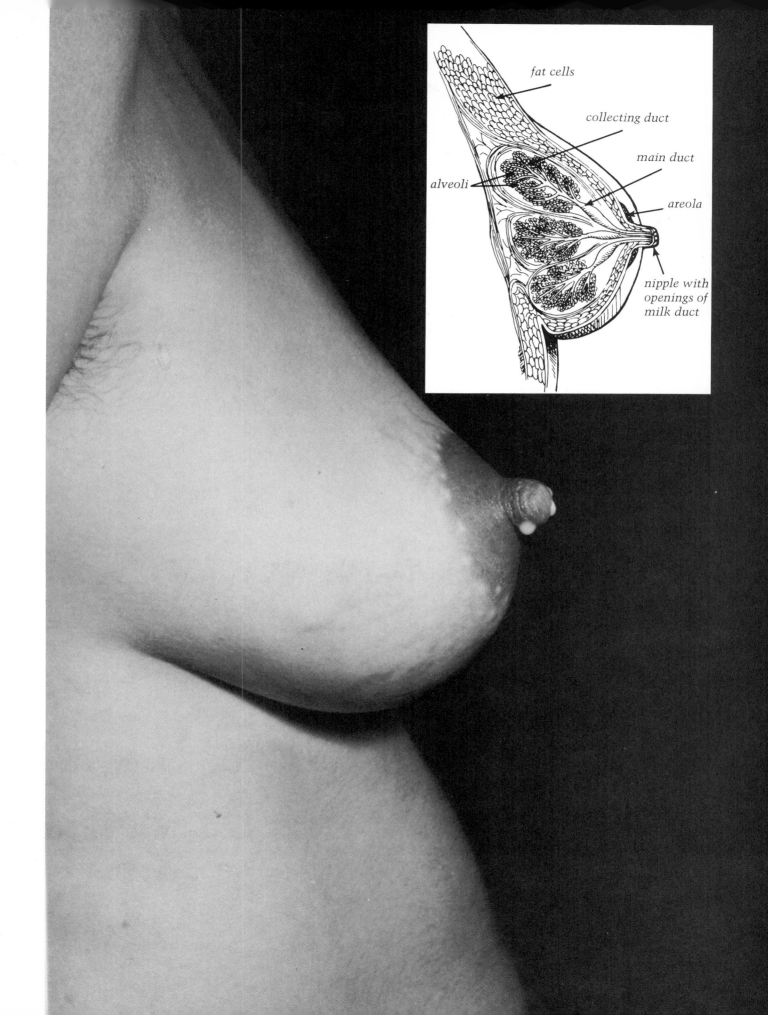

fat cells

collecting duct

main duct

alveoli

areola

nipple with
openings of
milk duct

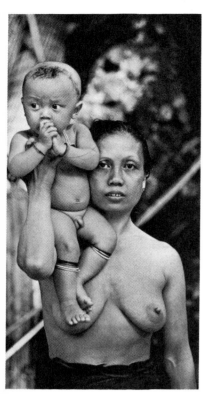

Borneo woman

• I didn't prepare my nipples beforehand and sure enough I had problems. The first week my daughter nursed, I was in agony. My nipples were just the sorest things. They *broke* and they were bleeding constantly. Every time she sucked on them, I'd go through the ceiling. It was *agonizing!* My breasts had always done so well in the sexual department, that I just assumed they would do well in this department, too.

I'm not unusual; this is a very common occurrence for women in this country. The reason is that in this culture we keep our breasts covered all the time so the nipples are ultrasensitive—unnaturally so, like cultivated flowers. They can't withstand the natural function of nursing. I mean let's face it, nipples are not supposed to crack. Obviously the way we live has something to do with it.

If we kept our breasts in the open air, exposed to the sun and wind, the nipples would not be as sensitive, and then when we nursed our nipples wouldn't bleed. The only way to heal cracked nipples is to leave them exposed to the air—not to wear anything. After my nipples healed and the nursing was established and proceeding normally, it was a real pleasure.

• My nipples were prepared and therefore nursing wasn't painful. I did the special exercises, like pulling and rolling the nipples between my fingers and massaging my breasts. And of course I religiously lubricated my nipples with lanolin cream for the last six weeks of my pregnancy, so they wouldn't be brittle later on. The fact that I go braless also helped—I think the roughness of clothing rubbing against my nipples toughened them up some.

Anne

Nursing was a nice feeling in the beginning and I was happy because I could be so close to her. But soon afterward my breasts became sore and I began to cringe whenever she came to me.

When the milk came in, my breasts became very, very enlarged and swollen. I had lots of milk and the baby could take only so much. You're supposed to start with five minutes on each breast and then increase it to seven, to ten, and to twelve, but I went up to fifteen minutes right away. Maybe I just did it too fast.

Pretty soon both my nipples were bleeding. The baby vomited blood that she swallowed from me, and that scared me. I became nervous and frightened and it wasn't good for the baby. She could feel how tense I was, so I didn't want to do it anymore. The doctor encouraged me to get over the pain and told me that the blood wouldn't hurt the baby, so I tried to continue. But it was so painful and the bleeding was so bad that I *had* to stop. It was excruciating pain, like knives cutting into you. I wanted to cry but I didn't want my husband to see me cry. He could tell how much pain I was in so finally he said, "If it bothers you so much, stop."

My husband had wanted me to breast-feed and often spoke about it while I was pregnant. I had been leery about it but I realized that it's better for the baby, and because he wanted me to nurse then I wanted to, too. He thought that breast-feeding brings the mother and child closer together and makes the family more united. He had also heard that breast-fed children are more intelligent—which I don't believe is the truth—and healthier. But I couldn't go through with it.

I was really sad about that at first, but the baby took to the bottle very well. The only thing my husband said about it was, "It's gonna cost a lot of money now," 'cause formula is so expensive.

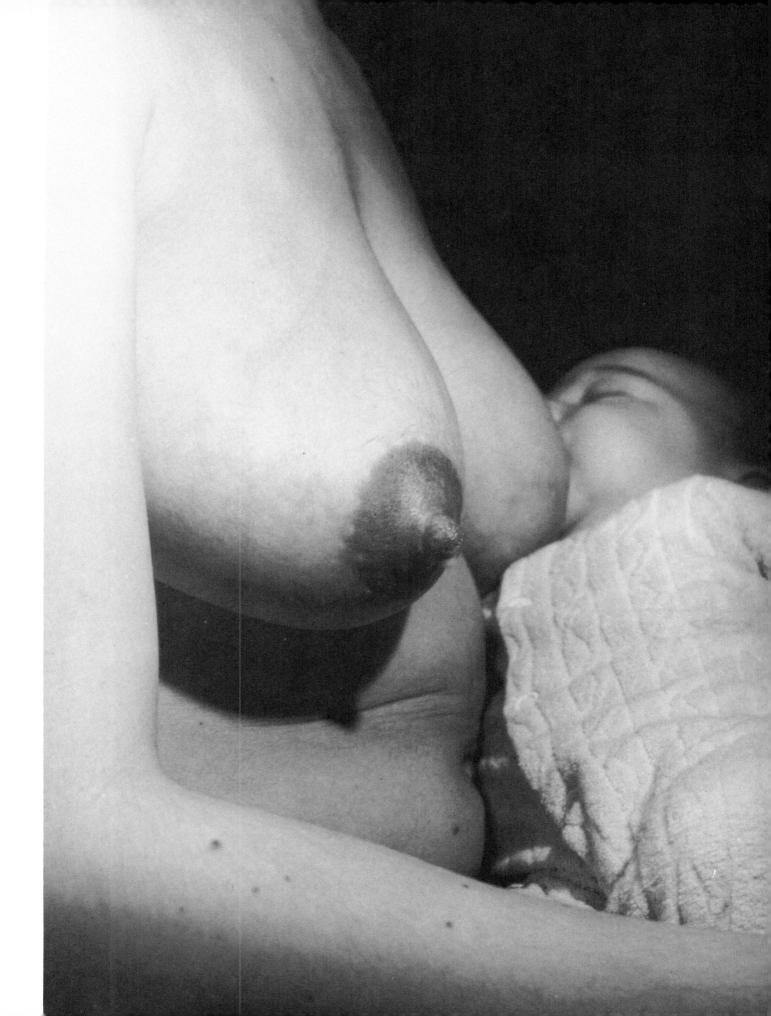

Why do you think your nipples cracked?

Because I didn't prepare them ahead of time. *After* I gave birth, I was told that I should have prepared my nipples before the baby was born. Maybe my baby just sucked harder than other babies. If I had prepared myself I probably wouldn't have had any problems, but I didn't realize I had to. I'm very disappointed that I wasn't told when I could still do something about it.

D: Some women who were interviewed feel that the reason women have difficulty with their nipples during nursing is because their breasts are covered up all the time and not exposed to the air. They say that in cultures where the women go bare-breasted they don't have to prepare their nipples for nursing—they are prepared naturally.

That's probably true because my nurse told me that I should expose my breasts to lots of sunlight and fresh air. I tried to explain to her that I live in a ground-floor apartment so I really couldn't stand in front of the window and lean out! (*Laughs.*)

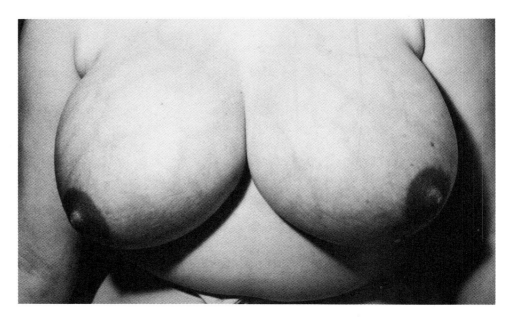

How did you get rid of the milk in your breasts?

I went into the shower and let the hot water run against my breasts and the milk came out. My doctor told me that the beating of the water is like a massage. I also took hot towels and wrapped them around my breasts.

I'm still engorged. It's taking quite awhile to get rid of the milk. It's still dripping! The doctor didn't give me any medication because apparently there's nothing you can do to stop the milk once you start breast-feeding. When you first deliver the baby you must tell the doctor whether you're going to breast-feed or not, and if you don't plan to, you get a shot. But once you have milk in your breasts, you must let it dry up by itself.

Before the nursing became painful, it was very sensual. Every time I breast-fed I could feel my uterus contracting. It was a completely different feeling—you can't imagine it. It's like making love. I felt so close to her. I felt so much love for the baby and I felt her love for me, knowing that I was her mother and that I could do this for her. I could give her whatever she needed.

●

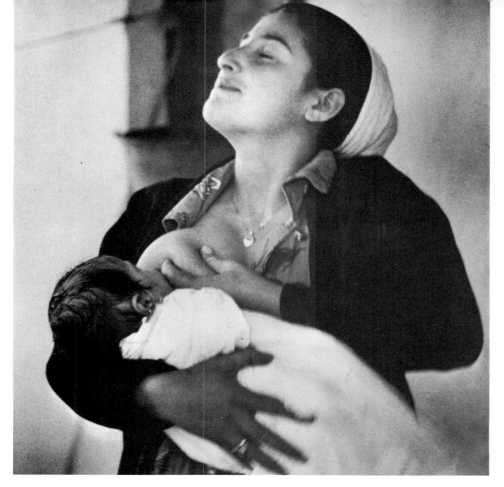

• *I read somewhere that Freud once said the most ecstatic orgasmic experience is having the baby asleep at the mother's breast. Milk running down, the mother looking at her baby—that is total orgasm, the highest moment of satisfaction.*

• *To me, the height of sensuality becomes spiritual. Nursing outdoors in some secluded place in the country, laying in the sun without any clothes on, surrounded by the beauty of nature, my baby's naked body against mine—that's a very spiritual experience.*

• *When I was growing up in the post-Victorian era, it was considered naughty to have sexual pleasure. "Nice" women were never supposed to experience it, only "bad" women. Yet I vividly remember breast-feeding as extremely pleasurable, and not just in a simple, superficial way, but in a very deep sense.*

As a doctor, I am aware that many women experience sexual arousal and sometimes even orgasm through their breasts, and that it is common for women to have the same reactions while nursing. I personally have never had an orgasm nursing, but I've met many women who have, and many of them are ashamed of it. I find that sad and an enormous waste of good human energy—it saps our spiritual and emotional strength.

I wish that women who experience pleasure from breast-feeding would realize that it's a most natural thing, and allow themselves to enjoy it. If a woman has an orgasm while nursing, she shouldn't think, Oh, I've been a bad person because I had an orgasm today when I was nursing my innocent little baby. It certainly cannot hurt the baby. I wish women would accept the totality of their erotic potential as women, for themselves and for their babies.

Was nursing ever a sensual or sexual experience? Describe.

• It's sensual, even sexual, but not in the regular way one thinks of sex. It's like a different department in my mind.

• Because I was sexually inhibited and frigid, I got more pleasure out of the baby sucking me than in having sex with my husband. For some reason I could really let myself go with the baby.

• I've talked to women who had sexual experiences during breast-feeding but I never felt that because I've disassociated my breasts from sexual arousal. I shut it out because I was afraid of that arousal in *any* circumstance. Denying myself pleasure was a set pattern with me, so even though I loved breast-feeding, I couldn't open myself up to enjoying it in sexual ways.

• Oh, nursing was very sensual, especially in the beginning. It was even erotic! I imagine that's one of the reasons women are uptight about nursing, because it's overtly sexual and a baby doesn't have inhibitions like the rest of us. A baby just has needs—pure yearning. They're totally into touch and feel and pleasure.

• There is nothing at all sexual about nursing a baby! That is one of the ugliest myths, one of the biggest lies, one of the things that makes me want to *throw up* it makes me so angry. Nursing is an ecstatic feeling of warmth, but it's not sensual. It's different. It's a feeling which is unique to you and your baby. It's like saving somebody you love from drowning. It's a good, human, spiritual feeling, just a purely loving feeling.

• Of course nursing is pleasurable and sexual. It was made that way by millions of years of evolutionary design in order to make *sure* that women breast-feed. The baby, besides satisfying itself, is making love to its mother upon whom its entire survival depends.

You literally *feel* a bond being created with the baby while you nurse, and each time it gets stronger. I don't know if it's love, but there's a need and I don't think it's just the baby's. As a mother, satisfying that need is incredibly pleasurable. I loved having my baby at my breast and I miss it very much now.

• Breast-feeding was *very* enjoyable in the early months, and I once even had a slight orgasm breast-feeding. The closest thing to it now, after one year, is when my breasts are very full. Then I feel a tingling sensation and a pressure in the front. If she sucks very hard, the relief is quite pleasant.

• I am always supremely relaxed when I nurse because it is so sensual. I think there is actually a hormone involved which works like a tranquilizer. When I'm relaxed, nursing is a fantastic high—the most beautiful feeling that a woman can have. With every swallow that the baby takes, you feel a world of pleasure and an amazing feeling of love.

• It felt fine. It wasn't earth-shattering but I must have really enjoyed it because I didn't really want it to end.

●

• It was strange, but even though I'm usually very sexually involved with my breasts, if my husband sucked on them when I was nursing, I didn't like it.

• I knew that there are some men who are just dying to suck the breasts of a nursing woman and I thought that was horrible. It was my bad luck that my husband turned out to be one of those types, you know, but I just couldn't *stand* it. I only saw my milk for the baby, not in any way as a sexual thing. I think my husband was very jealous of the baby.

• When I was young I wondered how would I feel if my husband wanted to suck my breasts, to taste the milk when I was nursing. I thought that was perverted and I didn't want it to happen to me.

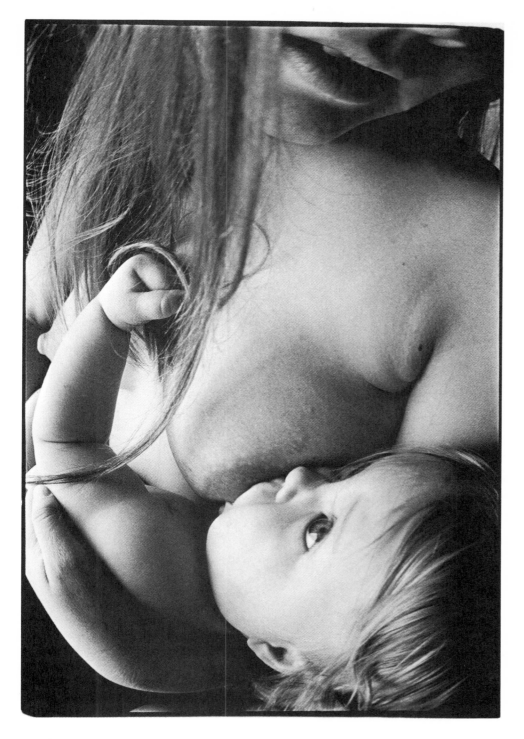

After my baby was born and my husband *didn't* want to suck on my breasts, I was disappointed. I thought, Isn't he even *curious?* I *wanted* him to do it! I love the feeling when my daughter nurses and I thought it might be very stimulating if my husband did it, too, but he never got into it.

• After my son was born, I had an affair with a man who was insanely attracted to the idea of my having milk in my breasts. He wanted to nurse and have the breasts close to him, and actual sex wasn't important to him at all. I was with another man a little later who never touched my breasts when we had sex. I think it was just a lack of interest. He'd seen babies breast-fed all his life, so the breast seemed to have lost its sexual role for him.—*Single mother.*

167

• *A Frenchman I know, who is a famous poet, drank a lot, and his driver's license was taken away from him so his wife did all the driving on their summer trip through southern France.*

One day she was driving, and even though she had just fed the baby, her breasts were full, dripping with milk, and it hurt her terribly. Finally, she said to her husband, "You'll have to suck my milk." He complained bitterly, saying, "Absolutely not!*" He was shocked by the suggestion. Meanwhile, the baby was asleep in the back seat of the car, and there was nothing she could do to relieve herself, so she finally said, "Since I am the driver, either you do it or we don't drive!" She turned the car off the road into the woods and parked.*

Well, she got out of the car and leaned against it, exposing her breasts. Grumbling and complaining, he bent down in front of her and began sucking the milk and spewing it out, and sucking and spewing . . .

While this was going on, she saw over her husband's head a young man on a bicycle coming down the path. She felt so good and so relieved that her husband was sucking the milk out of her, but she knew he would stop if she told him about the young man, so she didn't say a word. She assumed that the man would ride past quickly and go on. . . .

When he arrived on the scene, the young man got such a shock that he fell off his bicycle! Meanwhile, there she stood with her breasts exposed, laughing her head off. Her husband, on the other hand, was dying *of embarrassment and didn't know what to do with himself.*

Many years later, he told me that he lives in terror whenever he stops at a village pub or café that the men will be retelling the story. "I can imagine," he told me, "the number of times that young man is going to describe that scene during his life. It will be passed on throughout the French countryside, and I know that all the time the person being talked about is me!*"*

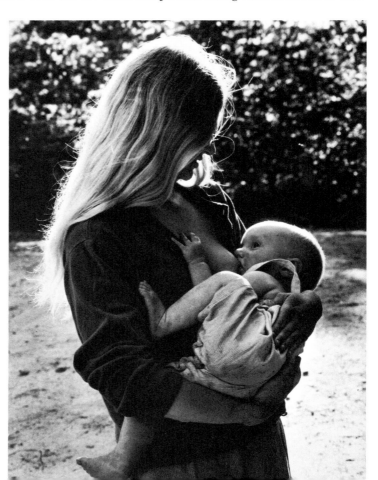

If you have children, do you think you'll breast-feed in front of relatives or friends, or in public?

• Maybe I would nurse in front of my mother, but my father—*never!*

• If I were smaller maybe I'd nurse in front of people. I'm so large-breasted that I've had looks and leers all my life, so it would make me nervous.

• There are certain parts of your body that you just don't show, and I'm sure my husband wouldn't approve of me breast-feeding in front of other men *or* women. In fact, I *know* he wouldn't approve!

He saw my girlfriend breast-feeding once and was so embarrassed that he just looked straight ahead. Everyone was sitting around the dining room table and she was breast-feeding in front of her six brothers and sisters, and her mother, father, and grandmother, when we walked in. My husband kept saying to her brother, "Oh, wouldn't you like to go into the other room?"

• I wouldn't nurse outdoors for health reasons—it's unsanitary! The air pollution, the dirt, the common city soot and the gawking people.

• I feel squeamish watching a woman nurse her child so I'm not sure how I'd feel about other people watching me.

• I don't know why, but I'd be embarrassed to breast-feed outdoors where I could be seen (*laughs*) . . . even though I've done nudes in magazines. There no one knows who I am—it's not *me.* I don't see the readers looking at me.

• I almost have a political belief about breast-feeding in public. If that's okay, then it should also be acceptable to walk around with our tops off. Otherwise, it's like saying that "motherhood" makes it all right to expose our breasts because that's good and dutiful and virtuous, but if it's for our own comfort, we can't because that's obscene and indecent. For the baby it's okay, but for the woman herself *never!* So I would nurse in public *only* if I walked around that way when I wasn't breast-feeding.

• I'm not sure. It would be nice if women did breast-feed in public and didn't think of their breasts as sexual tools. But then again, breasts do have more sexual possibilities than shoulders or elbows.

Did you ever nurse among friends or relatives, or in public situations? How did you feel? How did other people react?

• Once I made up my mind to nurse, I just *had* to get used to doing it in front of other people occasionally, otherwise I would have gone *crazy* hiding myself away all the time. But it wasn't easy at first.

• When I had the baby my natural tendency was to breast-feed anywhere. I didn't have the slightest hesitation about it at all.

• Dealing with family and friends was always a big factor. I have been continually shocked by people's reactions. I got endorsement from people who seemed conservative and repressed, and bad reactions from the most liberal types. Older people were usually better about it than younger ones. Shockingly enough, my grandfather told me that it was very important for me to breast-feed and to keep doing it, but my younger sister was *disgusted* by it. You just have no way of telling.

• When I was a little girl, my mother told me about one time when she was breast-feeding me at a family reunion. She took me into the bedroom and my grandfather accidentally came in. She was very embarrassed. But instead of saying, "Ooops!" and walking out, my grandfather sat down and with his sweet, old, Dutch accent said, "Darling, there's nothing in the world that you should be embarrassed about. One of the most beautiful sights on this earth is a mother breast-feeding a child."

• My father did not allow me to breast-feed in front of him. He would become embarrassed, excuse himself, and leave the room. One time he made an offhanded remark about "tits," and said, "Is the baby chewing you up?" Ironically, he felt strongly that breast-feeding was good but it was a little too much for him to see me open my blouse and expose my breast.

• My mother always walked out of the room when I nursed the baby because she didn't like to watch. The fact that I was openly using a sexual part of my body, no matter what the reason was, completely turned her off!!

• When I was growing up, my father was more embarrassed about my mother breast-feeding in front of company than she was. She was *never* shy but he wanted her to cover up if my uncle, who wasn't a blood relative, came over. They even had arguments about it!

• When friends came over while I was nursing I would turn away. I didn't have beautiful breasts that I wanted to show off. That little tiny head next to these huge breasts didn't look too great aesthetically.

• I think my nursing in front of my friends was somewhat of an exhibition on my part. There was one young man who simply couldn't keep his eyes off my breast, and that got a little embarrassing. Everybody's interested—I always was when somebody did it in my presence—but he was just glued to it. (*Laughs.*)

• A casual friend once came to the house when I was alone with the baby, and when I said to him, "I have to nurse the baby now," he said, "If you don't mind, I'm going to sit behind you because I'm not used to seeing it." I said, "Oh, don't be ridiculous!" But he said, "No, please. I don't want to." The whole time I nursed he sat in back of me where he couldn't see. I didn't agree with him, but I appreciated his honesty. Perhaps we have a false idea of men— that a man will always take the opportunity to get a look.

• I never breast-fed in front of *anybody*—it's shameful to take out a breast when men are sitting there. Whenever somebody came to visit, if the baby had to get fed I excused myself and went into the bedroom.

• I was watching a woman being interviewed on Johnny Carson once and she said, "Can you imagine? I went to somebody's house and she sat there breast-feeding her kid in front of the guests! Isn't that *disgusting?*" But I do that all the time, so I started to think that maybe I'm really offending people.

• A few weeks ago, we were with a group of pretty uptight people and I wouldn't nurse in front of them because I didn't want their negative vibes coming at me. When people think lurid things about me breast-feeding, it affects my milk and my concentration. The baby senses it and becomes upset, too. So I try to avoid places where it might be uncomfortable to nurse, which is pretty limiting.

• I practically live in restaurants and I never changed my way of life when the baby was born. I took her with me and I breast-fed her while I ate. Occasionally a loony old lady would give me dirty looks, but from the waiters and waitresses I got a lot of smiles and positive reactions. I found that the more expensive the restaurant, the better the reactions were. Maybe it's because you're paying more.

• When I've breast-fed in restaurants, I've often been told to "please cover up," or to go to another room and do it. So the only public place I nurse now is in movie theaters where it is dark. I can't do it in broad daylight because there's always a lot of violent hostility from the public—I can feel it in their looks.

• My neighbor saw me breast-feeding in the yard and she said, "You're a filthy cow with running udders! It's revolting!" I was horrified that another woman could feel that way. I'll never forget it.

• My friend got married recently and wanted to invite a dear friend of his, but she couldn't come unless she could nurse her baby in Temple. He said, "No, I don't want *that* at my wedding!"

• I was once asked to leave a courtroom in San Francisco because I was nursing my son to keep him *quiet!*

• Once I sat next to a woman on an airplane and when I started to breast-feed she jumped up, said, *"That's* disgusting!" and switched to another seat. What could I do? The kid was hungry.

• It was mostly men who were troubled by my breast-feeding. I remember one man—a perfect stranger—came up to me at an art show in a civic center lobby and said that I was really going to fuck my kid up in some Oedipal-complex way. He didn't even explain himself—he was just lecturing me, *scolding* me . . . *while* I was breast-feeding.

• When I nursed in the park, I once had some older woman tell me that it was going to make my son a homosexual if I nursed. Weird.

• Whenever I breast-feed in public, I try to be discreet. I hold the baby so that he's hiding under my blouse. You can hardly see what I'm doing. I would hate to have a strange man's eyes looking at my breast with dirty or sexual thoughts while I am doing this wonderful thing. It would be sacrilegious in a way—blasphemous! Breast-feeding is holy and sacred, if ever there was anything sacred. And I wouldn't ever want to belittle it or cheapen it.

• It's always nicer to sit in the park and nurse in beautiful surroundings than to be cooped up indoors. And I really *love* to nurse outdoors in the country, sitting on the grass near a tree. Then it is all natural, peaceful. Unfortunately, we don't get to do that very often.

• I heard that a group of women were breast-feeding their children in a park in Florida and they were threatened with arrest. The people there didn't think it was *decent!* But the police can't legally stop you from public breast-feeding. When I was an instructor for the La Leche League, prospective breast-feeding mothers would always ask questions about that—it was a real concern. Imagine if they could actually arrest you for indecent exposure? The poor kid's hungry and you have to go someplace where you can't be seen before feeding him. God, it's *bizarre!*

• I once worked for a pediatrician and maybe ten percent of the women were breast-feeding. Some of them nursed their babies in the waiting room. There were some children who had never seen this before and their mothers made them turn their heads away and shielded their eyes. I felt that they have no right subjecting everyone to such a sight. It should be done in private.

• Someone hassled me in Saks Fifth Avenue while I was breast-feeding in the ladies' room. I had to sit on the floor because there were no chairs. What the hell was I supposed to do, sit on the *toilet?* Society makes it impossible for women to nurse. If you can't face doing it in public, there's never any place in public bathrooms to comfortably nurse or change a baby's diaper. Mothers don't want to stay home with their babies all the time, but they are forced to become closet cases. It's very ironic to live in a society that tells us that women are supposed to be mothers to keep the race going, but makes absolutely no provisions for motherhood!

• Once I was nursing on the bus and a Spanish woman sat down beside me. She started talking about how she would be really embarrassed if she nursed her child in public so she was going to give her kid bottles. She said,

Mother Sues Over Ban On Her Breast-Feeding

A 33-year-old Long Island woman filed a $500,000 suit against the Village of Williston Park yesterday because she was not allowed to breast-feed her 3-month-old baby beside a community wading pool.

The woman, Mrs. Bruce Damon Jr. of 299 Houston Avenue, Mineola, charged in Federal District Court in Westbury, L.I., that pool officials had caused her great embarrassment and had violated her civil rights.

A spokesman for the village said Mrs. Damon had been the subject of complaints of some of the residents who used the pool. But she said she was not aware that anyone had objected although she had been breast-feeding her son, Michael, for six weeks before two lifeguards told her to stop.

"They told me I could use the bathroom," she said yesterday. "I refused absolutely, because that was not near the pool, where my other children were playing in the water."

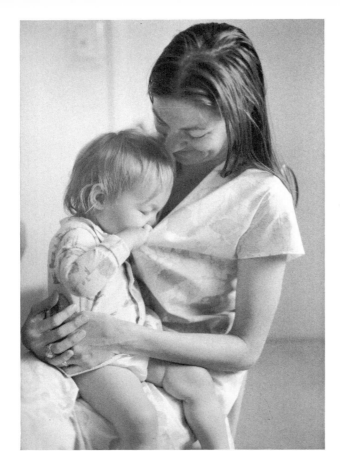

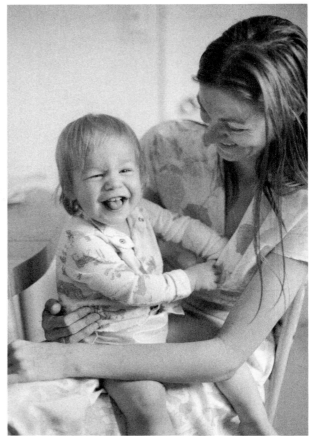

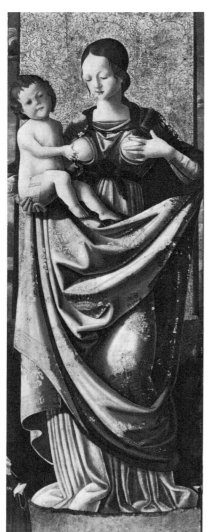

"Aren't you *embarrassed?*" Then it dawned on me why women are always slinging these bottles around with them—they're *embarrassed* to nurse!

• One day in the Paris subway my son, who was perhaps two or three, was sitting on my lap. He put his hand inside my blouse just as he had always done when he was nursing, and fondled my bosom. Of course, I let him. There was a woman sitting opposite me and her eyes nearly popped—she was scandalized. Finally, she leaned over and said, "Well, madame, your boy seems to be very *precocious!*" So I said to her, "Well, madame, you seem to forget that breasts were meant for children and not for men."

The reason she was shocked is because breasts have become sexual instead of maternal things. And on a deep level, when a man sucks a woman's breast he is both a boy and a man, so things can easily become distorted.

All over the world, women breast-feed their children in front of their fathers and uncles and grandfathers and cousins, and the whole bloody tribe! A Bedouin woman would keep her face covered out of modesty, but she would take out her breast in the middle of a bus and feed her baby because the breast is for the baby and the men don't relate to it sexually.

• Once while I was breast-feeding, a Chinese man came up to me and said, "Oh, I haven't seen anybody nurse a baby since I was in Asia!" It was really touching.

• It is one thing to breast-feed a new baby in public; it's another thing to do it with a two-year-old. When he was younger I was able to bear the social pressure, but at this stage I can't imagine letting my son nurse on me in the park—I'm too affected by what other people think. The bigger he gets, the worse the reactions I get—it has become really "dirty" to people. I think it's because most women who breast-feed do it for only three months or so.

●

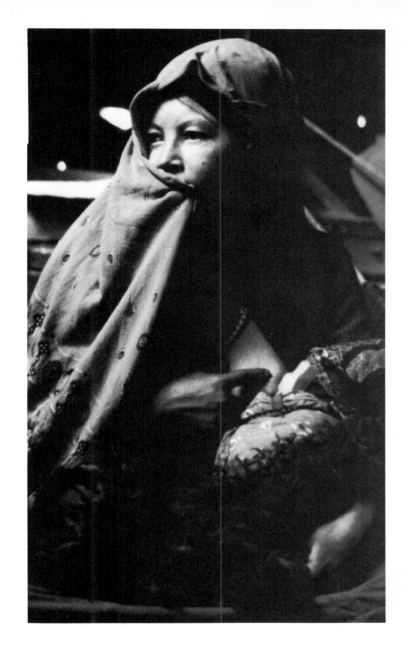

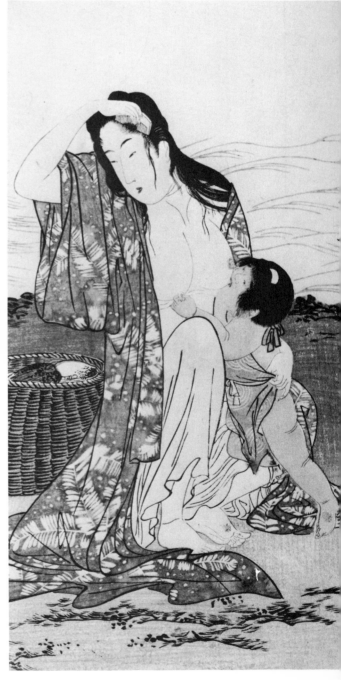

• I think breast-feeding is a personal thing—whether it's right for a woman depends on what she wants to do with her life. I've known many women who've gotten tremendous pleasure out of it, but for me it was just an annoyance. I was so sick of being debilitated for nine months that breast-feeding was really anticlimactic. I didn't like the idea of my daughter hanging on me all the time. I was ready to cut the umbilical cord as soon as she was born!

I remember having dreams about dying when I was eight or nine months pregnant. It was so clear that a part of me was dying for my baby. I was afraid that I would end up being a mother and lose myself as an artist, and that conflict came to a head right after she was born. Breast-feeding just got messed up in all those fears. It was more than I could manage—enough! I wanted to get on with my life.

See, she wasn't a peaceful baby. Some babies wake up and eat and go back to sleep. Mine had a lot of colic and cried all the time—all the time! Meanwhile, I was working in plaster, trying to get back to my sculpture, and every time she cried I had to come down from a huge ladder, wash my hands, and prepare myself. It was never-ending! I'd put her to sleep, and in half an hour she'd wake up crying hysterically. I felt completely overtaken by this being. My husband worked, so he was gone all day. It was very hard to be alone. . . . And when he was home, he wouldn't even change diapers!

*I could see that breast-feeding would be pleasurable if I were a woman of leisure, but I had to earn a living. I was teaching and going to school, and my husband wanted to go out at night. But I could barely manage to do **anything** except sleep! It was very hard. I breast-fed her for six weeks and then quit. I felt very guilty that I had weaned her, and about the way I weaned her. I just stopped cold turkey! She cried a lot and it was very painful, but I was determined that this was gonna end. That I would get back to myself and start making art again.*

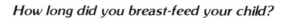

How long did you breast-feed your child?

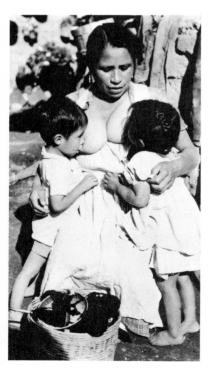

• I nursed the first two for six months, and then twenty years later, I had two more. I was forty-two when I had my last one and then I only lasted three months because my milk became a bit scanty. Interestingly enough, she was the only one of the four who was a thumb-sucker!

• I breast-fed my son for three months because I discovered with my first child that my postnatal depression set in at about three and a half months. I stopped because I became very depressed. Later I was told that if I had breast-fed longer it might have eased that depression.

• After six months I got pregnant again and I guess she sensed it because she didn't want to nurse anymore.

• In the beginning nursing was really satisfying, but after five months it got to be a nuisance lugging these things around—these milk bins—and pulling them out all the time. When I stopped, I felt as if my breasts were mine again.

• I breast-fed for a year and a half. I have known women who nursed until the next child came along to push it away. I don't think that's a bad thing. It used to be very common and still is in certain parts of the world. In some cultures breast-feeding goes on until the child is five or six. Until recently even in Europe babies were commonly breast-fed up till age two or three.

• Well, I'm not going to join La Leche League—they're wild, absolutely *wild.* I don't think my whole definition as a woman depends upon how long I nurse my baby. I certainly wouldn't nurse a kid until it was three years old like some women do. There is a terrific overemphasis on a certain type woman—"As long as I'm breast-feeding, I am the great, all-providing Earth Mother," even if the kid is ready for kindergarten. I couldn't get into that.

When my child was six months old, he was essentially out of infant dangers and was developing a tooth or two, and that's a good time to quit. When the baby bites you, you holler, and the baby thinks that's funny so he bites harder. You have to shake them loose like mad dogs.

• It's too much already. I can't stand this gnawing on me anymore. On his own, my son has no intentions of stopping. He's three years old already and I'm sick to hell of it. I *yell* at him whenever he wants the tit. I say, "Just get away! Leave me alone—it's *my* tit," and I don't even know I'm saying it. It just comes right out of my mouth. I am ready to quit. He's a big boy, a regular person. He doesn't *need* my breast anymore; he just *thinks* he does, so I let him run it out a little bit longer. But it's gotten to a stage where it's a joke. When he's bored and doesn't know what to do he says to himself, I think I'll get up and have a tit. So he gnaws me, holds onto it, and squeezes it, and meanwhile watches TV or plays with himself. This fiddle-farting around just to have something in his mouth drives me *nuts!*

• One of my students came to me teary-eyed the other day and said, "Today my son climbed up on my chest and started to nurse and we both knew it would be the last time." (Her son was eighteen months old.) He had been seeking her breast less and less frequently, so she started to give him supplementary bottles and her milk dried up. An experience they shared was ending—he was growing up. She cried and said, "I feel like somebody tied a knot in my breast." She felt that the experience they shared was unmatched anywhere in human experience, and it had ended.

• My daughter looks at my breasts as if she's never seen them before. She's curious about them and asks, "What are those?" It's really funny—these are the things that fed her for five months and she doesn't even recognize them. (*Laughs.*) Somewhere in her subconscious I'm sure she knows.

• I nursed my oldest girl till she was a year and a half and now, at four, she still remembers nursing. She's too young to express her feelings about it, but when I nursed her brother she was jealous at first. She asked me if she could nurse. I said okay and then she said, "Oh, I'm not a baby—it's not for me." If I had said no she definitely would have pursued the subject.

• Lisa and I weaned each other a month ago. Today as I lay in bed waking up, I discovered a drop or two of milk. This time two years ago I started expressing colostrum in preparation for breast-feeding. Two years in which I produced vast quantities of milk have passed, and I have become knowledgeable in one more aspect of life, an experience I can talk about endlessly.

Breast-feeding was as simple and direct as gardening—very basic, very warm, vitally here and now, as the whole experience of motherhood has been. Unfortunately, all along there was lots of pressure to quit—"She'll be too dependent" . . . "What if you get sick and are sent to the hospital or die?" . . . "Just a habit" . . . "It'll *make* you sick!" . . . etc., etc., etc. There was very little support, except from La Leche, to go on nursing until *she* was ready to stop. Fortunately, she was allergic to cow's milk and I hid behind that as an excuse when particularly nasty women pushed me.

Stopping came at the right time—we were both ready. Lisa breast-feeds her dolls and talks about "nipples" in the same delighted way as she exclaims over "tummy." I don't think there's any resentment.

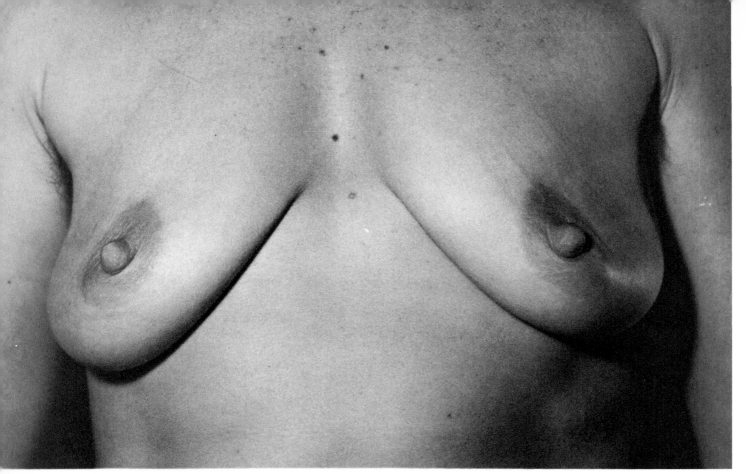

Age 36

• *I've nursed two children for almost four years, so my breasts look like two well-worn instruments. I wish they wouldn't sag like old women's breasts. I'm not proud of them anymore. All the vanity's gone. They're here and I'm glad, but they're not pleasing to me aesthetically.*

When I was younger, I had a twenty-one-inch waist and 32D breasts and I looked like an hourglass. I modeled for artists and for Playboy. *It was great to have such nice breasts—they were firm and really lovely. I wish I had a picture of* those! *When I see magazines today, I usually open them up to the centerfold and I get a little nostalgic.* (Sighs.)

How did you feel about your breasts after you stopped nursing? Did they change physically from the way they were before you became pregnant? If so, how did you feel about the changes?

• Before breast-feeding the left one was slightly smaller than the right one, but to my surprise and delight they sort of evened out.

• My breasts slope down a little more from the top than they did before. I'm not so crazy about that.

• They're bigger now—I'm thrilled about that—and I didn't get stretch marks. I swelled up from a 34B to a 42D and now I'm down to a 36C.

• I don't think there were any changes in my breasts after I no longer had milk in them.

• I can always tell by looking at a woman whether she has had a baby because once the nipple comes out it stays out, and the darker color of the aureole remains. My nipples got bigger and browner and darker and stood out all the time—they do now and always will.

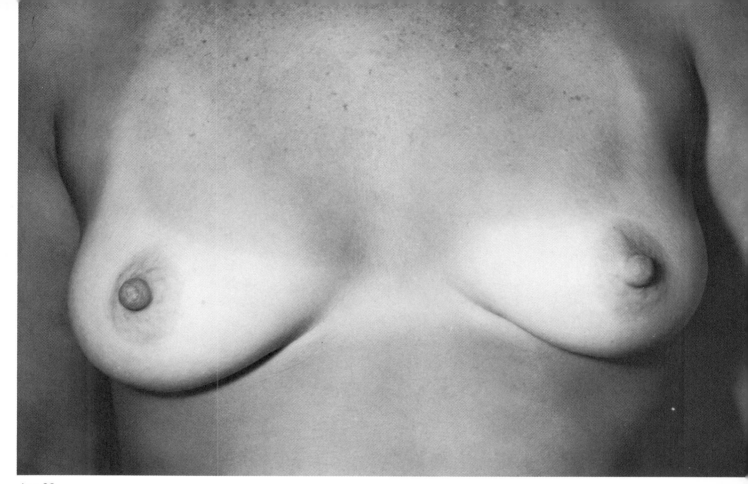

Age 30

Age 32

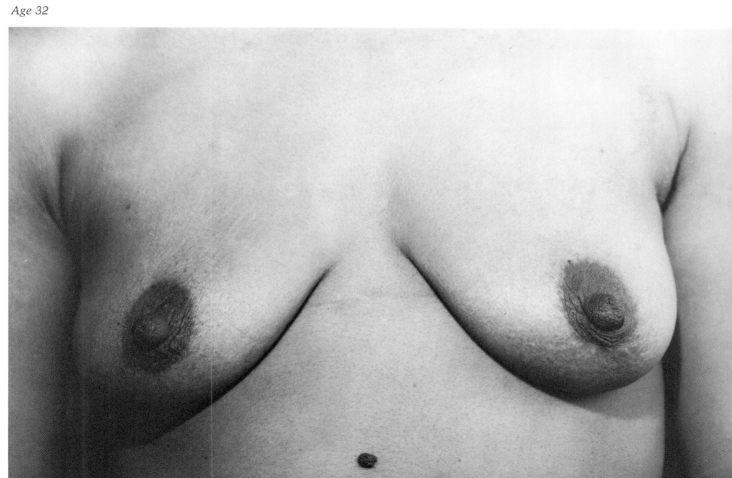

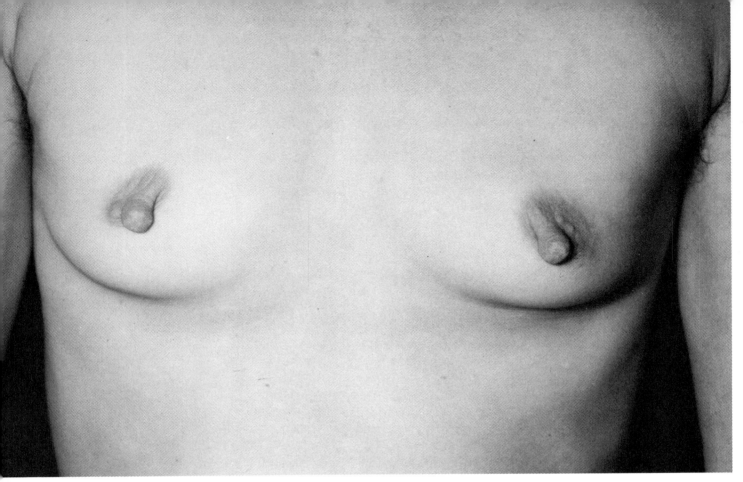

Age 32

• I didn't like the changes in my body and breasts. I had tremendous nostalgia for my old body—I thought it would *never* return. It took a year until it really changed back to the body I was comfortable with.

• Even though I'm unhappy about the way my breasts look—I mean they aren't what they were—I wouldn't trade the experience of nursing for the world. I got much more out of breast-feeding than out of having beautiful tits.

My breasts were not as firm after I weaned my child, but that didn't bother me because I always wore a good bra. My breasts got bigger and so did my bras. (*Laughs.*)

• The only change I noticed is that my breasts are not sensitive anymore before I get my period, which is a nice change.

• After I nursed the children, my breasts became much more of a turn-on sexually. That was a pleasant surprise. I thought it would be just the opposite.

• My nipples are somewhat desensitized since nursing. Before, the feeling in my breasts was a very intense part of sex. There were times when I felt close to coming just by touching them. Now I don't feel that intensity anymore. It may also be because I don't like my breasts as much since they've gotten so much bigger.

• My breasts have become much smaller and that's depressing. But I didn't get stretch marks on them—I got them all on my stomach! (*Laughs.*) Despite the "shrinkage," my breasts look pretty young for the amount of children I've breast-fed.

• I thought my breasts were really beautiful before I nursed—sort of the ideal kind to have. When I was pregnant my husband said, "Why on earth are

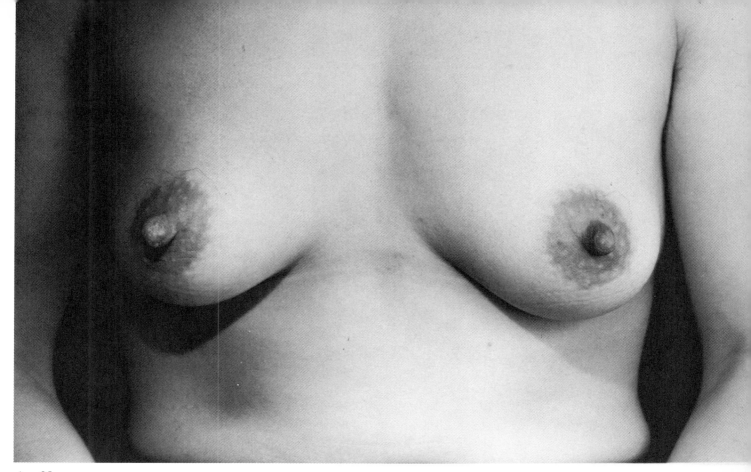

Age 35

Age 29

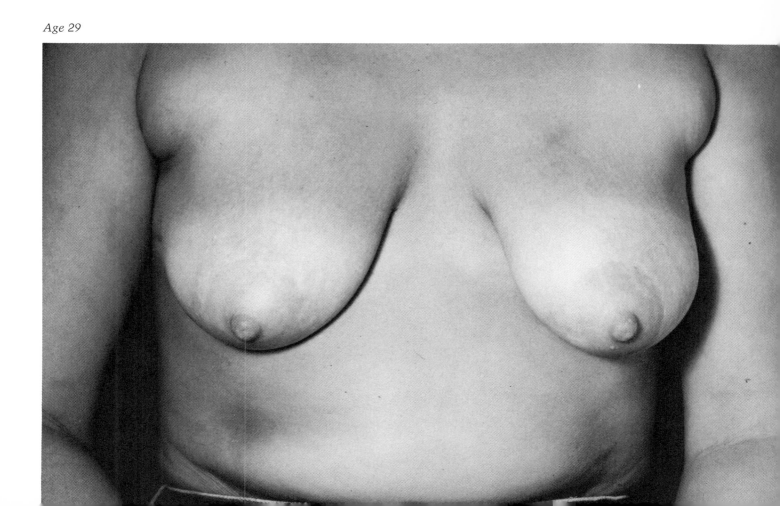

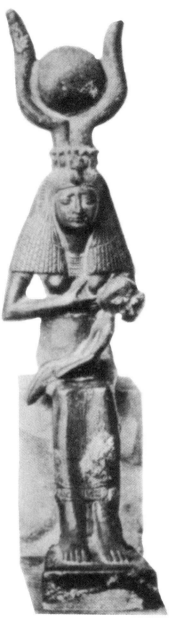

Isis suckling Horus;
ancient Egypt

you going to nurse? You're going to ruin your beautiful breasts!'' But it was too late, I had already decided. I felt that if your body makes milk, it's got to be the best thing for the baby. And he overcame his objections the first time I nursed—he thought it was the most beautiful thing he ever saw.

Yet after I stopped nursing I went through a complete identity crisis. My husband and I weren't getting along too well, and I thought, Here I am with these fat, droopy breasts. I would be embarrassed in front of another man. It bothered me so much that I started doing exercises for my breasts, which didn't help very much.

I used to be more upset about my breasts than I am now because my feelings about my body have changed, just as my feelings toward getting older have changed. When I was twenty-four I *worried* about it, but now at twenty-seven I look forward to each birthday because I realize I'm growing and expanding as a person. I feel that way about my body, too. It's been used; I've nursed two children; I've *done* things with it. Of course it's not unblemished. (I don't like the word ''blemish.'') It looks *used* because it has been and that's good. I *want* to have used my body—I don't want to stay the way I was when I was eighteen because life is a process of growth.

• I relate to my breasts differently now that I have breast-fed—I like 'em more! I am proud of myself for having nursed. I feel an almost mythological association with some female deities—the mother goddesses—for having done that for my baby. I'll feel good about it for the rest of my life. I associate my breasts with the most mushy, affectionate, protective, warm, milky, intense loving feeling that I've ever had.

• Breast-feeding was a fantastic experience! It was as if I reached another high point in my life just after the high point of the baby's birth. While I was breast-feeding I went through my Earth Mother phase and felt closely linked to the billions of women before me who had nursed their babies, fulfilling the chain of puberty to intercourse to conception to reproduction and nursing of the new life. That is a very great cycle to be part of, and I wanted to have every experience in it.

I felt a sense of honor while nursing—an accolade so to speak. It was as if nursing my child was one of the things for which I'd been born, one of the things that truly made me a woman. It was a very significant landmark in my life.

Woman nursing a baby;
prehistoric rock painting

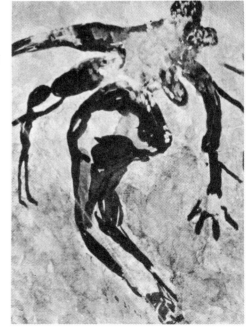

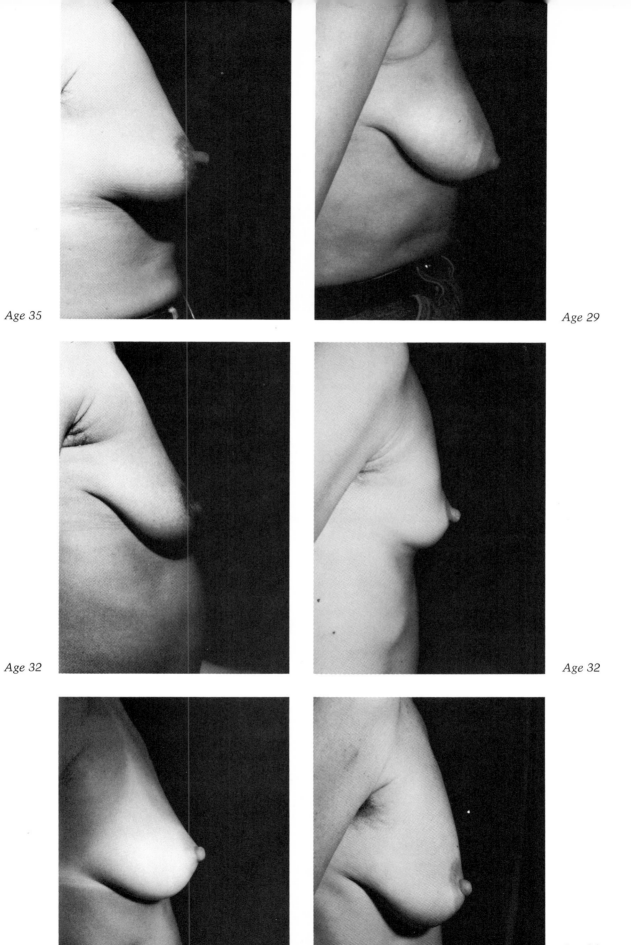

Age 35

Age 29

Age 32

Age 32

Age 30

Age 36

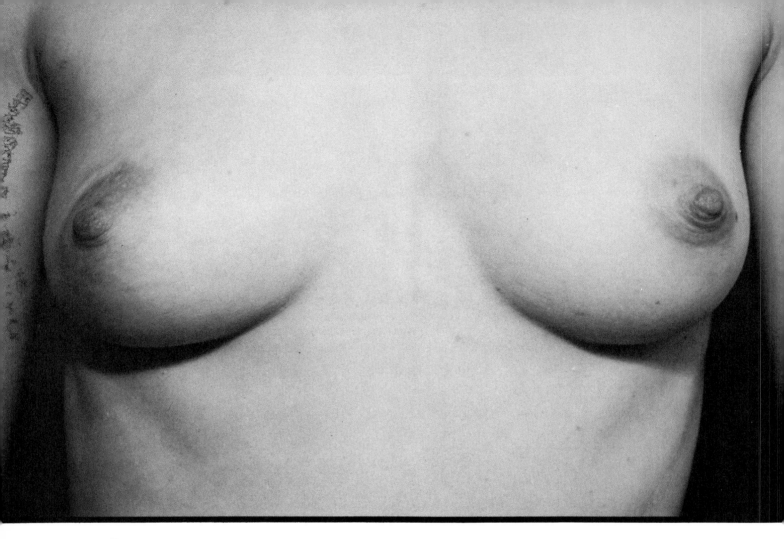

Jane   *Age 28 · Teacher · Mother of two*

If anything, my breasts have taught me about giving. I believe that we are all destined to develop our souls, and that we should learn to do so in the most natural way. It is almost as if breasts are given to us as a teacher and that by nourishing our children with them, we learn and understand how to nourish all human beings with love and sympathy and kindness.

I am a Sufi and Sufism—I don't like to call it an "ism"—encompasses all the world's religions. It is not a philosophy or a religion, but a combination of both. The beauty of Sufism is that it is based on personal experience. So my experience breast-feeding may have been very different from another woman's, yet there are bound to be very deep places where they are very much the same.

My mother had to stop breast-feeding me after a few months because she didn't have enough milk—it was right after World War II and she had gone through a lot of tension. My mother is European and experienced the war at firsthand.

The first time I came to America I was five. It was a culture shock, and as a matter of fact this is when I remember seeing baby bottles for the first time. I can't ever remember seeing them in Europe and I thought they were very strange.

My mother had bottles for my little brother and it was all so scientific and mechanical looking—like a chemist's laboratory. As a child I associated that with coming to America. I didn't understand how people lived here because it seemed very removed from life in a sense.

Many of my American friends tell me that there was a lot of physical uptightness in their families but that wasn't so in mine. We were a very huggy family because of our European background, and I can't remember any strange feeling about nudity whatsoever. There was a very natural feeling in our house.

I started developing breasts rather early—in the fourth grade. I had no awareness of sexuality to tell the honest truth. I liked my breasts and I thought that it was a very natural part of life. I didn't particularly *notice* it except that I thought they were funny because when I pushed them in, they bounced back.

When my breasts began developing I became a little bit shyer of my father. All of a sudden I was initiated into womanhood, so I had a very different kind of feeling—a natural withdrawal—and I didn't want my father to treat me like the boys anymore. I wanted him to consider the fact that my body was different now.

The development of breasts is an indicator of womanly function, whether one tunes into one's breasts as a sexual thing or not. Their actual development physiologically and psychologically indicates your womanliness and your nurturing quality. At the time of puberty I can remember growing very sensitive and inward and responsive, and wishing to nurture. It was a very delicate sensibility. The breasts developing are like an outward symbol of that nurturing instinct.

I tried to satisfy that nurturing feeling by mothering my brothers a lot because they were younger, and I also became very "caring" within my family. I was caring outside my family, too, but I didn't find much response because people were very awkward about it.

In Europe, when young girls went to school together, they'd walk arm in arm. But in America the minute you touched somebody of either sex it was considered to be something sexual. American kids had a really stiff attitude toward their bodies, but *I* was very warm and liked to touch, and that was frustrating because I couldn't share that.

My nature was really idealistic. When I was ten years old I was already wondering where my beloved was. I thought very warmly of him and wondered why I wasn't married with children. I loved climbing trees and playing with dolls, yet I distinctly remember wondering why I wasn't getting on with life.

I had a boyfriend in high school whom I really fell in love with, but I didn't understand petting. I thought it would be better if I married him so I could live with him and say, "This is it." In marriage I could have gone through the whole natural process of sexuality, rather than the petting game, which in its essence appeared unclean and unnatural to me. I thought that it would be better if people just went to bed with each other than to just do all that petting.

●

Now my breasts are a very sweet center of my body because I'm always nursing my babies. There is all this nurturing sweetness in them because they give out milk. Breasts really are an extension of your heart as a mother. They're very soft and sweet and I think that's why they're placed by the heart.

I love little birds; their undersides, so soft and sweet, are just like breasts. Babies feel like that to me, too. That sweetness is all contained right here. (*Indicates her breasts.*) When I imagine what my breasts look like internally, they are white. They give off a lot of light continuously and the light comes from my heart.

When I was pregnant, I took a very delicate and lofty piece of music that my teacher had introduced me to, and I listened to it every day. That was my meditation for my child. (It was a choir piece for Ash Wednesday—a psalm—very beautiful.) As I listened to it each day, it was my way of attuning myself to my child.

When my son was born, he just suckled a little bit and then lost interest. On the third day my cousin visited and since he is into music, I wanted to play this beautiful choir piece for him. When I put it on, my child heard the music and just started responding like crazy! Every part of his being, his arms and everything, began to move to the music. And then I knew that the concentration and attunement while I was pregnant had been *real* and that somehow it did have an incredible effect on his whole being.

Immediately he started nursing in earnest for the first time. It was amazing! As he suckled me to the music, I felt like the heavens had opened up and all the Divine Being was just poured down right through the top of my head into my breasts. Then, this complete richness of creation just flowed out of my breasts and into my baby.

It was like the paintings of Mary suckling

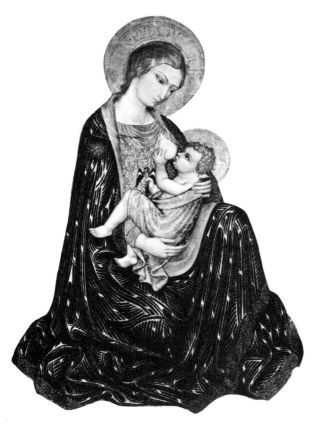

Jesus—they always have a halo above her head. She receives the Holy Spirit and gives it out through her breasts. The breast is really the extension of the heart overflowing with bounty. And that was precisely the feeling *I* had! It was just the most unbelievable experience, one of the highest experiences I ever had in my life!

I had an enormous amount of milk—an unbelievable abundance. I had so much milk that I didn't know what to do with it. I'd have to stand over the sink every once in a while to let it just pour out. It was so extreme, I could definitely have nourished two babies. I thought of my mother and her experience with me—not having enough milk and the tensions of war—and how utterly relaxed and secure I was. What a difference.

After a while the flow subsided and got into a more natural rhythm, which was good for me because such a constant outpouring is very depleting.

●

My Sufi studies helped me through the initial breast-feeding experiences because most mothers are very receptive right after they give birth. Frankly, if I'd had a lot of people around me saying, "Don't do this," I might have been influenced not to breast-feed. I doubt it, but it would have been painful for me. So I had the support of knowing the spiritual significance of breast-feeding.

Then when I actually experienced it, I understood beyond words what the real value of it was.

My baby was born to be nurtured by me in every way, and one of the most important is that he actually grows by being *nourished* by me. And so breast-feeding is an extension of the womb. When my child came out of my womb, the umbilical cord was cut. When I began breast-feeding, I can remember distinctly feeling that a second cord was formed—the pyschic cord—from my heart to the child's heart directly. It was almost physical—it was that strongly felt.

When you are pregnant, the child is nourished by you all that time, and then it gets too big so it comes out, but you shouldn't just cast it away from you when it comes out, which is what you do with a bottle. You should still hold it very close within your aura and your protection while you continue to nourish it from your body.

When a child is born, it's like a negative plate—*completely* receptive. If you feed the child formula or cow milk or whatever, you are pouring into your child all kinds of foreign impressions from just *anywhere* in the universe that the child shouldn't be receiving yet. My teacher has written:

While the infant is being nursed by its own mother the heart quality is being formed in it, and it is upon that quality that the feeling of the infant depends for its whole life. Not understanding this, people today have other methods of feeding an infant; and [it is] by these that the spiritual heritage and many merits and qualities that the child has to develop, become blunted. Mechanical food is prepared, and the child's heart becomes mechanical when it grows up. . . . Just as the flesh of different animals is affected by each particular animal's character, so with everything one eats one partakes of its spirit.

—*Hazrat Inayat Khan*

Now there is nothing more scientific than that, really, but people aren't used to hearing those things spoken of in such a manner. When people think about spirituality, they think it's some spacey, floaty kind of thing way out there in the East or someplace. They can't understand how the philosophical, the religious, and the scientific can come together. When my teacher talks about feeding your "heart quality" to your child, it's just as logical as someone saying two plus two equals four. People are going to discover this one day and they will be totally amazed.

If a woman really can't breast-feed, she shouldn't be discouraged either. The problem, when I talk about breast-feeding this way, is that if a sensitive woman who can't nurse her baby reads this, she will feel atrocious.

My brothers were both born by cesarean section and since we had come to America by then, there was a lot of pressure on my mother not to breast-feed. So she didn't and it was a pretty negative experience.

It was very hard for her, but her mothering quality was so strong that she did everything she could. When she bottle-fed, she held them close to her and cuddled them and kissed them an awful lot. She overcame not breast-feeding and my brothers are the most natural boys. My brother who is seventeen lies down and watches television with his head on my mother's lap without thinking anything of it. So real nurturing which goes beyond the physical breasts came through.

We must always maintain the broadest viewpoint so that women who can't breast-feed don't feel terrible or transmit unnecessary guilt to their child. But, if a woman can breast-feed and doesn't—it is a crime!

●

When my daughter was born the nursing experience wasn't as powerful as with my son because with him it was the *first* time and it felt like the whole opening up of the motherly function. With my daughter that function was continued, because once it opens it never really stops.

If you are still breast-feeding your previous child while pregnant with the next, doctors may tell you that the milk turns sour during pregnancy, or that it will just stop and the baby won't get any and he'll turn away. Well, it's not true—it doesn't turn sour and it also doesn't have to stop—my breasts *never* dried out. The milk flow definitely grows less during pregnancy, so the nursing child must make an adjustment.

My milk grew less and less while I was pregnant, but there was still enough to make my son happy. Everybody adjusts a little bit—I fed him more often and he nursed all the way through. The day I gave birth to my daughter the milk stopped for three hours and then the colostrum reappeared and the whole process started all over again.

When my daughter was born, I still breast-fed my son so he realized he wasn't being excluded. He was still young and I thought it would be too much of a shock to stop him abruptly. Sometimes I even nursed them at the same time—one on one breast and one on the other—and he appreciated

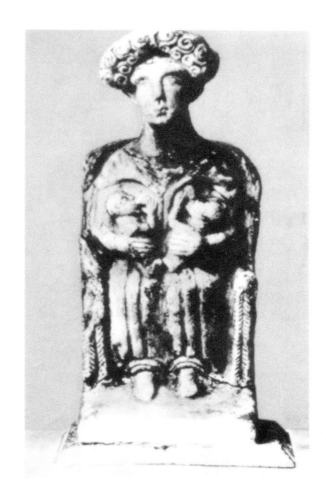

it. They loved cuddling with each other and with me, and now there is very little jealousy between them.

Nursing them together made me feel like the Goddess of Plenty for a little while. But soon after, I stopped nursing him regularly because it was a little too much for me. By a very natural process, I could feel my body going "no," almost like an animal mother.

I nursed my son for two and a half years and he is completely satisfied orally. You can see it—he barely ever sucks his fingers. I never said no to him when he wanted to nurse, so he nursed himself crazy, to complete fulfillment. When a child can walk away from you at his own desire, when he weans himself, then he is satisfied.

Nursing my daughter was a very interesting experience because I learned that there is a much different feeling whether you nurse a boy or a girl. It was almost like she understood this function very well because she was a little woman, too. She was very civil and less demanding, whereas my son was very active and liked to nurse a lot and lustily. Her whole being was different—she was more refined and her nursing had a different rhythm.

I think it is real important for the first months of a child's life to spend as much time as you can holding it without clothes on, to have that contact. Even now that my children are older, I take them in the bathtub with me from time to time, just so they can remember that I'm flesh. Because we are dressed so much of the time they just forget, or *you* forget, the warmth that comes from physical contact—like that first contact when you nursed.

It's a treat for them. They get all excited and crawl all over me, cuddle in my arms and examine me and take me apart. My daughter examines every part of my body. And my son just immediately sees the breast and "Aaaah"—that's it! I think mothers should be intimate with their children a lot because they *need* it—they need the physical magnetism more than anything else.

●

Believe it or not, many people couldn't understand why I would want to breast-feed my babies. And I don't believe in provoking people's unnatural reactions if I can help it, so whenever I nursed in public I always wore a shawl or something, which is not ideal because it limits the skin contact between you and the baby.

When I was young I read a book, which I remembered vividly when I was nursing, about a Chinese family coming to America. In the book,

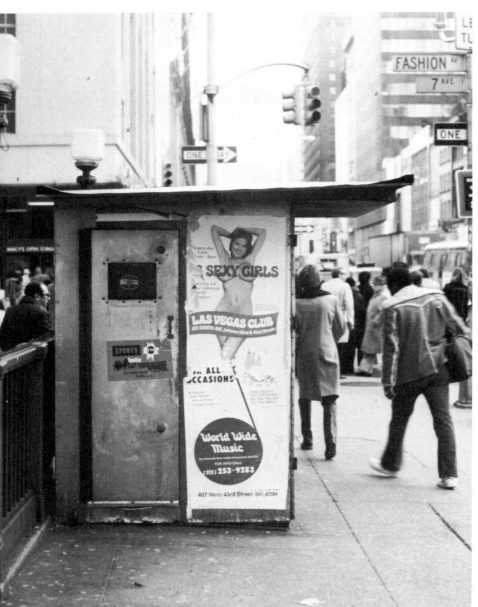

Since all the moralists and purists support Las Vegas as the entertainment capital of the world, one would assume that the attraction at The Star Dust is *The Passion Play* or a Monet exhibit or the New York City Ballet with Eugene Ormandy conducting. But, no; what *is* the big attraction?

"Tits and ass."

I beg your pardon?

"Tits and ass, that's what the attraction is." . . .

Just tits and ass? . . .

"That's it, tits and ass, and more tits and ass."

Do you mean to tell me that *Life* magazine would devote three full pages to tits and ass?

"Yes, right next to the articles by Billy Graham and Norman Vincent Peal." . . .

Soon they will have just a big nipple up on the marquee and maybe that's why you want to have FOR ADULTS ONLY because you're ashamed to tell your kids that you're selling and exploiting and making an erotic thing out of your mother's breast that gave you life.

—Lenny Bruce

the mother nursed her baby in a public place and the American people were all aghast. It horrified her. She just didn't understand their attitude at all. Then the Chinese family was riding along the street and they saw a billboard. On it was a very sexy lady displaying her breasts in a bra—that was the advertisement—and the Chinese family was in shock—*mortified!* They all blushed and didn't know *what* to think of such a thing.

Now *their* attitude was the healthy one. We don't get upset when we see women advertising lingerie and propping up their breasts, but we get upset when we see a woman nursing her baby.

I nursed my baby in a restaurant one time. Even though I was all covered in a shawl, the waitress told me, "You can't do *that* here!" I thought to myself, What? I can't feed my baby? I was totally stunned and defenseless. Well, I just left everything, got up and walked out. I couldn't *believe* it! The unnaturalness of the society struck me completely. I felt just like that Chinese family.

In my opinion, there's too much emphasis on the sexuality of breasts in our culture and there must be a balance. After all, a breast is a breast and you have to get past the point where it's always so exciting. Breasts *are* a sexual center because nursing a baby is sexual, too, but it's part of a *total* sexuality and to draw it all out of proportion is wrong and unnatural and unhealthy.

People should be able to see the body without always thinking in sexual terms, but when a society thinks of women's breasts as being exclusively sexual, then women have to hide their breasts. A mother should be able to pull out her breast anyplace to nurse her baby without anybody paying attention—she shouldn't have to think twice about it. Then the child—particularly boys, since they don't have breasts—will consider it a completely natural sight when he or she grows up.

I think a breast that has been used is really beautiful. And breasts don't have to get com-pletely dilapidated from nursing. On the contrary, nursing *helps* keep them in shape. Breast-feeding can strengthen the breast. I have a grandmother who nursed all her children and she has the most beautiful breasts I have ever seen. They're nice, firm, fine little breasts. It is also important how you carry yourself and what you eat. You don't have to fall to pieces because you breast-feed your baby—*I'm* not falling to pieces!

My teacher used to say that in some instances disease, like cancer, is a form of greed and selfishness. On a large scale it's like the pollution of our environment. On a personal scale, it's like worrying about me, myself so much that the possibility of your breasts becoming misshapen prevents you from nursing. Biologically, nursing is a deep and intense instinctual desire of the mother, and if she doesn't give in to that desire, she may experience some consequences.

Sickness is just the logical outcome of an unnatural process—something tries to flow out of us and we say no and send it back the other way. It gets all dammed up in there somewhere! And it's not just milk that gets dammed up, but also the energies of creation and growth.

Nature gives you this perfect function to use—everything is like clockwork. The baby gets born, you put your baby to the breast, your womb contracts, everything comes together, and it's all *given* to you—that's what is so amazing. There are women who have real problems with their breasts *because* they didn't use them. Breasts are the natural teachers of giving, and if you don't use them you are really depriving *yourself.*

When my baby wanted to nurse day and night, when my whole life's rhythm was turned upside down, I *had* to learn to accommodate my baby and it was hard. But this experience made me strong. Breast-feeding taught me true selflessness. It was really an endurance test on the path of the heart, a natural lesson from which to learn to extend my love even further.

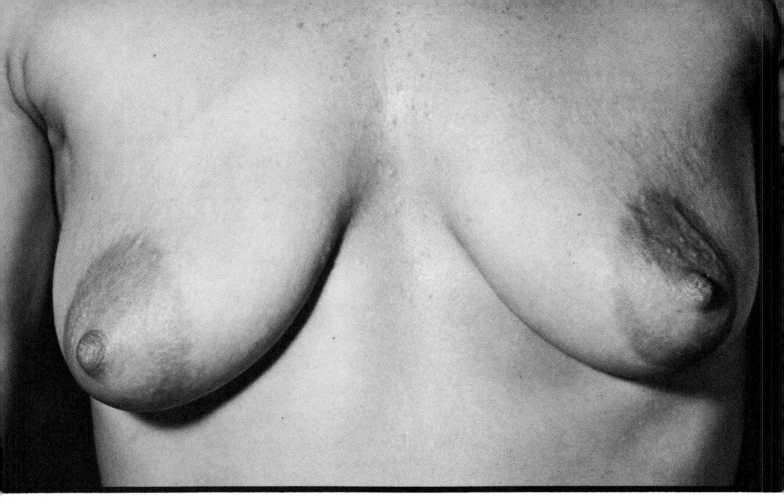

Brenda

Age 28 · Raised in the Midwest · Homemaker · Mother of one

Every Christmas when I was very young my grandmother would hold me in her lap as she sat in her rocking chair. I liked to snuggle against her breasts and stuff my face between them because they were so big and warm, like pillows. My memory is of **mammoth** *breasts. Oh, it was lovely! And you know, that saddens me with my son. He's never going to have that experience with me—big, warm breasts to snuggle up into—there's just not enough there!*

When I was in college my breasts were very nice and they provoked **lots** *of attention. The man who taught me scuba diving just loved my breasts! We've remained friends over the years and he recently called to say he was coming out to visit me. One of the things he said on the phone was, "How are your breasts?" So I said, "Well, they're not the way you remember them," and he said, "Then I don't think I want to come out and see you. I just want to remember those beautiful breasts the way they used to be." He was kidding, but he was also telling the truth. Anyway, he didn't come!*

He remembered me in a leopard skin bikini that I used to fill out completely! My breasts bulged over the top—it was gorgeous! I still have that bikini but when I put it on now, I can grab hunks of material. It upsets me remembering how it used to be. . . .

When I was little I remember visiting a friend and we were all sitting together—my girlfriend, her baby sister, and her mother. All of a sudden her mother pulled out her breast and started nursing the baby, and I jumped up and *ran* out of the room. I felt embarrassed and frightened. I remember her mother saying, "That's okay, Brenda, you can stay." But I just made furtive looks—I was *afraid* to look.

When my breasts began to grow I never touched them because I was afraid of them. They grew large very quickly, so at a very early age they drew lots of attention. That was nice, but there were drawbacks.

In class, boys would pass around notes saying things like: "There's so much milk in Brenda T. you could almost hear her moooo." There was a lot of joking and snickering and pointing, which made me very uncomfortable and self-conscious about my breasts.

I was nicknamed "B.T.," my initials. Boys would always say, "Hey, B.T.—how are you doing?" Later on I realized that what they really meant was "Big Tits," and that was *awful!* I really stood out! (*Laughs.*) Not only was I big, but I was one of the first to develop and I was miserable during that time.

Once when I was eleven or twelve, I was in a shoe store and the salesman pulled me in the back. There was a kind of rape scene and he was feeling me all over, particularly my breasts. I screamed and ran out and my mother went back and told the manager. The guy was fired—it was a bad scene. My breasts have gotten me into a lot of trouble.

There was a time in high school when army-navy turtlenecks were very popular. I wore them like everybody else, but there was an incredible commotion over that. I was a cheerleader and it was considered unacceptable for me to wear such a tight sweater by some of the flatter cheerleaders. The head of the cheerleaders got together—I can't believe this! (*laughs*)—with the Student Council president! I don't know how *he* got involved, but they actually had a *meeting* about my breasts. It was insane.

One of the girls was loudly complaining about me and she had on the same turtleneck, but she was flat. They asked me not to wear tight clothes to school anymore because they felt it reflected poorly on the school. The entire thing was a terrible embarrassment.

I think my sister, who was four years older and not as developed as I was, was jealous of me. I remember overhearing some discussions in which she told my mother about an article in one of the ladies magazines about some girl who had *eleven pounds* of her breasts taken off! After that my mom made remarks to me, saying that if my breasts got any bigger I would have to have one of those operations. She scared the shit out of me!

From the very first I realized that my breasts were something that the opposite sex was attracted to—a sort of sexual object. I got the notion that they were important since I was always noticed *because* of them.

I started wearing bikinis at a very early age, and the head of the swimming club always wanted to take me for rides in his boat. I was a twelve-year-old punk and he was an older married man. He always said things like, "You really have *beautiful* breasts!"

As I got older I wore tight clothes and low-cut things. I was very sexy and I was into it but it was also a problem. For example, one night I came in late—I'd gotten lost—and my father called me a tramp and accused me of pushing my breasts around. In his better moods, he used to say I was a little Liz Taylor.

My breasts made me very popular and I was always asked out on dates. But all the guys wanted to do was *feel* me! I got so ticked off because everybody went after *that* instead of wanting to be with *me*, and in some way that still hangs over me now. . . .

My husband just grabs my breasts *all the time* and he pisses the hell out of me! I really get angry about that. I'll be doing the dishes and he'll come up behind me and grab my breasts when I'm not interested in sex at all. It just ticks me off and I tell him to stop. Then he says, "Well, they feel so good, I want to feel them," and I'll say, "Yeah, but if you're trying to be loving, it doesn't feel good to *me*." I'll say to him, "Stroke my back, touch my head, do *anything*, but leave *them* alone!"

It is very aggressive on his part, because after eight years of marriage he ought to know better. I mean, that's pretty *dumb!* Basically, I guess he just doesn't give a shit. Meanwhile, I can't stand it—particularly now that I'm more self-conscious about my breasts than ever. It makes me so angry!

If I was single—which may be sooner than I think (*laughs*)—it would be a sensitive area with any guy who wanted to get to know me. If he was too fixated on my breasts I'd immediately get turned off. He would just have to blend in with all of me and not make a particular fuss about that part of my body.

●

When I was pregnant my breasts got *gigantic* and I used to *hate* having them hang on my stomach. They were so *big!* I didn't breast-feed because I didn't want to look at them that much. I didn't want to be reminded of them that many times a day. So after I gave birth, I had a shot to make my breasts go down.

When my mother came into the hospital she gave me a big, long lecture about how *awful* it was that I wasn't breast-feeding, and didn't I know the terrible things it would do to my son? Wasn't I ashamed of myself? Meanwhile, my husband's mother was quietly sitting right there and she suddenly piped up and said, "*I* didn't breast-feed Bernie [my husband] and *he* turned out okay!"

So I didn't breast-feed my son—I didn't want to. Now I don't feel good about that at all. The whole subject of breasts is sensitive when it involves my son. He's seven now and awhile ago he asked me what breasts are, and I showed him a picture. I don't feel very comfortable around him. He does see me sometimes but I tend to cover up.

●

I think my breasts have always been a real point of identity for me. In the past they had a lot to do with the type of person I was. Now I feel very uncomfortable about my breasts because there was a traumatic change when I had my son—they just went kerplunk. They used to be much fuller and now they sag and they've got stretch marks. Now that I'm on birth control pills, they are even *smaller!* They're kind of flat—almost like someone took the air out of them! My breasts are the saggiest, most untaut part of my body. Basically I hate the way they look and sometimes I have the feeling that my body would be attractive if it weren't for my breasts.

There was a period when I was a real fanatic about not wearing a bra, but then last year I became really bothered by the fact that my breasts were sagging so much. I thought it was ugly, so I started wearing a bra and I've gotten used to it again.

I always had a lot of gas from my mother when I went braless. She got sick of looking at me and she'd say, "Ugh! Ucch! You look *awful!*" and she'd make horrible faces. And she used to give me a hard time about my breasts sagging—"They're so *ugly!*" she'd say. "They just hang so badly."

It was the *damned breasts* again! She didn't talk about the rest of my body, which is in great condition, she talked about something I couldn't do anything about. I don't think there's any way you can correct sagging breasts. If the tissue is stretched, it's stretched! Even with the bras that I wear now, a friend said to me one day, "Look at you, Jesus! Your breasts really *hang!* Go get yourself a good support bra—you'd look *much better.*"

I don't think my breasts are ever going to be a point of pride at the rate they're going. I imagine they will become more pendulous, and I'll have to come to terms with that. My breasts are aging faster than the rest of my body. They've let me down! (*Laughs.*) I know there's nothing I can do about them—like I can't change the length of my fingers—but they could have hung in there a little bit longer!

●

My breasts are a constant reminder of aging . . . of impermanence . . . of nonacceptance of myself. In that way they're a universal symbol. I look at my sagging breasts and I think to myself that they're so terrible I can't possibly accept them, and then I remember that everybody else in the world does not accept something about themselves. I still get *lots* of compliments about my looks, but when I hear them I think that little do they know how ugly I *really* am. There are war victims who have been *disfigured,* and the aging of my breasts is very mild in comparison, and yet here I bitch. In fact, there are times when I've even *cried* about them!

I used to believe that my breasts would *always* be beautiful, and that I could rely on them. But they taught me that you can't ever expect things to stay as they are. I couldn't expect to be a kind of Playboy bunny forever. So every time I see myself in the mirror it is a lesson—a reminder that I can't hold onto any part of my body or any relationship or *anything* for that matter.

Intellectually I know that any peace of mind or sanity does not come from clinging and craving . . . like craving better breasts. I want to be prepared for *anything* that could happen, even a mastectomy. So I've got to accept myself *totally* the way I *am*—not just my breasts, but my whole being. My breasts probably are more symbolic of *that* than anything else about me because they are the most difficult part of me to accept.

You know, if I had speculated ten years ago (*laughs*) . . . well, there was *no way* I could have imagined that my breasts would ever be the way they are now . . . or that I would ever feel the way I do.

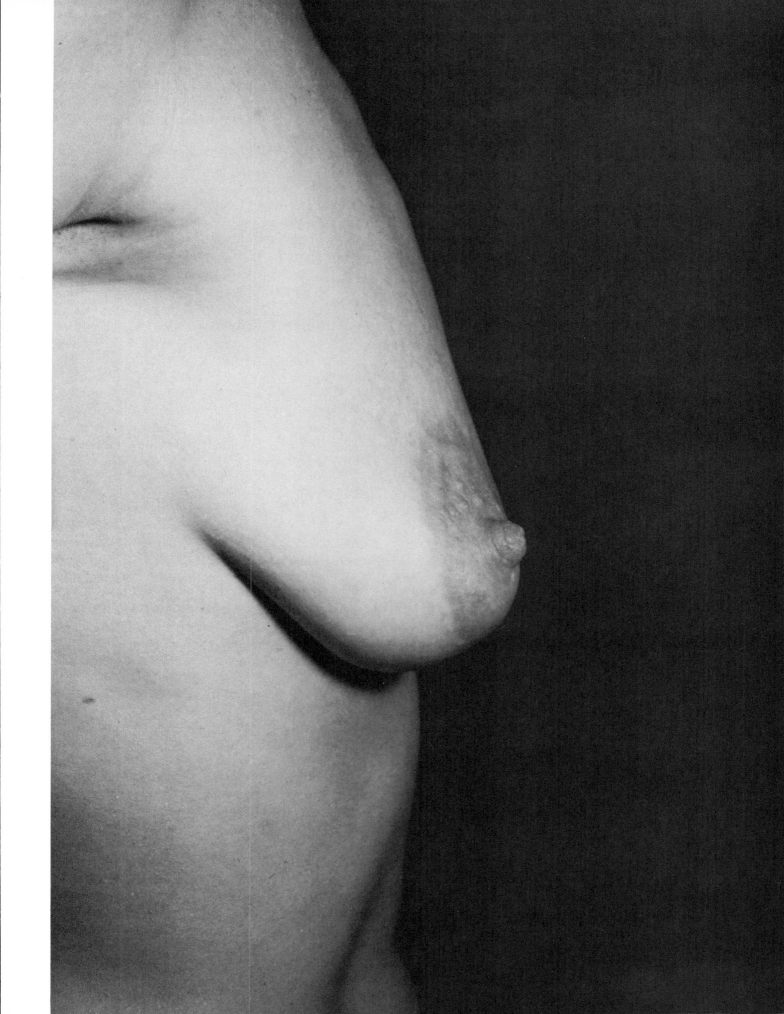

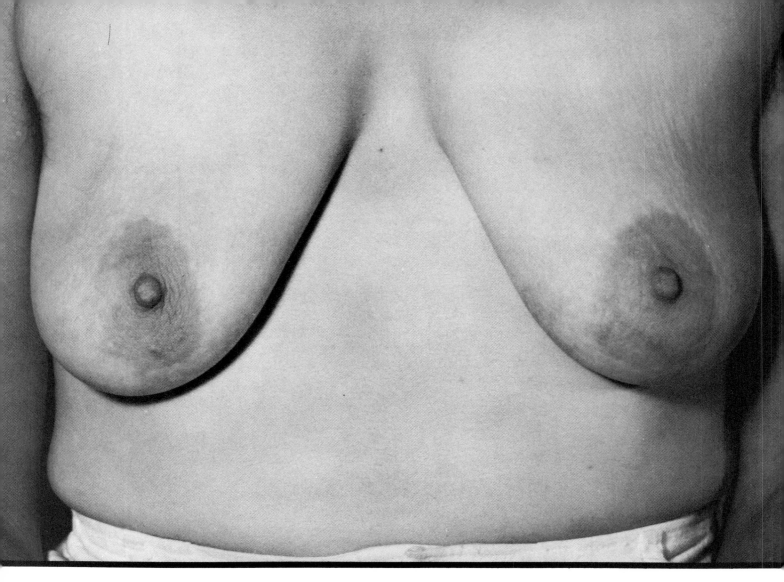

Maria
Age 32 · Raised in New Mexico · Chicano · Nurse · Mother of one

I like my breasts now. They're pretty funky! They've been through a lot. After I no longer had milk in my breasts, I realized that they had changed incredibly. The skin really stretched out and there was less fat tissue, so they were a whole lot baggier. But it didn't bother me because I don't remember how they were before very well—I mean it was such a repressed thing.

During pregnancy I felt really good about my breasts and their size for the first time in my life! And for the first time they were sexually sensitive. My feelings about my breasts were completely transformed after I breast-fed.

When I say that I think of my breasts as functional now, it's not as unemotional as it sounds. Breast-feeding was an affirmation, as much as motherhood was, of my being, my sexuality, and my feminine energy. For the first time in my life, I appreciated these breasts—these functioning breasts. Now breasts make me think of bearing fruit . . . milk.

My parents came from a rural, Spanish-Catholic, super-uptight-about-sex culture, so *breasts* or anything to do with the body were a really sensitive subject. My mother didn't breast-feed me and that's kind of funny because in the culture we came from, it was very common to breast-feed. But my parents wanted to be upwardly mobile and they were trying to identify with the Anglo values, so they rejected their minority culture—breast-feeding was a lower-class thing to do. Proper ladies *denied* their breasts!

The fact that I wasn't breast-fed reflects the whole repressed attitude about sensuality and sexuality that was my total environment. I just now remembered one time when I was really young—barely three....I was sitting in my mother's lap in some waiting room and I put my hand on her breasts. Well! She really gave me *hell* for doing that in public. In fact she pushed my hand *away* and told me *never* to do that again! (*Pauses.*)

I guess *that* was the first awareness I ever had about breasts. God, I'd completely forgotten about that. It's amazing delving back in time like this....So I guess I was taught about breasts by being pushed away. I pretty much ignored her breasts after that—I was forced to.

When I was about four one of my friends had a really *zaftig* mother who had big breasts and I really liked this woman. I have a vivid memory of her leaning over at my friend's party to light the birthday candles. I remember seeing her cleavage and being *turned on* yet totally *frightened* about looking. I *knew* I wasn't supposed to so I felt real guilty. There was something very exciting about it and I became incredibly curious about women's breasts. Once or twice I tried to get a peek! (*Laughs.*) But I didn't get much opportunity to see them.

I'll never have to teach *my* son anything about breasts because exposing my body has never been a private thing. He's seen me and a lot of other women continually so he's gotten that kind of education. Even though he's six, he still remembers being at my breast. You know, sometimes he wants to touch my breasts and look at them closely...and I let him. Why not?

I hit puberty really young—I was around eight when I started to develop. It was horrible because I didn't know what was happening. I was afraid of the pain and thought that something was really wrong and that I was going to *die!* I was afraid to tell my mother. It was a great *relief* when another friend confided that her breasts were hurting, too.

At a certain point, I remember a lot of competition about who was developing and who wasn't, almost like a race. I *won* the race, but it never felt like a victory to me 'cause instead of a nice, gradual adolescent blooming, it was *ploop!* There I was with a *"mature figure"* way before I could handle it! I won the race and got the "booby" prize but I felt like a freak.

By around eleven I was completely physically mature. I was ready to breed. It ran in the family, you know. One of my grandmothers had twenty-two kids and she started at age fourteen. Later when I was in nursing school, I read that there were ethnic differences—Mediterranean and Indian peoples tended to reach puberty earlier than Scandinavian and Northern Europeans. If I had gone to school with children of my heritage, puberty probably would have been a lot easier to deal with. But I was sent to a school where there were mostly late-blooming Anglo girls.

My mother wouldn't *recognize* that I had breasts. In retrospect, it really messed me up. When she finally got me a bra, it was a C cup! Getting a bra was a relief because it was good to have that floppiness under control, but even so, it felt uncomfortable—like a horse being saddled.

I always wished my breasts were smaller and I'm sure that had to do with our whole denial of sexuality. I would rather not have had breasts at all!

Sexuality was totally denied at convent school. We wore really frumpy uniforms. I developed a certain posture with my forearms. It was an unconscious fig leaf position which I *still* do when I'm feeling insecure—a certain closing over with my arms, kind of caving in my chest and hiding the breasts. I used to wear baggy sweat shirts and *layers* of clothing to hide my breasts as much as possible. I felt awful about girls or *anybody* looking at me.

Having breasts made me feel so out of control ...as if I was falling *apart*...sort of falling *out* into the world...I thought I couldn't handle it. I did everything possible to prevent drawing attention to my breasts and *denied* it if it happened.

I was once accosted at my job in a public library when I was about fourteen. My boss cornered me in a back room and ripped off my blouse. It was a Saturday and we were doing inventory so the library was closed. He was really *pawing* my breasts and holding me and kissing me and stuff. It was very breast centered—you know, like he didn't rape me or anything. But I just wanted to *kill* him!

I remember hitting him—it was an incredible

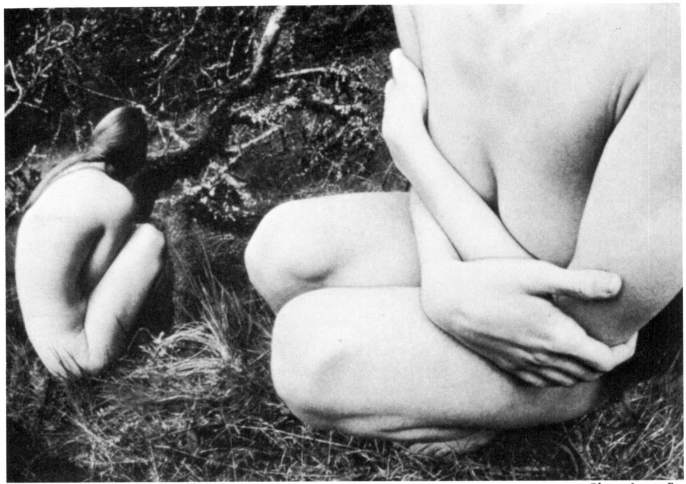

Photo: James Fee

physical struggle and I finally got away. I went running home with my torn blouse still on one arm, falling off my shoulder.

I felt *guilty* and was afraid to tell my parents because they would think that in some way I had provoked the situation. But I was in such a state that they knew something was wrong. So I finally told them what happened, and I remember it took me a long time to get it out. This subject was all very taboo (particularly with my father) and I didn't know what the ground rules were. Luckily, they took the attitude that "a bad person accosted our daughter," and he was fired.

When I think of it now, that experience must have had a lot to do with reinforcing my repressive feelings about my breasts and my sexuality.

I didn't date in high school. It was an all-girls school, so I didn't have any contact with boys at all. I didn't go through any kind of social or sexual interactions during adolescence. Finally in my freshman year of college I went from never been kissed to screwing in a couple of months.

I had many ambivalent feelings, not only about my breasts, but also about being sexual at all. The first time my breasts were touched, even with clothes on, I was *overwhelmed* with guilt! After, I almost wondered if my roommate could tell. (*Laughs.*) Sure I got pleasure from it, but it was like forbidden fruit.

As long as my strict Catholic background held up for me, its whole moral structure of sin and guilt held up, too, and made me a *wreck*. When I finally threw that away, in a very short space of time everything, and I mean *everything,* changed! When I was eighteen or nineteen, I once ate a hamburger on Friday just 'cause we weren't *allowed* to eat meat on Friday, and then I *puked!* In my mind I wanted to challenge it all, but my guts were still really tied up with it for years. I wonder . . . does one ever really untie oneself from that kind of upbringing?

Even when I began having sex I always denied my breasts. I tolerated being touched because men liked it, but I was doing 'em a favor. You know, you do that or they'll split, right? That's

194

what's expected. I often feigned being turned on by my breasts in order not to disappoint my partners. I feel shitty about it now and I don't do it anymore.

Now when I'm in bed with somebody, if my entire body is aroused as part of a lovemaking sequence, then my breasts become aroused, too. But I have to be turned on *before* my breasts are touched; otherwise it doesn't work. If somebody tries to turn me on by touching my breasts then I just turn off. It just doesn't work for me and I'm sure that's also a result of my repressed upbringing.

●

I breast-fed my kid for two years until he just self-weaned.

Before I breast-fed, I wished my breasts weren't there, and now I have a very functional attitude about them, by and large. Breast-feeding undercut a lot of my uptightness about my breasts, and that was a lot for me to overcome.

Since I breast-fed, my breasts seem smaller, or at least they don't have much fullness anymore. They're half the size of what they were and they've sort of baggied out. (*Laughs.*) My general image of my breasts now is that they're not sexy, but I don't think I ever felt that they were. And I certainly don't think that they're particularly beautiful. Fuller breasts are more beautiful. That image, you know, of fullness . . . fatty tissue! (*Laughs.*)

I stopped living with my ex-husband about four years ago. The first woman he was with after we separated was a good bit younger than I was. Then we went to bed together in a reconciliation attempt. Well, he commented—which was sort of a way of getting back at me—that I was *old*, that my breasts weren't firm anymore. I wanted to kick him in the balls! (*Laughs.*) Before the separation he related to my breasts really positively, so I'm sure that this wasn't an expression of his real feelings about them. That was just a powerful way to get to me, knowing that it was my most vulnerable area. . . .

Actually, I feel better and better and better

about aging. It's funny—I don't think of my breasts as aging anymore after the breast-feeding experience. Breast-feeding had an aging effect on my breasts and then they stabilized. My breasts were the *first* thing to develop and the *first* thing to go. They've always seemed like separate and autonomous things that had nothing to do with the rest of me, as if they had their own life separate from the rest of my body.

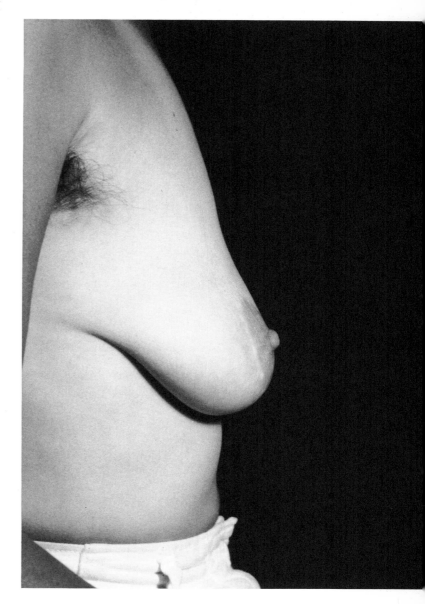

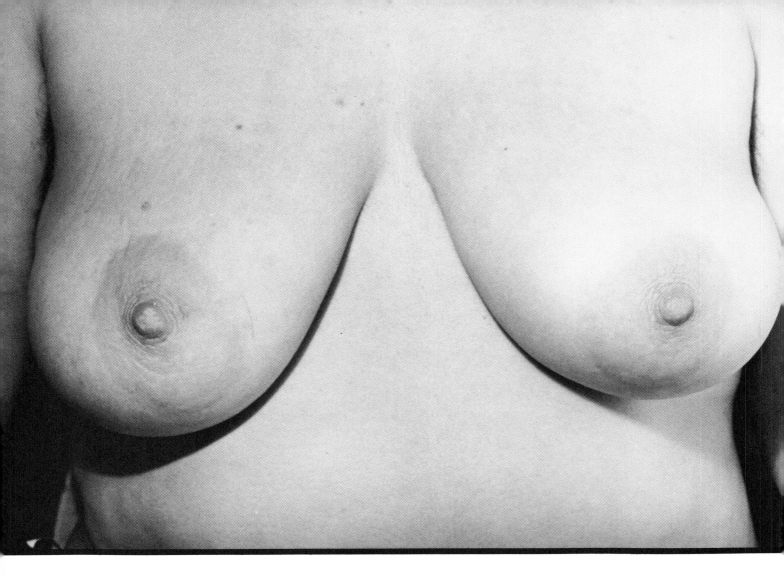

Sharon

Age 29 · Raised in Arkansas · Broadcasting

It's funny, when you asked me to do this interview, I thought about the fact that I really never gave that much thought to my breasts until fairly recently. And realized that for most of my life I have had a tendency to repress thinking about any sensual parts of my body. I didn't think about breasts negatively—they were just not in my con-sciousness! That's *a very strange thing.*

My breasts are not as important in my sex life as they're "supposed" to be, and I have always wondered if that means something is wrong with me. I like to have my breasts cuddled, but I have never found that sexually arousing.

Sex has always been problematic for me. I don't get aroused very easily. I guess I'm just not a very sexual person. A long time ago, I read an article which said that breast-fed babies grow up to be healthier people. I was not breast-fed and I wonder if my whole relationship to sex would have turned out differently if I had been!

I have never felt incredible erotic sensitivity in my breasts, and as a

*matter of fact, I have some ambivalence about having my breasts
sucked. I don't know if it has anything to do with my not having been
breast-fed, or whether that is just the way I am. I have no idea.*

*But I am more comfortable about the appearance of my breasts than
about other parts of my body. Often, when I stand naked in front of
the mirror, I cup my breasts in my hands and just cuddle them a little
bit. I guess on some level my breasts reassure me about something in
myself.*

*There was a long period in my life when I was very unsure of my
own sensuality, sexuality, and everything like that. I couldn't even
put myself in gender! So my breasts kind of told me, "You're a woman,
and a neat woman at that!" That was very reassuring.*

I'm really sad that I wasn't breast-fed. I *really*
wish I had been. I remember one incident very
strongly. At some point early in my adolescence,
I crept into my mother's bed one morning, desperately wanting to suckle her breasts! I must have
felt that it was something I missed. Well, she was
horrified!

I was *struck* with a vivid desire to crawl into
bed with her and suck on her breasts, and I was
aware of her strong conflicting feeling that I was
too old for that. Then I was confused and guilty,
feeling that I had done something shameful. Perhaps she thought my motives were somewhat
sexual and maybe in a way they were! (*Laughs.*)

My mother bought me a bra long before I ever
needed it. I also remember her fitting me for
Kotex before I got my period. She was always very
involved in showing me what was going to happen so I would be prepared. And she always told
me that it was all going to be wonderful and natural and lovely. You know, all this "what it
means to be a woman" bullshit—"all these wonderful things are happening to your body and isn't
it lovely to grow up to be a woman?" Of course,
when you get out into society, you realize that
not everybody reacts the way my mother did and
this *progressive propaganda* has no relation to the
real world.

When I was eleven I once slept over at my best
girlfriend's house. In the morning her brother,
who was about fourteen, came into the room
where I was sleeping and got into my bed. When
I was a kid, everybody was always getting into
bed with everybody else and it was the most normal thing. I had baths with other kids and my
parents were very open about nudity and stuff
like that, so at first my reaction to him was completely normal. But then it suddenly became apparent that he had something else in mind.

The first thing he did was grab my breast and
suck on it! I was *appalled!* I realized his intentions were totally prurient. It certainly wasn't,
"Hey, isn't this beautiful?" like my mother had
said becoming a woman would be. He was really
skidding very heavily into his own sexual fantasies and here was an opportunity for him to play
with breasts, right?

Well, I reacted very negatively to put it mildly.
I freaked out and got *hysterical!* That was the first
time someone ever touched my breasts and it was
awful, and it was a long time before I let it happen
again.

Throughout high school I didn't really have any
relationships and I didn't date much. Around that
time I began slouching a lot and my parents always yelled at me to stand up straight . . . and you
know, it just occurred to me that that probably
had a lot to do with my having breasts.

Of course I wasn't really conscious that I was
slouching then, or why, but now it's clear to me
that I did my best to hide *anything* that would
make me sexually attractive to others because
that was just too threatening.

As a result, I consciously made myself unat-
tractive for large portions of my life. I wasn't
aware of how much I was doing that—slouching
and letting my hair fall over my chest so that no
one would see my breasts—until years later in
my consciousness-raising group when it was
pointed out to me.

●

When I was growing up, I used to look at pictures of African tribal women with long, hanging
breasts, and I recall being *amazed* by that. I was
also aware that my mother was somewhat embarrassed about *her* very long and saggy breasts—she
always blamed them on the bad bras she wore in

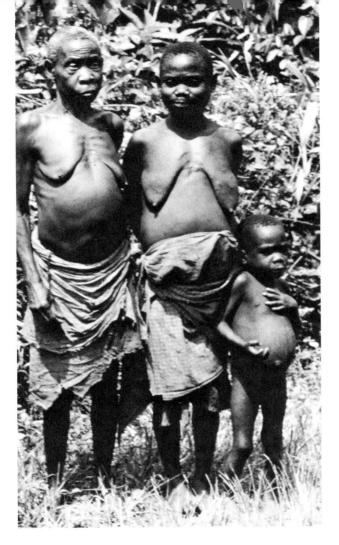

tracted to are those that fit the conventional standards of beauty and I have never *really* been able to wean myself from that. So I'm always amazed that people ever want to be with *me* because I obviously don't represent those standards at all. (*Laughs.*)

A few years ago I went through a stage where I felt a tremendous amount of confusion about my sexual orientation and I didn't know what to do about it. I was having a lot of trouble with men and I didn't know whether I was gay, but I didn't have fantasies about women either. I just couldn't figure out *what* I was. Finally I decided that the only way I could come to some understanding of myself was to make love with a woman. But I wasn't really attracted to anyone except a woman I worked with who was a lesbian. So I just made a proposition to her and she accepted.

She was the most *gorgeous* woman, even by conventional standards. She had a gorgeous figure and long dark hair—even longer than mine—and she was just beautiful. When I made love to her I remember having the feeling—and it was kind of freaky—that I was making love to the *me* that I wanted to be! She had the figure that I wanted to have, and her breasts were firm and pretty ideal in the conventional sense. It was so strange because the whole time I felt as if I was making love to an idealized version of myself.

When I was still totally confused about my sexuality, I went out West to visit a dear friend of mine. As it turned out, she and her man wanted to share themselves sexually with me. They thought this was the most natural, beautiful thing in the world and I, never having experienced that, was really shocked. She was a woman of forty who was not attractive at all, and he was about thirty and gorgeous, one of the most beautiful men I have ever seen! I was amazed at her strength in having a younger woman who, however attractive or not, was still more attractive than she was share the bed with her gorgeous lover and not feel at all threatened.

When she took her clothes off I was also amazed to see that one of her breasts was very tiny and the other very full. And I thought that here was a woman who was a little freakish by all the standards, and still she had no problems with her own nudity and sexuality. I couldn't believe it! But it was very hard for me to find her sexually attractive. I had been so steeped in traditional attitudes about what was or was not attractive that the different sizes of her breasts really *bothered* me.

The next morning she said to me, "You know,

her youth. So when I saw pictures of those African women, it provoked a whole bunch of ambivalent feelings. On one hand, the pictures were obviously beautiful even though the breasts were kind of long and saggy. On the other hand, in our culture it was considered ugly. And even though I never made the connection at the time (I wasn't a Stone Age primitivist the way I am now!) there was something about those photos that really affected me.

My breasts were just beginning to appear then, so I still didn't know what they were going to become. They could have turned out like my mother's. I had no idea whether I was going to be blessed or cursed, in the traditional sense, so there's a subtle and generalized anxiety about your breasts when they're developing. On one level I felt that the bodies shown in those pictures of African women were all right, that it didn't matter *how* your breasts turned out, but I wasn't yet decultured enough to *really* accept that. Now I think that those women are a strong symbol that the natural body is beautiful in all different states.

But the culture did a good job on me—I'm still not entirely deculturated in terms of my aesthetic values. The men and women that I'm most at-

Sharon, when you finally become really mature, you won't feel that this so-called 'attractiveness' is what *really* attracts you sexually to another person." She had obviously picked up on my feelings 'cause I hadn't said anything. I was devastated by that observation.

I visited her again last summer, but this time my reactions to her—to her breasts and to everything—had undergone a change. I spent a week there this time and got very close to her, and suddenly I was able to actually see her breasts as rather lovely, rather unique, rather neat. This woman has had a great effect on my life!

There have only been two women whom I've ever made love to, and in both cases I was very happy that they had breasts. I enjoyed fondling and kissing their breasts, particularly the first time. The one "problem" in making love with men is the fact that they don't have breasts! (*Laughs.*) I mean breasts are a very nice thing to have on the side.

What is it about the breast that you like so much?

I'll show you. This beautiful sand dollar really looks like a breast to me and it has everything wonderful that a breast has. Of course, it's not as soft as a breast, but there's something in the shape. It's got a certain kind of soft, undulating flow, like hills and valleys, not straight and narrow and pointed like buildings. It's like the country and the land—it's nature. And there's something about the shape of the breast that's found everywhere in nature.

●

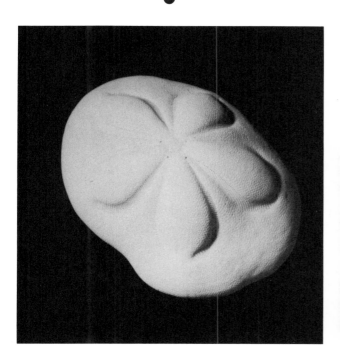

In the past month I've had several dreams in which I was breast-feeding a baby. In one, my milk was drying up and that was scary. In the other, it was an ecstatic experience of me suckling a baby and there was *lots* of milk this time. In fact, I had the dream again last night, which is very interesting since I knew I was going to be interviewed about my breasts today.

I've also recently been visiting a woman who was suckling her baby a lot, so I saw breast-feeding happening in a way that I had never seen before. I was amazed at what a beautiful experience it was for the mother. As we talked she'd just lie down and open her blouse. And the minute the breast came near the baby, all the baby's attention turned to it . . . as if the goddess had arrived! It was the most wonderful thing for the little baby —pure ecstasy—and I was really envious of that baby's experience. Suddenly my feeling is that breast-feeding is something I'd like to experience, but I don't know if I want to have kids, which is a big problem. (*Laughs.*)

●

My present lover really loves my breasts and it makes me feel so good. He constantly says, "Oh, you have such wonderful breasts!" When he heard about this interview his reaction was, "You've got such wonderful breasts—of course they'd interview you for them!" And then he said, "Are you going to answer the door with your breasts showing?" . . . as if it was the most natural and normal thing in the world to do.

I must confess he thought it was a little funny to do a book on breasts, but he said, "If anybody's breasts should be included, *yours* should be!" So I get a lot of positive reinforcement these days about my breasts and it makes me feel really good inside.

Acorns

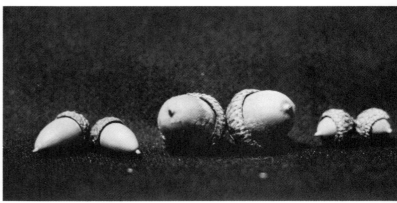

Audrey
Age 33 · Raised in Brooklyn, N.Y. · Homemaker · Mother of two

I want to know what it's like to have nice-looking breasts. Is it really going to be as great as I think it is? Is it thrilling to be able to go braless? I think it must be because I can't. If you've never had my problem, you might take it for granted.

I have a girlfriend who says she learned through her religion that the only thing breasts are for is nursing babies. Then there are some girls who think breasts are there to please their husband or boyfriend. But after the experiences that I've gone through, as far as I'm concerned breasts are good for nothing!!!

When I was six months old a pediatrician told my mother that there was milk in my breasts. He said that it might be a gland problem, but that nothing could be done about it until I was at least six or seven. A few years later I was diagnosed as having an endocrine gland problem. My sex glands were overactive and developed very early. So at seven years old I had my period, and while everyone else was wearing undershirts with bows on them, I was wearing a brassiere!

For two years, from age seven till nine, I was treated for this glandular condition, which involved weekly visits to the hospital for shots and tests. It was a *horrible* experience! I was a medical curiosity, so to speak. For several weeks in succession, I was displayed in front of, oh, anywhere between thirty and fifty doctors. I remember standing there naked and the doctors would say, ". . . and from this angle and that angle." I was embarrassed to *death!* It was terrible! They sat there writing, not paying any attention to me. I wasn't a person, I was a *freak.* I was a little girl who was not only fully developed but also had one breast *twice* the size of the other. That was my introduction to breasts.

Naturally my parents were very upset about my condition, but they never made me feel badly for it. They never hid me, but it was never discussed fully either. They are yesterday's generation and I guess they were embarrassed. It was very hard for them, because along with the physical development, the sex glands affected my emotional makeup, too. I was oversexed, so I had certain feelings and desires that could only be satisfied through sexual activity, which at nine years old I knew nothing about.

My condition lasted for two years and then it stabilized because of shots and treatment I was getting. When most girls were *beginning* to develop, I was *ending.* I had to have bras made to order because on one side I was a B cup and on the other side I was a C.

Throughout school I was kidded and taunted, which made me very conscious of my breasts. I remember one boy in particular who teased me all the time in a singsong voice—"Oh, *Audrey,* your falsies are drooping," or "Can I have a glass of milk?" I once beat the shit out of him—I almost *killed him!*

In a way, I think my large breasts made me less feminine. I was never very dainty, I always had a loud voice, and since my large breasts were *always* on my mind, I attribute it to them. I blame myself for being teased as much as I was because if I had been a shy, quiet little girl, maybe no one would have noticed me. And if I was so self-conscious about my breasts I should have worn loose blouses, but ironically I always wore *sweaters!* Maybe subconsciously I made myself suffer more for it.

After a while my breasts sort of evened out, and as a teenager the attention they provoked was much more positive and I began to like that. I had something that other girls didn't. If you had to go by personality and facial looks, the boys bypassed that very quickly! I was always the "sexy" one, and I learned to use it. As "the girl with the big tits," I wasn't the freak anymore . . . or was I? (*Laughs.*)

My husband always says, "You underestimate yourself. I didn't fall in love with you because you had big breasts. I fell in love with *you!*" Of course, *now* I don't think he's in love with me because I have big breasts, but as a teenager you don't have anything else to judge your own worth on because you don't have a real relationship with anybody. So you can't say it's because I'm compassionate

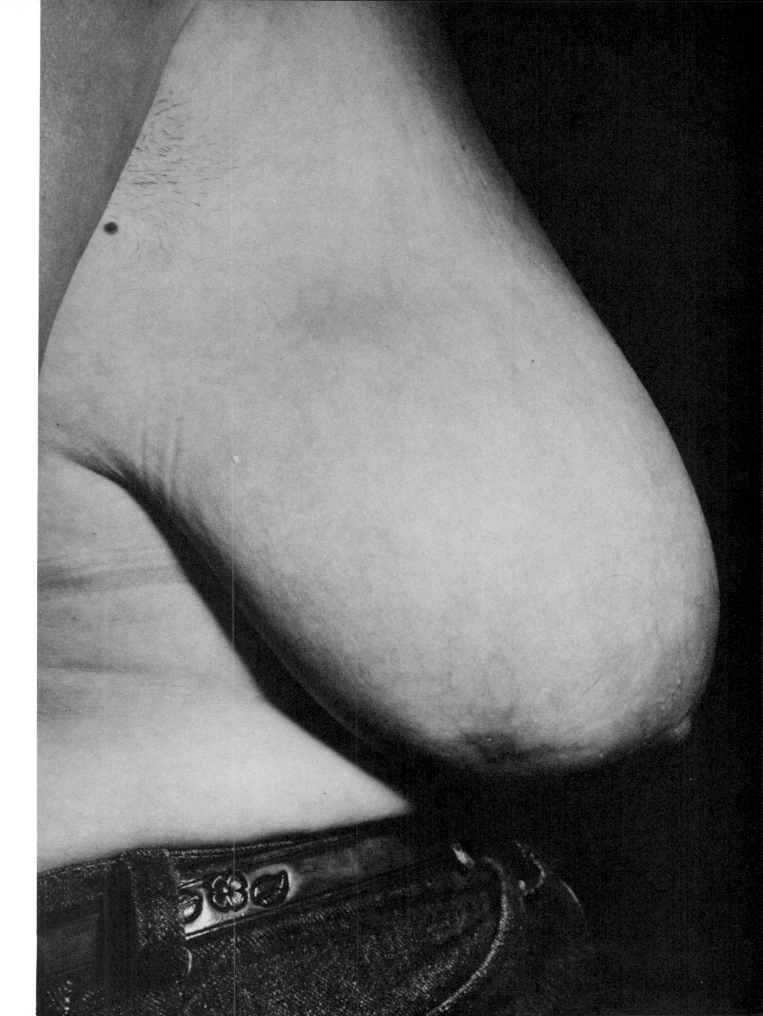

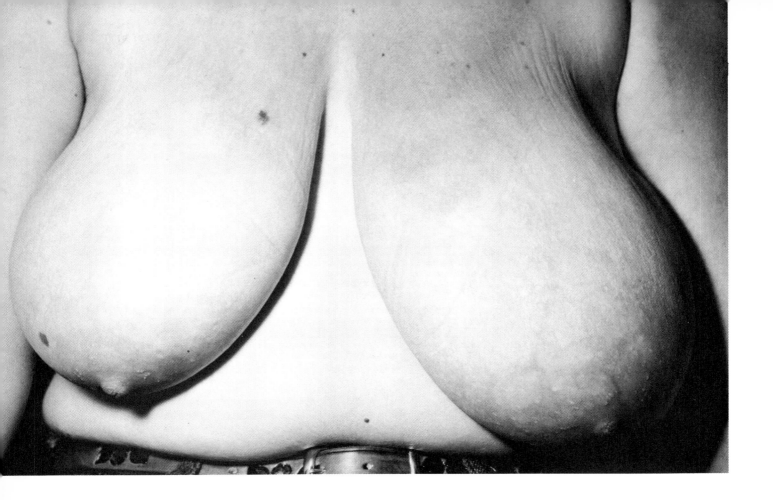

or good-natured or nice to talk to. Nobody thought of those things in those days, right? It was simply the girl with big busts.

I always preferred petting from the waist down rather than from the waist up. As far as I was concerned, breasts didn't *exist* sexually. I didn't like having my breasts touched. The fellas couldn't understand because *that* was supposed to be the big thing with the girls, you know, *that* is how you are supposed to get girls excited. If they wanted to do it I said, "Well, all right, what the heck?" but it never meant anything to me. My breasts attracted fellas and I petted when everybody else didn't, but I was one of the rare women who was a virgin when she got married!

For the first few years of marriage, I hated having my breasts touched, and unless I was very excited, they couldn't be. It annoyed me—it really bothered me. For a while, after my second child was born, my breasts were very stimulating, but then that went away.

I was a 36C when I got married. With padding they *looked* reasonably normal, but the two different sizes bothered me. And for some reason I made *sure* I would tell everybody. It was absolutely a state of mind.

In fact, when I first started seeing my husband, before we even got to the petting stage, I told him that I was lopsided. It came out very quick and harsh—kinda like a confession—and he didn't know what the hell I was talking about. The poor guy! It took him about two weeks before he got up the courage to ask me. Since then, I've always had a Chinese name for them—"One Hung Low."

●

My breasts almost *never* stopped growing! When I was pregnant, they got so big so quickly that I had to wear maternity clothes in my second month because none of the other clothes *fit*. And my belly never hit the blouse because my breasts always made it stand out so far. My breasts threw me completely off balance! Oh, my God, I don't know how I *walked . . .* how I didn't fall over on my nose.

When I had my first son, I went up to a 36D and never went down. I never *considered* breast-feeding! When I was pregnant with my second child, I had terrible headaches. I went from one specialist to another. First they thought it was sinuses. Then it turned out that my breasts were so *heavy* they were causing a strain on the back of my neck and *this* is what was giving me the headaches. They wanted to put me in a neck brace. I said,

"Get lost! I have a little boy at home. It'll scare the life out of him!"

After I had my second child, I went up to a double D and never came back, and that just added to my disgust. It was like stretching out bubble gum and leaving it there. Supposedly I don't have Cooper ligaments, which are muscles on the sides that make breasts stand up. So I began to get really *worried* that my breasts were just going to keep on stretching until they would be hanging *down to my knees!*

One thing about having big breasts is that you can be singled out, prejudged, eliminated, or accepted without opening your mouth! When I think of physical appearance, I can only think of breasts. Somehow, I am always the center of attraction—uh, my breasts are. In a group, I am the one that the men like to dance with at parties, even though I am married. Oh, and the comments! If I wear a sweater and then take it off, there is one friend in particular who always says, "Oh, shit! Come on over here!" I've always gotten reactions, and as soon as I learned to laugh and joke about it, then it was all right. That's what I've been doing ever since.

But I have this attitude that goes way back— the more I knew people were looking at my breasts, the farther I stuck my chest out. Some people would hunch over, but I figured no matter how much I hunched over, I wasn't gonna hide them. My husband doesn't like it when I do that, and he gets annoyed at me, so I say, "You know, when large breasts were in, they were *fine*, but now that they're out, I can't stick them under my armpits. There aren't any hidden pockets that I can drop them into! There aren't any false-bottom bras. My breasts are *there* and that's that!"

My brassieres are like two big football helmets. And the bigger the bra the higher the price. I can never buy a bra for three or four dollars—I always have to pay eleven dollars or more. So it's really *expensive* to have big breasts.

I've always had to wear underwires, which choke the life out of me, and I've always had pain in my shoulders from the weight. I have ridges in my shoulders, so I wear special pads that hook onto the cotton straps. When I take my bra off at night I really *feel* it. I have to take my bra off slowly, otherwise I'd break my neck! Once I remember my bra strap breaking and it was a disaster. I could never hide it because it was like a mountain caving in! (*Laughs.*)

I *never* go without a bra—I have to put one on as soon as I get up in the morning, and a lot of times I sleep in one. I'm most comfortable with

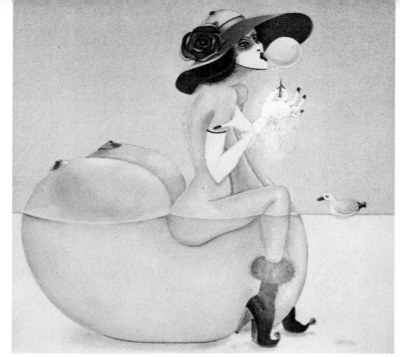

Illustration from National Lampoon

my breasts when I'm lying on my back, and the only time I'm really happy with them is when I'm sleeping and I don't know they're there.

My breasts are ugly and fat and they have no shape. Well, they have two different shapes. One of them looks like a long salami and the other is wide and flat. I've always *hated* my breasts—it's been a very hostile relationship. I've always felt that they were *disgusting!* I'm one of those women who won't share a dressing room when the big department stores have their sales. I'd *never* take my bra off in front of anybody except my husband. When you photographed me, it was the first time I ever showed my breasts to anybody aside from my husband and my doctor.

●

When I was about fifteen, a doctor said to my mother, "If she wants to be glamorous you could let her have plastic surgery," but he certainly didn't encourage it. He was an old-fashioned doctor.

I never thought seriously about plastic surgery until after I was married. My husband would do anything to make me happy, and he knows how unhappy I've been, so he says, "Why don't you go and have the operation?!" But there were just too many inhibitions—you don't go for an operation unless you have a disease! There is a certain stigma about this drastic kind of cosmetic surgery.

Last summer I had a very bad pain in my left breast—it was a beauty mark which turned out to be a benign tumor. It was removed in the doctor's office and I had to be nude from the waist up. The surgeon was really adorable and his associate was scrumptious looking, and I just *died*—laying there with my breasts exposed. Then they put a sheet around me to expose just the one breast. The doctor would say, "All right, Audrey, turn all the way on your side so it can fall *this way*," and if I lay "this way," my breast fell *that* way, and every time I turned, it flopped the *wrong* way. Oh, it was just a terrible experience! Every time I go for an examination it's humiliating.

Anyway, about six weeks ago, I started getting pain where the tumor had been removed—bad pain. When the doctor examined me he said, "Audrey, the breast is perfectly normal. You have this pain simply because your breast is so heavy it's pulling on the incision from inside." And when he tried to take the stitches out, everything popped open and I started to bleed, so he had to clamp it up again.

Then he told me, "You are cystic prone—you have cysts and growths in your breasts. A lot of women do, but because you're *so large* and *so heavy*, the chances are that these cysts will pop up every couple of years, and they'll have to be removed. Also, within ten years you'll be in constant pain from the weight of your breasts."

A few days later I went to a clinic for a breast examination and I was *too big* for the X-ray machine! They had to use a special table! That's when I broke down and got hysterical. I told the doctor everything about my background and how I felt, and asked him, "Can anything be done?"

He said, "Of course, honey. You see I'm a little bald. I don't want to be bald. I don't want to look older than I am. I'm a doctor, you know, and I'm not ashamed to tell you," and he showed me that he had hair transplants. "Honey," he says, "judging from the way they sag now, they'll sag even more. They'll say you *used to be* a good-looking woman." Meanwhile, I was having pain in my breast, in my armpit, and down my arm. So I went into the waiting room and told my husband, and that's when I made the decision.

I think if my parents had had this surgery for me when I was fifteen years old, I wouldn't have gone through what I did for the last eighteen years. At age thirty-three I'm finally doing it by myself. I cannot really afford the operation, but even if we have to borrow the money and pay it off, it's going to get done. It is going to be listed as a "partial amputation and reconstruction of the breast due to growths and cysts," and hopefully we will be able to get insurance coverage for it.

To make me feel better about the cost of the operation, my husband figured it out to X amount of dollars a month. He said, "Over the next thirty years it will cost us four dollars and fifty cents a month for you to be happy!" He knows how desperately I want it.

Truthfully, I could do without the operation (*says guiltily*). I'm not *enormous* enormous, because I've seen pictures that the doctor showed me. There was one girl, my God, I don't know how she was walking around on the face of this earth! I'm not going to die if I don't have the surgery, but this is my *chance*. The doctor said, "Do it—it should be done—don't wait! You won't have pain, you'll be a different person," so I'm taking advantage of his advice.

Everybody thinks I *have to* have this done, because I wouldn't open myself up to ridicule from people who'd misunderstand and think that I am *crazy* to borrow money and put myself in debt to make myself "pretty." Certain friends kid me about the surgery. The women say, "Can you have the leftovers molded into new ones, so I could use them?" But the men can't understand why I want the operation—"What are you, crazy?"—because they think that large breasts are just wonderful. Of course, they've never seen me without a bra—they've always seen my breasts under clothes, propped up.

During the first consultation with my plastic surgeon, I sat in his office for over an hour and asked a million questions, and when I went home I thought of a million more. I thought of all these crazy things: what if they still hurt me afterward? I'll feel guilty that I spent the money for an operation—I'll punish myself and drive myself crazy! What if they look like plastic fakies? So in a panic I called the doctor up and asked him whether they would look normal. He told me, "I'm not going to paint them or anything—they're going to be *your* skin."

I thought a lot about it and the next time I saw him I said, "Look, I was *cheated* the first time around, so if I'm going to go through this already, I want a *perfect pair!* I want them to *stand up!* I don't know if you're going to put in silicone or something to make them stand up, because they don't stand up now. Is *that* going to make them look phony?" You get these *terrible* thoughts! Finally, I said to him, "Listen, you must be careful to make the nipples point in the right direction. I don't want one pointing one way and one the other way." So he said, "Look, honey, I won't be able to match you up with every month's *Playboy* centerfold, but you'll compete against most of them."

Right now I'm very conscious of breast sizes. If I'm friendly enough with a woman and I like the way her breasts look, I ask her what size they are. I figure, maybe I'll take that size, you know, "Give me one of those." The surgeon didn't give me a choice of breast size. He just said that it's according to my size and build, and he will let me know. So I told him he better not make me an A cup—I don't want to look like a bump on a log!

There are different kinds of breast reduction operations. In one, the nipple is completely severed and transplanted. The doctor asked me if I had much sensation in my nipples because this type of operation would take away the feeling. I've never associated touching my breasts with pleasure, but I said, "No, I don't want *that* done," because I am hoping to have a completely different attitude after.

I don't think the doctor likes to discuss surgery at length until the day before the operation. That's when he'll measure me and see how much he has to cut. If it is too much he might have to sever the nipples, to prevent them from winding up on the bottom of my breasts or on the side or something.

Of course I'm looking forward to not having pain in my breasts for the first time in my life, but I have so many fears about how they're going to look that I constantly have to remind myself that this man does cosmetic surgery all the time. That's what he does every day of his life. So of course they're going to come out beautiful! Naturally there will be some scarring but it'll depend on how I heal. I don't care what the scars look like under a bra—I mean, nobody has seen my breasts all these years, so nobody *has* to see them afterward!

●

I am very excited because I've been told that the operation is going to change my personality. My husband gives me lots of encouragement—he's one in a million! He says he's really privileged to be the only man married to two different women—you know, two different versions of the same woman—in one lifetime.

My biggest and best fantasy is that I'm going to be gorgeous, naturally. My breasts will be up and out and bouncy. People will finally be able to see that I have a waist. I'm expecting to lose weight from not eating in the hospital and to come out looking absolutely magnificent.

I've asked my husband, "Will you still like my breasts when they're smaller—you're used to such big ones?" He says I'm the most attractive woman that ever walked around anyway. He grabs me in the supermarkets and even at my mother's house when I'm cleaning off the table, if nobody's looking. He says that men will be after me all the time and that he'll go *crazy* if I go braless. We both have these wild fantasies—we're thrilled that it is going to be done, and we are expecting the absolute best out of it.

You see, I'm in a transition stage which is hard to describe. In a couple of weeks my breasts are going to be completely different, and I'm looking forward to being a completely different person. It's such an expectant feeling. . . .

Two and a Half Months After the Operation

I was *petrified!*

The doctor met us in the waiting room at the hospital. It was very nice—just like on television. He put his arm around me and took me up to the room. I asked him a lot of new questions that I had saved up. I was very frightened but I never wanted to change my mind.

He gave me a full physical examination and measured the breasts and marked them with something that looked like a black magic marker. He had to make a road map—it's really more like a sewing pattern—of the lines that he'd follow. He was going to cut under each breast, then from the middle up to and around the nipple—like making a keyhole—in order not to sever the nipples.

It's a four-hour operation and I had been told that the anesthetic kills more people than the operation, so I was absolutely panic-stricken of the mask going over my face.

When they woke me up, it seemed like a minute later. The anesthetic had put me out so heavily that I felt like somebody hit me on the top of my head with a sledgehammer. They were slapping my cheeks, saying, "Okay. It's over. Take a deep breath." I took a deep breath and *nothing* went in. I felt no air, no oxygen! Then they started shouting, "Okay, hurry up—onto the table to recovery—oxygen—give her oxygen!—take her pressure! Hurry up!"

My blood pressure had dropped very low during the operation and I'd lost a lot of blood and they had to give me a transfusion. The normal recovery time is two and a half to three hours—I was in the recovery room for six and a half hours! It took them a long time to stabilize me, and I was very nauseous from the anesthetic. So the anesthetic, as I feared, was the worst part of the operation.

●

The first time I saw my breasts, I *fainted!* I was going into the shower to bathe the incisions, so I took my bra off and as I walked past the bathroom mirror, I caught sight of my breasts and passed out. After all, I was weak and only six days post-operative. I didn't see the actual incisions for a month because they were underneath my breasts . . . and I was *afraid* to look.

It's funny, but in all our discussions and preparations about the operation—what was going to be done and the results and everything—I never realized that the wounds had to be dressed and cleaned two or three times a day.

I had two hundred and six stitches, and my doctor and I had one session where he took out fifty stitches in one night. He knew how badly he was hurting me because he was wiping the perspiration from my shoulders and head. He's marvelous, but he's a strict man. He doesn't go for hysterical antics, so I didn't yell and cry and scream. When it was over, he bent over and kissed me and patted me like "you were a good girl." Sometimes he doesn't answer my questions as directly as I'd like, but maybe he can't. Over all, he has made me feel very comfortable and very secure.

There was never any definite commitment from the doctor on the length of time to recuperate. In the beginning, when I asked he said, "I'll have you washing floors and walls in two weeks," which was, of course, just to pacify me.

Before the operation, I really didn't think beyond that date, about what was going to happen. But it isn't just having the operation and coming home and it is over. The laundry and the shopping have to get done and the house cleaned and the kids have to eat three meals and get taken to school. Everything has to go on as it did before. I don't know what I was thinking—that the house would get vacuumed by itself? That the food shopping would get done? I don't know why, but I didn't think of any of these things.

My mother was here for a month and my friends helped out, but my house was upside down, which drives me out of my mind! I went crazy watching my mother and my husband trying to fold laundry. My kitchen counters were messed up. Things were laying all over them. My oldest boy didn't like the French toast Grandma made—he only likes it *my* way! (*Laughs.*)

But for a solid six weeks I did *nothing.* In the very beginning I was just barely able to brush my teeth and put on a little eye makeup. After about a month, I could fold some laundry, and now, two and a half months later, I am doing everything except lifting heavy grocery bundles.

●

Am I happy with my breasts? Well, there's a lot of different answers to that question. Whenever I thought of my breasts being different, it was in terms of how I would appear in clothing—in a bathing suit or a sweater. And I am *thrilled* with that aspect.

I am very happy with the size. They are exactly what I asked for—they are up and out and there is no sagging. They are firm, yet they move and jiggle, so they don't look fake. Before I was a 36DD and now I'm on the small C size, closer to a B. In comparison, what used to pop out of my bathing suit before is now my entire breast! I can tell because they're completely suntanned now. There's one thing that really gives me a charge—the left breast used to be so much larger than the right (forty-five percent larger according to the doctor's measurements) and now the right is slightly larger than the left!

But I don't like the appearance of the actual breasts *yet.* My right breast is almost healed completely, but the left breast is still very red and scarred and ugly-looking. It looks like a messy Frankenstein forehead. I'm somewhat unhappy because we aren't finished yet. There are some complications.

The part of the operation that involved moving the nipples is like transplanting a new plant. When you transplant nipples, the nerve cords have to remain attached. If they are severed, the nipples no longer function—there's no sensation and they are just decoration. The hazard with the procedure I had is that if the nerve cord is stretched too much when the nipples are repositioned, sometimes a nipple will be pulled in, inverting it, which is exactly what happened to me.

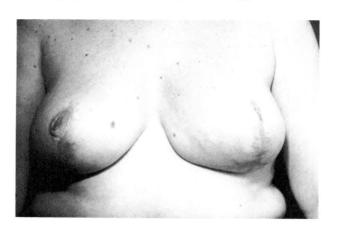

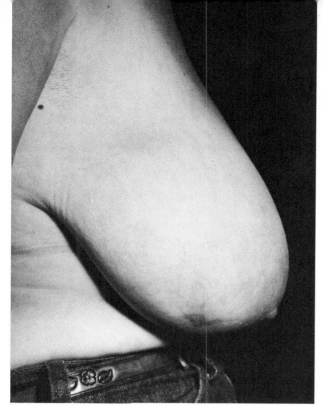

Before

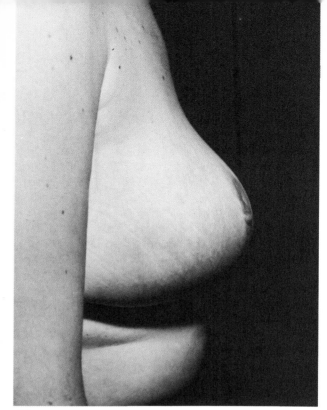

After

So on the left side the nipple is completely inverted, and on the right side, it's slouched—the nipple is only partially out. Other than that, the right breast came out perfect. The left breast—the one that was twice the size of the other one—is the one that has all the problems because the nipple had to be moved up a greater distance.

Usually, the patient is completely finished in three months except for a once-a-month checkup. But I need some corrective surgery done. I've almost got to start all over again. As soon as I'm healed, I'll go back into the hospital. The doctor describes it as a simple procedure—just eliminating a piece of skin around the nipple area, pulling it out and stitching it up again. That's for the nipples. Then there's a little piece of skin underneath the left breast that has to be tucked in—it's like molding clay. It could have been worse. In the procedures where they sever the nerve, the nipple is just sewn on a different part of the breast like a patch. And sometimes, according to my doctor, they fall off! (*Shudders.*) That sounds horrendous!

I haven't shown my breasts to anyone because most people are squeamish and it's hard to take. A lot of people are afraid to even ask about the operation. So most of my friends don't know the details—the stitches, the pain, the complications.

I went to a party Saturday night and I was braless. Everybody was complimenting me on how I looked, and one woman naively asked, "Are there any scars?" I laughed to myself, but I realized from her position, looking at me clothed, I looked perfectly normal. So I suddenly thought to myself, "What if I just whipped up the top of my sweater? Everybody would scream and run!" It really is quite a shocking sight. I would have loved to do that—I really would.

Sometimes, if I'm in a giddy mood, I'll say to my husband, "Wouldn't it be wild if somebody raped me now? Boy, would they be surprised when they ripped open my blouse!"

This woman (age 54) had breast reduction surgery 25 years ago. Her nerves were completely severed so that her nipples can no longer become erect.

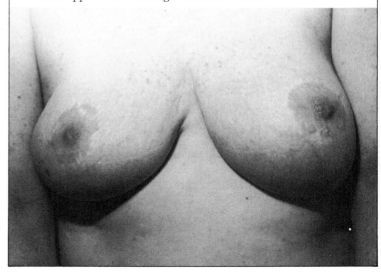

I wore a bathing suit for the first time two weeks ago, and I didn't have to lift my breasts up and make sure they weren't popping out of the top or slipping out from the bottom of the cup. Imagine, I can even bend down to pick up a towel and jump into the pool! I sink a little faster though—I lost my floats! (*Laughs.*)

There are a lot of little things that have changed. I get dressed much faster. I definitely feel lighter. And I have absolutely no pains in my breasts at all! Not even when I get my period. Before, when I turned over in bed, I would have to take my breasts from underneath and pull them up so that I wouldn't roll over on them and get *tangled.* I still find myself behaving, just out of habit, as if I still have my large breasts. It sounds ridiculous, but at one time if I was wearing a nightgown and I wanted to pull it up, I would tuck it under my breasts to hold it up. It was a habit and I automatically did it this morning in the bathroom and of course the nightgown didn't stay! (*Laughs.*) There are a million different things to think about. I have to completely recondition myself that I'm not "so-and-so with the *big tits.*"

For the first couple of months I didn't feel anything—my breasts were numb! Then I had the feeling that my nipples were down where they used to be. If my breasts were being caressed up above, I felt it down below. But as the months passed I've had more and more sensation in the proper places.

My husband loves it! He is absolutely thrilled out of his mind! I see the same look on his face now, six months later, as the day I came out of the hospital—a look of pure love and admiration. To him I was beautiful before I had the operation, I was beautiful the day he saw me cut up with two hundred and six stitches, and I am just as beautiful now when my breasts can be *manhandled!*

I don't think I'm more sexually attractive to him now, but I am more *something.* He loves the way I feel about myself. I feel better, therefore I act differently, and when I act differently, it affects him. So it is just unbelievable in every respect. It's made a difference in my own personality—what's projected outwards—and the responses I get from people. There is absolutely no area in my life that it isn't different!

My older son is nine and he's completely aware of the operation. His biggest reaction was that my breasts used to hang "down there," pointing to my midriff, and now they are all the way "up here." The little one knows that I had an operation on my "breastis," and ignores it most of the time, except he asks me every once in a while when I am going to be all better so he can jump on me. I really am just about able to start hugging my sons again. They used to hug my arm because they couldn't get their arms around me; very soon they are gonna be able to really hug *me.* I can't wait!

I'm almost at the point now, six months after the operation, where I feel completely natural. Most of my friends tell me that it seems as though they've always seen me this way. People seeing me for the first time since the operation think that I've lost about a hundred and twenty-five pounds. They don't realize right away what the difference is. They say that it's unbelievable—it's beautiful! But there have been reactions from some friends that hurt me very badly, even though I expected it.

A couple of people didn't accept the operation as a medically necessary, cosmetically advantageous operation. They think it was done completely and purely for vanity. I'm sure they'd accept it if I told them that I had cancer and that was why it was done. I interpret their reactions as jealousy, pure and simple, because as the words were coming out of their mouths, no matter what they were saying, it sounded like, "I'm jealous, I'm jealous, I'm jealous. . . ."

And they *were* jealous because both of these women are very large-breasted, and what we had in common before were the type of "harnesses" we wore and the gossip when one found a new type of bra that doesn't cut into you—that type of thing. One girl hugged my husband and said, "See what it's like to hug a big-breasted girl? Do you miss 'em?" Since then I'm not friends with her anymore.

One of my friends recently remarked that before the operation I had something very attractive, and no matter what I looked like or how I was dressed, men would look at me. She said that I don't have *that* anymore—that edge, so to speak—and that sort of shocked me. I guess I was hoping that people didn't *really* think my breasts were my major attribute.

But I've been on both sides of the fence. I enjoyed what large-breasted women enjoy, and I suffered, too. But I feel much better about the way I am now. As much as people used to look at me for having huge breasts, now they look at me because I go braless. My breasts jiggle when I walk. They're free to move as they please. (*Laughs.*) I feel more attractive because I can go braless and I know it's stylish and sexy. There's nothing bad about being the size I am now, so I am enjoying all of it.

I was recently in a unisex barbershop. The owner was hiring new people, so I asked him if they needed a receptionist. All the girls who worked there were really sharp-looking and they were all braless and fairly large-breasted. I mean the barbershop was *known* for having girls with big, swingin' boobs. Well, the owner looked at me, and he was not ashamed to say, "Oh, I'm sorry, you can't work here, you're too flat-chested." It was . . . like a dream or something. I was speechless! I only wish I had a tape recorder so that I could just keep playing it back to myself.

Several Months After the Corrective Surgery

Today is exactly two years since the first operation. Two of the major scars have turned white, but the ones down the center of the breasts are still reddish. You know, I don't even look at the scars. They don't matter to me.

The second operation went okay but it did not completely correct what it was supposed to. That was just an unavoidable pitfall of this procedure, which I was not fully aware of. I'd say it's eighty to ninety percent better. The nipple that was completely inverted is now a little slouched, and the one that was slouched is much better. So they're both improved.

The corrective surgery left me with a new scar in a spot that was previously untouched and that upset me a little bit. It comes up quite high in the middle of my breasts and it healed in a very puffy ridge. So in a very low-cut bathing suit or top you can see it—it's in the cleavage. That's the one scar that really bothers me.

Now when I meet people for the first time, if we talk about dieting and losing weight, they say, "Oh, you don't look like the kind of person that could ever be heavy. You're so slim. Everything about you is *small*—you're small on top, you're small on bottom." And I think to myself, Oh shit, if they only knew! (*Laughs.*)

I was at a party on Saturday night and a buxom girl in my crowd who was supposedly smaller than I used to be was there, too. She looked *disgusting!* If I *really* was bigger, thank God I did

what I did! I never thought she looked disgusting *before* the operation, but now I said to myself, My God, if I was *that* big . . . I mean, I was *known* for my breasts! I found myself staring at her breasts and then I'd look away because I was ashamed that she might catch me staring, but she was *tremendous!* God, she really looked disgusting!

The other night my husband had a nightmare that we were at a wedding or some big affair, and I told everybody I was going in for breast surgery. Everybody got very excited, and the first thing they said was, "Well, it must be cancer." And all the people in the dream went to my mother and offered their condolences saying, "This is terrible, what your daughter has." My mother came over to me and got very upset. Then I got hysterical and I died—because I thought I had cancer—from the *thought* of it.

Now that nightmare is tied into a couple of things. First, my husband's mother died when she was thirty-three, which is how old I was when I had the operation. Second, the day after I came home from the hospital, I fainted in the shower. My eyes went back up into my head and for a moment my husband thought I was dead.

The weirdest thing is that I had a nightmare at the exact same time. When he poked me and said, "I just had a nightmare," I said, "So did I. I dreamt I had an abortion and it was a girl." Isn't that strange?

Before

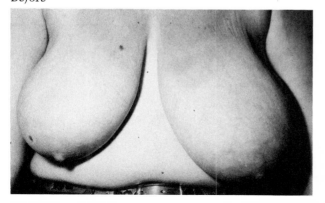

Two years after surgery

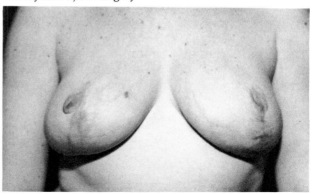

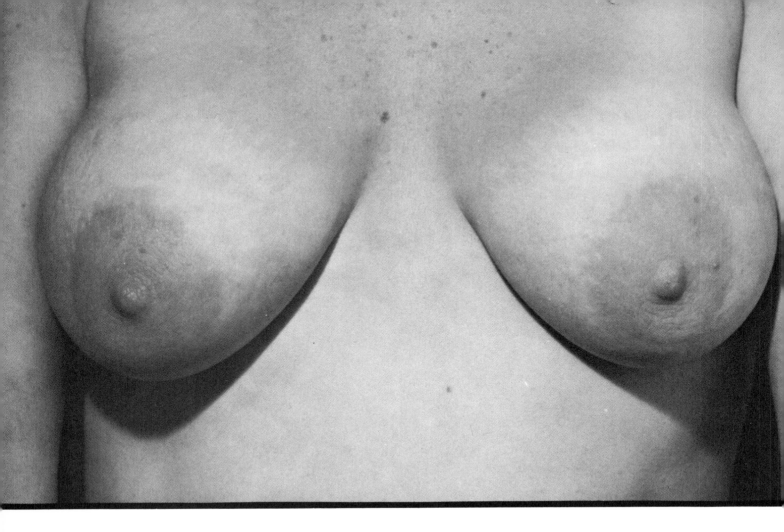

Vicki

Age 35 • Bronx, New York • Mother of teenage daughter

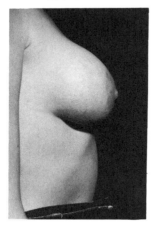

I've never really been fixated on my breasts, and even though my story gets a little bizarre as we go along, I never thought of my tits as something to entice men with. I've always considered myself intelligent rather than attractive, and hoped that if I attracted anyone, it was because I was a nice person and not because of the way I looked. In fact, for a long time I played down the glamorous aspect of myself.

I didn't have bad tits to start with. I was a full B cup and they weren't saggy. They weren't as firm as an eighteen-year-old's, but they looked all right. I wasn't unhappy with them.

My second husband was the "booby man"! He was the one who was hung up with my breasts. He talked me into having them enlarged and he paid for it. On my own I would never have had that kind of surgery done to me! And not because of economics either, but because of where my head was at. I just was not into my tits—I was never a "tit girl"!

As it turned out, having my breasts enlarged didn't enhance our relationship much. He didn't touch my tits any more than before. As a matter of fact, we remained married for only six months. And once he left, I was pissed off. Here we were divorced, and I couldn't give him back his tits!!!

210

I subscribed to *Cosmopolitan* at the time, and the magazine was always around in the house. My husband was reading the latest issue one night, and there was an article about breast implantation that showed photographs of before and after. He asked me to read the article. The impression it gave was that the operation was relatively painless and simple and did exactly what one hoped it would.

My husband was entertaining the idea of getting a hair transplant because he was thinning on top. He was quite vain obviously, and I guess he projected his vanity onto me. Obviously he was a "tit man"—my tits didn't please him so he used his money to improve them before going ahead with his hair transplant, which he desperately wanted.

He thought it would be something nice, you know, like, "Wouldn't you like to have big tits as a present? And have them raised up, too?" And I thought, "Geez, if he wants to *give* me something like that, it sounds like a pretty good deal." I didn't think much about having the operation. It was a very superficial thing to me. I thought I'd look better in clothes and they would hold up longer than they otherwise would. Within a month of reading this article, I had it done.

I went into the hospital the night before the operation. Of course, all the people there were genuinely ill, and I felt guilty that I was there just for cosmetic reasons. On top of that, there was a chaplain making his rounds and he stopped at my bed. He asked me what was wrong with me, and I was truly embarrassed to tell him that I was having my tits enlarged. But I couldn't lie to him either. He asked my *why* and I told him the truth and he said he hoped that it made my husband and I happy. So then he blessed me—I had my tits *blessed!* (*Laughs.*)

When I first came out of the anesthesia I was absolutely horrified because my breasts were at least three to four inches higher than they are right now . . . and very *swollen!* The surgeon warned me that it would be several months before they would look the way they're supposed to ultimately.

When I had it done, I weighed about twenty-five or thirty pounds more than I do now. Consequently, the surgeon gave me certain-sized implants based on the proportions of my body *then.* Now that I am much thinner, I look inordinately top-heavy in certain clothing.

Breaking up with my husband had to do with

our sex life. I'd like to believe that the operation had nothing to do with it, but then again, you never know. It's very possible. . . .

Because my tits are large now, I run into a lot more "breast men" than before. I have to weed them out. Men are always talking to me and staring down at my breasts.

Since my divorce, most men I've gone out with know that my tits have been augmented. They can feel the difference. My breasts are still a turn-on for me in sex. I feel sad for women whose breasts aren't. I'm pretty shy when I expose my breasts for the first time to a man. I'm very romantic and I still like to be made love to like in the movies—the old movies.

●

Now I have ambivalent feelings about my breasts—it bothers me that there's something in me that isn't real. I don't eat red meat or pork for both health and moral reasons. You might think it's kind of odd for someone who feels so strongly about certain things to have something so unnatural done to herself, and I am *sorry* that I had it done.

If I had it to do all over, I would not have it done. I'm not happy with the results. My breasts are uncomfortable sometimes. I'm thirty-five, and for thirty-two years I didn't have big breasts, so they're still newer than anything else on my body. Frankly, I've even seen doctors about having them undone.

Last September I went to a breast clinic because with these implants, I can't examine myself. I don't know where *I* begin and where *they* leave off! My mother died of cancer, I've been on the pill for twelve years, and with the implants, I worry a lot about breast cancer.

After a thorough examination, I was advised by the doctor that I'd already fooled around with my breasts as much as I should have. To have the implants removed was just tampering with nature even more and I should just leave well enough alone.

Do you have any advice for women who may be considering having their breasts enlarged?

Be very careful! Check out several doctors and shop around. Make sure you're going to the right surgeon. Most important of all, be sure *that's* what you *really* want to do. If a woman thinks her breasts are going to improve her lot in life—if that's her only reason—she had better do some heavy internal searching before she goes ahead and does it.

Helen
Age 38 • Raised on the East Coast • Filmmaker/Teacher

When I was thirteen my breasts came out and I really enjoyed them. I became aware that they were very sensuous and began touching them a lot. I also started masturbating then. I really liked the shape my breasts turned out. I blossomed! They were *beautiful.* Until then I was sort of an ugly duckling, and then I got these great tits and I was a *prize!* I became aware that I was "sexy." My sister's boyfriends were all interested in me and she envied me. I became aware of my "powers" as a woman.

I had a cousin who got teeny, long, hanging ones with big nipples at the end. We would show our breasts to each other, but mine were *great* and hers were terrible. She knew it—I didn't have to tell her.

I looked very sexy and men were always making passes at me. But actually I was more interested in developing myself than in exploring men. I wanted to be an artist. I began studying dancing *because* of my great body. It was real body narcissism.

When I was seventeen, I fell in love and suddenly lost my virginity—that was it! I went to extremes. Up to then I was waiting for the great Lover to walk through my door! My first love would write poems as I slept naked. He adored me and my body. He would say I was "holy" and my breasts were "holy." He was Catholic and I guess it was his way of telling me they were good. It was very beautiful. I don't remember ever feeling hung up about being naked in front of a man.

My breasts were round and high and stood out, and the nipples weren't too large. I liked my body, but more than any other part of me, my breasts gave me a certain assurance and sensuality. They were very important because they gave me power! I was free and strong and beautiful.

In my twenties I *always* wore very low-cut things and no bra—*never* a bra! There were certain guys who always noticed my breasts and would kid around with me about having the "best tits in the art world." It was a kick for me. On the most basic level, my breasts cleared the way for me.

Wherever I went I'd think, "Well, I have these *great* breasts!" and I'd go in and sort of knock 'em dead. It was like magic! My breasts gave me power in the battle of the sexes. Rather than be used, *I* would use. I chose a young and beautiful lover. I saw him for the first time at a party. I was

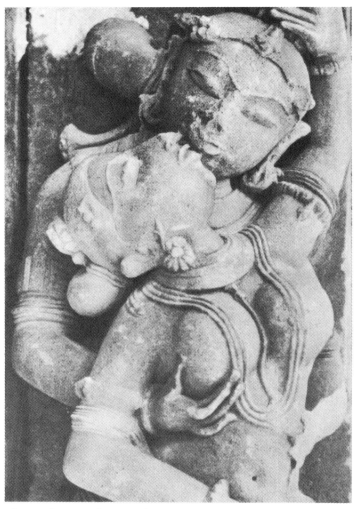

Khajurāho temples in India

wearing a low-cut dress and no bra. I feigned dozing and was leaning over quite seductively and that's how we met—he was attracted to me *because* of my breasts!

●

I feel that breasts are an integral part of female eroticism. A woman's sexuality, unlike a man's, is in her whole body. In a man it's localized in the penis, but with a woman, sexuality is not localized just in the vagina and the clitoris, which are internal. It's the whole sensuous experience of her body, and breasts are the external manifestation of her sensuality.

In the films I make I emphasize the naked body and its eroticism. I think eroticism is very "high" and beautiful—almost religious. The ancient

212

Greeks were erotic, and the Indians, too, celebrate the beauty of sexuality in their temples and Tantric cults.

It's strange, but underneath it all, Americans are still very puritanical. Take porno films, for example, where men have to degrade women to feel hot for them. Pornography is strictly for men, and it turns most women off because it is done with vulgarity and exaggeration that is grotesque. It's *ugly* instead of beautiful or sensual in the romantic sense, and it has *nothing* to do with eroticism.

The difference between porno films and the films I do is in approach and attitude. It's *how* something is done, not *what*. I've filmed erotic scenes which involved the caressing and sucking of breasts, but I don't treat it the way pornography does. It's *how* the breasts are framed—the body as a divinely erotic subject. *My* films are not commercial—they're shown in museums and art festivals.

I haven't made an erotic film . . . since my mastectomy. . . .

How did you first discover that you had breast cancer?

I had mastitis over the years, and I had two nonmalignant lumps taken out before. Every six months I went for a breast checkup. Once they found another two lumps. They said, "Let's wait a month and see if they dissolve." This was in August.

By September the lumps *hadn't* dissolved. I called the surgeon who had operated on me for cysts previously and he immediately put me in the hospital. He removed the lump that was on the outside, and then told me I was all right, to go home and forget it. He felt that the remaining lump had gotten smaller and didn't have to be removed. My brother-in-law, who is a doctor, was concerned about this, and got me to the cancer center a month later, where they spent a couple of weeks making tests. *They* said they suspected a malignancy.

My brother-in-law and I had heard about all the new nonmastectomy treatments, and we wanted to have just the lump removed—a "lumpectomy." So he recommended me to a surgeon. I had been treated by a female doctor who wrote a letter to the surgeon supporting my wish to have a lumpectomy rather than a radical mastectomy. It was a long four-page letter saying, "I would recommend, since I think it is early . . ." and so on.

When I walked into the surgeon's office, he said, referring to the letter, "Oh, the woman who believes in this nonmastectomy bullshit is a *whore!*" That's what he called her. Well, he's of the old school, but he's also the *head* of breast surgery, and firmly believes that this doctor was risking the lives of her patients. That upset me and I burst into tears. Then, as soon as he touched the lump, he exclaimed, "It's *cancer!* You're a young woman, and if you don't let me do a mastectomy, you are risking your life!" He threatened and bullied me, and I got hysterical!

I was scared. By now two months had passed since the first lump was removed. Everyone was certain that the remaining lump was cancer. I was afraid that it might spread, but I still wouldn't give him permission to do a mastectomy. I only signed the release papers for a lumpectomy, which is what he did. When I woke up out of the anesthetic, he was standing over me droning, "You have cancer, young lady, and unless you let me do a proper operation, blah . . . blah . . . blah. . . ."

Meanwhile, the surgeon spoke to my brother-in-law, whom I really trusted, and convinced *him*. My brother-in-law came into my room and said, "Well, you have two choices—life or death. It was too late for the lumpectomy, it had started to spread." I felt that I no longer had any choice in the matter.

The surgeon didn't prepare me in any way. He just put a lot of pressure on us and acted super-righteous. It was like when you are a little girl and they scare you. He didn't even tell me the alternatives. Now, three years later, there is much more publicity and information and we know more about the consequences of removing your pectoral muscle. I didn't know how much he was going to remove. He just said I was *only* losing my breast!

One of the things he did tell me, though, was that *his* mother had had breast cancer but she didn't have a mastectomy and she died. I suppose that's why he became a breast cancer surgeon—a hero—to save all women from the fate of his own mother.

So I signed permission for the second operation—the radical—but again it was because I really trusted my brother-in-law. I am very close to him, and he *knew* how upsetting it would be. He knows me and my life-style—how important freedom and sex are—and how traumatic it would be for me. But this surgeon told him that he really didn't think I would live without the radical. I think this is the operation that women fear most and a lot of women do choose to *die!*

●

When I woke up after the operation, one of the first people who came to see me was a Reach to Recovery * woman. She sat by my bedside looking totally sexless and said something like, "Can you tell the difference? Which one is it?" *What?* All I could think of was my gorgeous lover—ten years younger than me—whom I was mad about and I knew I wasn't going to be able to keep him. So what the hell was she talking about? It would look the same in *clothes!!*

Oh, it was so *painful!* I cannot tell you. I woke up in searing pain. Not just my tit was in trouble; it was like they blasted a hole in my chest. And all the nerves . . . It's like when they amputate someone's arm and the person still can feel the arm there. It's so strange because I'd feel the breast and it wasn't *there!* And I was in such pain!

The Reach to Recovery women are very noble and they do help some women. They have classes where they make you do exercises, and those are very helpful. Then they have counseling groups where you are *supposed* to talk about your feelings. The whole psychology of these traumatized women is like sheep, and everyone was supposed to say in so many words, "Oh, I'm fine." But I said, "I don't know about all of you, but I'm very *angry!* I know that my surgeon saved my life, but, God, I'm furious with him. I'm sorry, but I'm not so happy this happened."

Reach to Recovery was helpful for the older women, since they weren't into conscious sexuality anymore. There were practically no young women, and nobody like me. A couple of women said, "Well, my husband didn't marry me for my body, anyway. I'm the mother of his children."

Meanwhile, my young and beautiful lover showed up while I was still in the hospital, looking totally ashen and pale, and then he *left!* He really got frightened by the whole ordeal. I almost never saw him again.

After I left the hospital, I had to have radiation treatment for two months. Oh, God, it's just *horrible!* It makes you so ill and nauseous. It's a nightmare! One of the worst things about a mastectomy is that recovery takes so long, and you become extremely weak. For two years I went to work, came home, crawled into bed, and that was it. I had no energy.

Psychologically, it was the biggest trauma of my life. I lost my lover and I lost my life-style. I went to a therapist who told me I was really strong not to have gone mad because of the per-

* A volunteer program of the American Cancer Society, run by women who have had mastectomies and who are trained to help others through the initial period of adjustment.

sonal trauma that I felt. I didn't think I would ever have a sexual relationship again.

I have a lover now whom I would never have looked at prior to my operation. I wouldn't have found him attractive before. He is in his fifties, not really sexy, and has had a heart condition, but he happens to be a really gentle person.

I knew him before—he was my teacher. Someone told him about the mastectomy and that's when he first called me. He found out that my ex-boyfriend had deserted me, so he wanted to take care of me. He told me he once found a dog who had a broken leg and he took care of it, so I guess he is attracted to things that are wounded. Also he probably thought that I wouldn't be very demanding or threatening to him sexually, compared to the way I was before the mastectomy.

He spent about six months just taking me out to eat, but I wouldn't let him or anyone near me. The relationship is working out because it's more like a companionship.

My young lover came back once when I was still really sick and healing, and still on drugs. He jumped into bed and tried to make love with me, and it was so painful I couldn't take it. Once or twice he tried to put his hand *there* and I just went bananas and got hysterical.

Even with the older man I'm seeing now, I can't take it! At first, when he went to touch me, I started crying and got very upset. Yet he's been very patient with me. Sexually, the relationship is just now starting to work out, but I never remove my bra while having sex. It's not his fault; I simply can't deal with it. I'm only comfortable during sex when I'm lying on my side, so just the remaining breast is exposed and that part of me —the wound—isn't. I *always* keep my bra on, but he can reach into it and touch my breast. In fact, I don't even let him do that very much, but sometimes *I'll* hold my breast, not sexually but in a nurturing sense, for reassurance and security.

Before the operation, I was *very* breast oriented, and I'd get turned on sexually first by my breasts. After the operation, my whole sexual system didn't respond for two years! It really took a beating. And now my menstrual period is much more painful. My whole chest is just beginning to feel again, and positive sensation is just now beginning to come back in the remaining breast. I've even just started to have orgasms again. That's a great thing for my whole system. Before I was terrified and thought, Oh, God, I'm *never* going to have an orgasm again!

The *worst* thing that can happen to a woman is

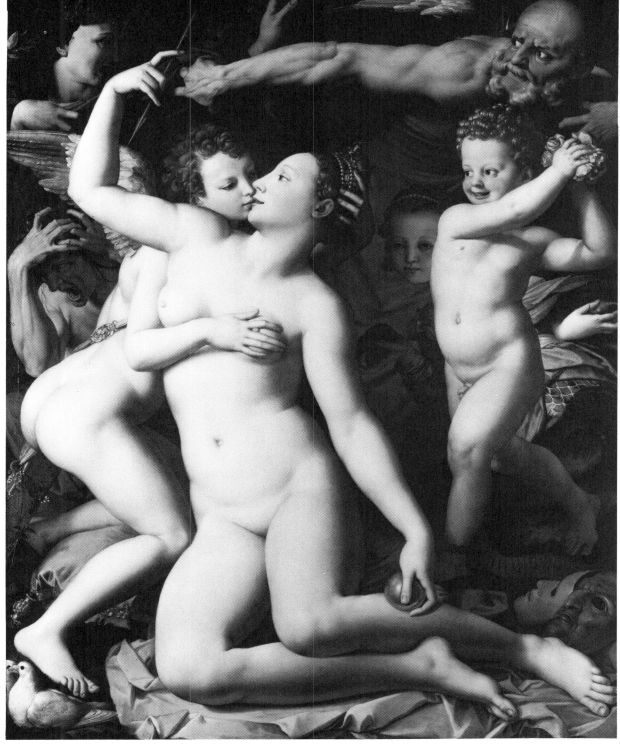

"Venus, Cupid and Time (an Allegory)" by Bronzino. The National Gallery, London

to lose a breast. If you are into sex then you're really in trouble, but if you're a nun, well . . . It depends on your personality—your body narcissism. I have vivid memories of my own eroticism with my breasts. To me, breasts are the doorway to a woman's whole arousal. They are so very sensuous, warm, and nurturing. They remind you of sucking and feelings of arousal and warmth throughout your body.

When someone's making love to you, the first thing he does to turn you on is suck your breast. The sensuous image of a woman nursing her child is always subconsciously recalled, and then you become aroused.

There is a sense of nurturing that you have from your breasts—a sense of giving and warmth and mothering and loving . . . to everybody, to yourself, as part of your sensuality. I used to be really in touch with that feeling. Now I am unable to nurture.

The man I'm seeing now nurtures me. He takes care of me, whereas before it was the other way around. I had a young lover whom *I* took care of. The roles are reversed. With my students also, I now resent having to nurture and I don't like being in a position where I have to give out more as a teacher. This is something new for me—I've changed.

●

The mastectomy has affected my work drastically. It has destroyed my energy and my ability to compete in a very competitive field—my colleagues are just stronger than I am. After the operation, I was so crippled that I couldn't even pick up a camera. It was like that for two and a half years and I am *still* not all right. I can *never* again lift heavy things, and meanwhile everyone else is out there rushing around, hustling, and making films.

Before, whatever I did had a quality of leadership and self-assurance—I used to do these far-out "happenings"—but now whatever I do is interpreted as being very "defensive." So the mastectomy has become a stigma for me. Whereas before my erotic films were considered "daring" and "original," now everyone says "Oh, she's a little strange." So *whatever* I do now, people believe that it *has* to be motivated by the mastectomy.

I think people treat you like this because of our culture and all the fuss that is made in America about youth and beauty. I've been treated very differently by people since the mastectomy. At first they went out of their way to be super-sympathetic. Then, suddenly, they stopped calling. It's a *stigma!* You've had *cancer!* You've had your breast cut off! You're a *freak!* So they treat you in a certain degraded way that they reserve for people who are mutilated or cripples.

I once heard a story . . . In a henyard, one hen was attacked by a raccoon and it crippled her. After that, when the crippled hen came back to the henhouse, all the other hens tried to kill her! That's sort of what happened to me.

People have been very abusive. On jobs, colleagues have treated me as a servant. Several times, women I work with have screamed at me—blown up and ordered me around. These are people who would never have *dared* to talk to me that way before. I think the mastectomy really upsets them. It upsets their own sense of security. It's a fear they have that it could happen to them. I'm a threatening image, like a messenger with bad news.

Someone whom I worked with at school told one of the younger teachers about the mastectomy. I was her supervisor, but as soon as she found out about it, she never listened to anything I said. She treated me in a really abominable way. So I've laid down the rule that I don't want *anybody* to know.

After the mastectomy, someone tried to get me fired. Only recently I found out that it was a *man* who protected me when a woman tried to get me out. She was just so insanely threatened! It's incredible, but I've heard these kinds of things about other woman who've had mastectomies. I met a woman who was fired from a copywriting job after having a mastectomy. Until you live through the actual experience of it, you don't know how very brutalizing it is. You just don't know what it's like!

●

I'll say one good thing about Reach to Recovery—they brought me a little bra to wear in the hospital that was very loose and knitted, and on the mastectomy side it was stuffed with cotton. Well I *still* have it. When I get home, I take off my regular bra and put the soft one on. I have to wear a bra to hold my prosthesis in place. The prosthesis is a form shaped like a breast, made of rubber with silicone inside, and it is heavy and uncomfortable, but I look better in it.

Using it really helps me, not only in terms of how I appear, but also how I feel, because it balances the weight. I also like the feeling when I wear it because the nerve endings in the brain come from *two* breasts, whether one is removed or not. And it's strange but if someone touches the prosthesis there is almost a sensuousness there because my brain is still receiving messages about two breasts! It almost feels like that's me.

I can't even *sleep* unless I wear an artificial breast! Falling asleep, especially in the beginning, was very hard. I had a horrible feeling of being a war victim whose entire chest had been blown off. I'd go to sleep and wake up in the middle of the night with terrible nightmares, feeling a sense of mutilation. So to this day, I still sleep with a bra. If I feel the fullness where my breast should be—if I feel the presence of two breasts—I feel whole.

I did a Rorschach test with my therapist about a year after the mastectomy. One of the main things they saw in it was imbalance. The mastectomy did something so incredible to my head as to make me *imbalanced!*

●

I think *daily* that if I had known how it was

Radical Surgery Is Questioned In New Study of Breast Cancer

N.Y. TIMES 1/29/79

A biologist who has been ?
results of follow-up surveys
try and abroad has raised a?
tion of whether radical s?
most effective treatment
the breast.

His conclusion, as summ
Massachusetts Institute ?
where he is a professor
molecular biology, is that
"no more effective than
tive, less mutilating trea?

His study will be ?
Friday's issue of the
American Medical Ass?
scribed in an M.I.T. ?
author, Dr. Maurice
on his findings in a ?

THE NEW YORK TIMES, WEDNESDAY, NOVEMBER 24, 1976

Belief in Limited Breast Surgery Is Supported by Cancer Research

WASHINGTON, D.C., Nov?
various approaches?
ncer continue to s?
sive surgery may ?
dical mastectomy ?
th early breast ca?
hus far the ?
erence ?

...nse. In such high-risk
...xtensive

THE WALL STREET JOURNAL, Monday, Sept. 19, 1977

Breast-Cancer Screening Project Finds Some Women Had Unnecessary Surgery

WALL STREET JOURNAL Staff Reporter

The federal govern-
...plagued breast-
...run into seri-

...be-

that routine screening X rays should be restricted to women 50 year?
those 40 to 49 years ?
used only if the ?
cer or if th?
For ?

...tory of can-
...sters had cancer.
...ted only if they had a his-
...cer. Current National Can-
... are the same for women 40
...tly less restrictive for
...r. Arthur Upton, in-
...d the recommenda-
...rce.

...tion program, a
...ican Cancer So-
...en involved in
...start, som
...a prope
...te an
...gne

IS BREAST SURGERY REALLY NECESSARY

New and Better Breast Cancer Treatments

TODAY: Breast cancer outranks all other forms of cancer in America.

...DAY: Most American breast surgeons perform radical mastectomies.

...erican women are kept in the
...bout cancer treatment.

... must learn the facts
...the decisions.

Many women think a diagnosis of breast cancer carries an automatic sentence of disfigurement or death. Not so. The picture is a lot more hopeful than many commonly held myths would indicate

WOMAN'S DAY/NOVEMBER 1976

viewed 506 an?
cancerous and ?

The unnecessar?
pected finding in a
with the initial contro?
in the project—exposur?
to X ray. Critics have con?
years that there isn't any h?
women under 50 ye?
younger wom?
devel?

TOMOR?

Instead, the only plan
...vate doctors with a rec?
...biopsy in cases where
The ?
...was to turn those women ov?

NEW DAWN

...deal
...nger w?
...arisen
...ded ?
...had detected ?

going to affect me, I don't know if I would have had a mastectomy. But if I had said no, I don't know whether I would have lived or not.

Every time I take my clothes off and look at myself, I get very angry. The whole area is so painful that I still can't really touch it yet—neither the skin nor under the arm. They have to find another way to solve this for women—a better way, a less mutilating way. They can't keep on doing this to women and saying that it's normal and it's okay, because it's a horrible, nightmarish thing. It's a castration!

I've heard that if they leave the muscles, there is a way they can reconstruct the breast. A female surgeon whom I've spoken to believes that during the operation they could scoop out all the tissue inside the breast, leaving the nipple and the outer skin, and then just put a silicone sheath underneath. They are also experimenting with taking part of the other breast and implanting it so it would be actual breast tissue, which is much safer.

One of the things that infuriates me about the mastectomy is that so much of my muscle was removed. Since I have recently considered the possibility of having breast reconstruction, that really is a problem. If they don't remove the muscle, it is possible to lift and stretch the skin and then put the implant in, but in my case it would be extremely complicated. If I knew before as much as I know now, I would *never* have let them take my muscle out—*never!*

I'm *still* trying to straighten out exactly what happened to me. I have seen all my medical reports, but they are very conflicting. Certain things were told to my brother-in-law, but *other* things were written on my final medical reports. So . . .

If only the original surgeon had removed both lumps in the first place 'way back in September. . . . I am suing him for malpractice, for not removing the lump that was on the inside. Had it been done then, the cancer probably wouldn't have spread, and I wouldn't have been forced to have a radical.

●

For two years after the operation, I couldn't do my film work. Psychologically I couldn't deal with nudity and sexuality. But recently I did some camera work on someone else's film. We were filming a wild party scene where one woman gets very drunk and takes off her shirt and dances. As I was filming her I couldn't help but focus on her breasts, wherever she danced, whatever she did.

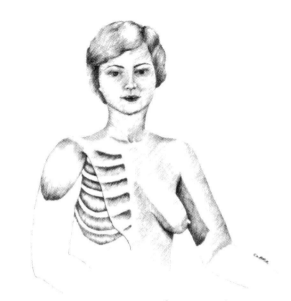

RADICAL MASTECTOMY: *this operation removes the breast, the entire pectoral muscle and the armpit nodes. Swelling of the arm and restriction of movement must be treated after surgery. The lungs remain vulnerable throughout life.*

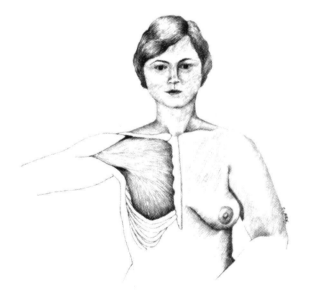

PECTORAL MUSCLES *provide support for the breasts and are necessary for many arm movements.*

Perhaps, soon, when I get stronger I'll try to make another film about beautiful, poetic lovemaking.

Nakedness is very beautiful because the human body is beautiful. That goes back to what the Greeks believed. But Americans are so hung up about nudity and sex that they think the human body is sinful and shouldn't be enjoyed and that's so perverted! I don't know . . . but maybe, in some way, *that's* the origin of this whole obsession with chopping women's breasts off as if it was some holy mission!

●

Almost two years after the interview took place, Helen was contacted for a follow-up statement about why she would not be photographed:

I didn't want to be photographed because the way I cope with life, the way I survive at all, is by just denying the mastectomy. I get dressed every day, and I *always* wear the form [prosthesis], which is really (pause) . . . a denial of it. You know, I avoid touching myself or even *looking* at myself. I *can't* look at myself! And since *I* can't look at myself, then obviously looking at a published photograph of myself would just be a constant reminder. I couldn't bear it! It would be too painful!

When you're living in the daily moment, you really tune out and pretend you feel you're normal. You have to, otherwise. . . .

Recently at a cocktail party, I met a man who told me he had a male mastectomy. He said, "Well, I guess you know how I feel." So I said, "How did you know about *me?*" And he said, "Oh, *everybody* knows about you!" That felt like cold water thrown in my face. I said, "Oh, geez!" and then started laughing nervously. He broke my balloon . . . which is to pretend.

Then he said, "Oh, I can't stand it—this hole in my chest." He told me it has affected his sex life and he's *self-conscious!* Here's a *man* telling me all the same things . . . it was really strange.

The mastectomy *still* affects my life in all the ways I talked to you about—my eroticism, my personal life. Now I'm more used to it 'cause of the time that has passed. I feel that I've come a bit more to terms with living without *sex!* Without a lover! Without being in love! And it's more true now than ever. Maybe I'm better off. (*Laughs.*) Men are difficult. And you're really better off by yourself . . . but what a way to find out! Being alone is still not something I would choose.

The man that I was seeing after I had the operation . . . we're not lovers anymore, just friends.

When we were lovers, it was very difficult. Making love just made me more aware of the mastectomy. No sooner do you make love, then you become aware of your mutilation. So without sex I can still deny the mastectomy.

Aside from the fact that I have no personal life, no love life, the rest of my life is okay. (*Laughs.*)

How does one live with no "personal" life? It sounds so bizarre!

It does . . . I know. I'm sorry to sound so sad and depressed about the mastectomy. I would love to give you a big, wonderful "happy ending" story, but I can't help it, I *hate* it!

There's no way I'll *ever* come to terms with the mastectomy. It's an *abnormal* thing, so why should I? I really hated it then, and I *still* hate it! I can't *force* myself to overcome the mastectomy. Reconstructive plastic surgery would probably be the best thing for me, because of a lot of things that run deep inside me about my body and my self-image. But I don't have the money, and I won't *ever* have the money unless I win this malpractice case.

I can't see myself coming to terms with the mastectomy any other way. I can't ever really be . . . what's the word? . . . *Naked!* I can never be naked again unless I have some kind of reconstruction. It's my only hope. I'm too wrapped up in the image of who I . . . was.

●

I remember that during the interview I was able to communicate with you—I was able to really open up and tell you what I was feeling and going through. That is something I was not able to do with any of my peers, only with my therapist.

Unfortunately, the mastectomy is not something I can go around and be open about *and* be accepted. On the contrary, I better keep it a secret as best I can. I have to actually seem stronger than I was before . . . and better than I was before. I'm *constantly* being *tested!* So I can't say how I really feel . . . to *anybody!* It'll soon be five years. . . .

When Helen was first approached over the telephone about doing the interview for the book, she immediately said yes and then began to pour out her experiences with her mastectomy. Her urgency made it clear that she really needed to share her traumatic experience and unburden herself. I felt badly interrupting her on the telephone to say that we should save it for the interview. It is tragic that Helen has found that she must keep her mastectomy a secret.

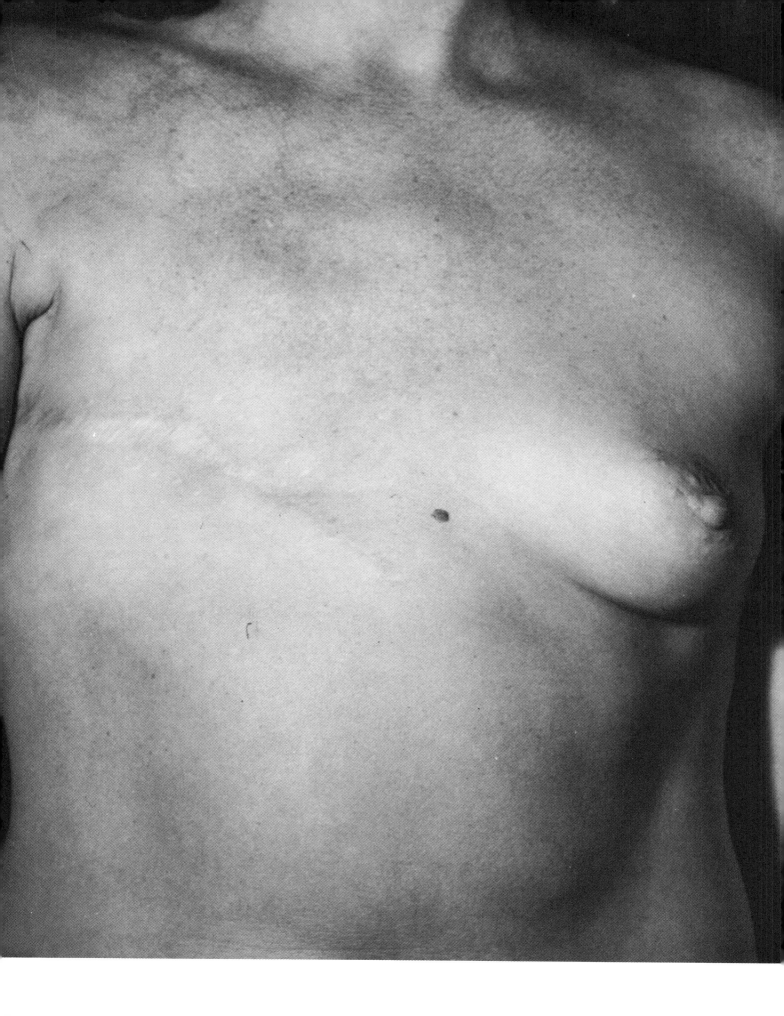

Elizabeth

Age 42 · British · Anthropologist

I tell people quite openly that I have lost a breast, partially for the educational value for them, and partially because I think women should make people aware that one breast more or less isn't going to make or break them as a woman! That's not where they are invested as a person.

I also think that women can take something negative and turn it into something positive for themselves, if they will recognize their strength to do it. It is inside you. You're the one who has to transform it and transcend it; no one else can do it for you. You can use it as a positive influence in your life. And this isn't just true about a mastectomy; it is true about any potentially negative experience you confront.

The first memory I have of my breasts was when we lived in Egypt—I was thirteen. We had during that time a houseboy and one day he picked me up from behind, with his hands over my breasts, just to lift me over something. I had a tremendous reaction to it, and I complained to my parents that he had touched my breasts. They wisely said, "Oh, well, I'm sure it was quite by accident." *He* probably didn't even realize that I had any breasts to touch, but *I* was very aware of it.

I never went through the same teenage syndrome as people in this country did because the English community was different. The emphasis was on keeping girls young, not having them grow up fast. I think that's good because kids should have time to be just kids. I never really thought about my breasts while they were developing.

I used to sunbathe in the nude all the time if no men were around. I thought of my body as a whole and I loved being in the nude. In one place where we lived we had a beach miles and miles long for ourselves, so I was always in the nude, even around my father who went nude around us. Since then, I have been a confirmed nudist all my life.

I don't know whether I was rationalizing or not, but I've always been glad that I didn't have large breasts. It would've made all the different things that I've done, like horseback riding, so difficult.

After I finished studying anthropology in university, I went to Mexico. I lived in the jungle with a tribe of Indians which was becoming extinct—quite an experience at the age of nineteen. The entire time I was there, I never wore a bra because of the oppressive heat. Had I been large-breasted I couldn't have done that. This was twenty-three years ago and it was very daring not to wear a bra then. I was a hippie long before the word was ever invented.

My breasts were never large enough to attract a man's attention to me sexually, until I was old enough for him to be attracted to all of me, if you know what I mean. I was fond of my breasts. I would have liked them to be a little larger for aesthetic reasons. I didn't like the idea of being out of proportion on top, but I was not in the least obsessed with it. Never having considered myself a raving beauty, I always depended more on my personality and intellect and warmth in attracting men to me. I always thought of myself as a person first and a woman second. I had a good strong body, with which I used to climb mountains and go swimming, but I was never into the sexual aspects of my body alone. If a man didn't want my body simply as a good human instrument—forget it! This attitude was a big help when I had the mastectomy, because I did not have a large emotional investment in my breasts.

How did you discover that you had breast cancer?

It was a cold December day. I was standing naked in the bathroom waiting for the water to run into the bath. I stood with my hands sort of tucked under my arms and over my breasts, and I felt a lump on the side of my right breast. I thought, Huh—that's strange. I had a friend who was dying of breast cancer so I thought, Oh, my God! When my husband came home a little later, I said, "Will you please touch me and see if you feel anything?" He said, "Yes, I do," so I was on my doctor's doorstep at nine o'clock the next morning. He told me he was fairly sure that it was malignant and that I would have to have it operated on. This was seven years ago, just before Christmas. I was thirty-five.

He sent me to a young doctor who gave me a very rough examination. My breast hurt for days afterward. He is probably very, very bright, but he was also the sort of doctor who pats you on the head and says, "Everything will be fine, don't ask me any questions, I'll take care of it all." I told him that I didn't like that attitude. It was *my* body and *my* breast, and I wanted to know *everything* that was going on. He said no, I should leave everything up to him. So I decided that I was not going to have him as my surgeon.

I wrote him a letter and explained very explicitly that I had a *right* to know what was going on. That if it was cancer I wanted to know what stage it was in, and if I was likely to die, I wanted to know that, too! He wrote back and said something about how they had found that it wasn't good for patients to know too much about their illnesses because they imagined things and they didn't have the training to interpret them, and this and that, and I thought, Bullshit!

I set out determinedly to find a cooperative surgeon. This was long before women's lib began to influence medical practice. I had to do it all on my own common sense. After some investigation, I got the name of the head surgeon in a local hospital whom I went to see. He was sixty-five and rather conservative. I just told him straight out that I had a lump that had to be operated on and I knew it might be malignant. I wanted to ask questions and get answers. He hemmed and hawed and harumphed a bit but finally said, "All right." But the bastard decided that if I could be tough, he could be tough, too.

The day before Christmas they operated and removed the tumor, not the entire breast. I wouldn't sign for the whole mastectomy because I wanted to make sure that it was necessary. I wanted the biopsy first. The surgeon put a little pressure on me and I said, "Listen! If I don't want to sign, I'm not going to sign—it's *my* breast!" I don't threaten easily!

When I woke up after the operation, the first thing I asked was if it was malignant and nobody would answer. All the nurses would say was, "Oh, you have to speak to your doctor." So I did a little yoga and deep breathing and got myself out from under the anesthetic very quickly. I wanted to go upstairs where my husband was waiting, but they wouldn't let me. The nurses

were all standing around talking about their dates and ignoring me—it was Christmas Eve. Finally I said in a very loud voice, "If I'd known you were going to keep me here so long, I'd have brought a book," which so astounded them that they immediately tried to get the doctor.

Eventually I was sent upstairs, but that damned doctor kept me waiting all the next morning and half the afternoon. At about three o'clock he finally telephoned. I immediately said, "Well, what's the verdict?" And he said, "Not so good." I said, "You mean it was malignant?" And he said, "Yes." I knew I would be operated on the day after if it was malignant, so I said, "All right, see you at seven o'clock tomorrow morning." He hung up.

I was furious at the deliberately cold, brusque way he handled it. He could at least have come and told me *in person!* I decided that if he thought he was going to break me down that way the hell with it. I could be, at least on the surface, just as tough as he was.

Anyway, I spent that Christmas Day in the hospital. My mother called from England and my family called from all over, and everyone was very upset, except me. I just decided, "Well, if it's got to happen, it's got to happen."

There was a bandage over my breast where they had removed the tumor, so I wrote little things on it, like—"Dairy closed for the duration" and "A stitch in time saves nine." I remember the night before the mastectomy I was in the bathtub and I looked at my breasts and I thought, Well, it's the last time you see yourself with two breasts. Good-bye breast.

The next morning when they came to get me for the operation, they couldn't find me! It was 6:30 in the morning and I was doing pushups behind the bed! When they came around and saw me, they said, "What on earth are you doing?" and I said, "I'm getting ready for the operation." (*Laughs.*) I also wanted to see what they were going to do—see the instruments and talk to the doctor—so I took a bath at the crucial moment when they came in to give me the injection to make me sleepy. They couldn't give it to me until I was ready to be wheeled out to the operating room. I was perfectly awake as I'd planned. I sat up on the operating table and asked questions and then finally lay down and said, "Okay, you can give me the Pentothal now."

I tried to be the boss. I've been told that the way I behaved was defensive, and looking back I'm sure it was. But I still think it was a healthy kind of defensiveness, much more so than lying back frightened and letting people do what they wanted.

Meanwhile, I had also found a lump in the other breast, so when I woke up from the mastectomy, the first thing I said was, "Was it one or two?" Thank God the nurse said, "Just one." If the second lump had been malignant, they would have removed both breasts and *that* would have been very hard to take—a double radical would have been hard, psychologically hard. But a single you can live with—no problem.

My husband said something very marvelous to me. "Of all the parts of your anatomy, *that* is probably the most expendable. If I were a woman, I would certainly rather lose a breast than say an arm or a leg or a finger or a toe or an ear or anything," and I thought about that, and he's absolutely right. That was really a wonderful thing to say. He was very supportive and helpful about the entire thing, and very unemotional about it. He said it didn't make any difference to him and that he's not a "breast man," anyway (even though for other reasons we later got divorced).

After five days, I called the doctor and said I wanted to go home tomorrow. He said, "You can't possibly go home for another week." I said, "I'm healed enough," and he said, "You can't be!" I said, "Come and look at me." So the next day he came and he couldn't believe it. He said, "You are as healed as if you had been here for two weeks. I can't think of any reason to keep you," so I got out of the hospital in six days. They had never released anyone in less than *ten.*

It was because I lived on health food. I wouldn't *touch* hospital food. I had my husband bring in all my yogurt and wheat germ and vitamins. Also, I kept the nurses out at night because I opened my windows for fresh air. Since all the nurses were from the West Indies, they weren't about to walk in when it was nineteen degrees out! (*Laughs.*) I slept in my sleeping bag.

I couldn't figure out *why* I got breast cancer because I was always such a health nut. I believe my tumor was probably caused or triggered off by the birth control pill. I had been on them for five years and I was taking too high a dose. Now they use much, *much* lower doses. Also, I wasn't taking them regularly, so I could've upset my pituitary gland. But you see, all this was twelve and fifteen years ago, before we knew very much about the pill. Knowing what I know about them now, I would *never* use them.

I went to stay with my aunt who lives by the sea, and when I came back a month later, my doctor gave me a big song and dance about having cobalt treatments. I said, "They told me there was no implication of the lymph nodes—the cancer had not spread or metastasized—so why should I have cobalt treatments?" He said, "Well, I just think you ought to." This went on for an hour or so. Finally, I said, "If I were your daughter, what would you recommend?" and he said, "I would *insist* that you have cobalt treatments."

From there I went straight to my surgeon's office. He looked at me and said, "Did you hear about your slides?" I said, "What do you mean?" He said, "They had lost two of the slides. They just found them and they showed that two of the lymph nodes were indeed implicated." It *had* metastasized!

Well, my own doctor knew this but hadn't told me, not wanting to scare me. Instead, he just tried to persuade me to have cobalt treatment, without even telling me *why.* When I heard this, I absolutely blew a fuse! I was as angry as I have ever been in my entire life.

I went flying back to the doctor's office and had it out with him. I really gave it to him; I said, "It's *my* body, and *my* operation. You promised to tell me the *truth!* Why the hell did you *lie* to me?" "Well," he said, "I didn't want to hurt you." I said, "You hurt me ten times more by trying to shield me. I'm not a child. If I have to die tomorrow, I can stand the truth and you bloody well tell me!"

He was so upset that finally I said, "All right, I forgive you, but don't you *ever* do that again." And as I walked out the door, he said, "You know, people like you belong in the jungle." So I turned, looked at him, and said, "Well, remember I used to live in the jungle!" And I stalked out. Oh, I was angry!

So I went and had the cobalt treatment. It made me feel weak and miserable, and then I got a reaction. The lining around the outside of my spinal cord swelled up a little, and every time I put my head forward, I'd get a tingling, dizzy feeling. The treatments only lasted for three weeks, but the reaction went on for almost a *year!* Finally, I got over it but I never quite had the energy that I had before.

Meanwhile, my friend who also had breast cancer died. She didn't do anything about it, so by the time she finally went to the doctor, she had an open sore and she was riddled with cancer. Cancer is nothing to play around with. I have been involved with different types of nontraditional healing practices, but I would still prefer to be pretty conservative about treating cancer.

At the time when I had my mastectomy, there was no sanctioned medical procedure other than the radical. Given the fact that my tumor was in the upper-outer quadrant of the breast, today I would probably not have to have a radical with removal of all the muscles underneath the breasts, but only the breast itself. It's too late to feel sorry about that now.

As I began to live with my mastectomy, I learned what it's like to live without lymph nodes. The circulation of fluid in the affected arm is impaired and there is a tendency for the arm to swell. I always have trouble finding dresses with wide enough sleeves to protect my arm.

God, I'll never forget . . . a year after I had the mastectomy I went to get a flu shot. They gave it to me in my right arm but I should never, *ever* have an injection in my right arm. That damned flu shot made my arm swell up for three weeks, and the silly bastards—they never *told me!* My arm is in a permanently swollen and fragile condition and will be for the rest of my life. A sunburn or even a wasp sting can be so dangerous that I could lose my arm!

●

I will never forget the one night I broke down and panicked. For five days I lay there waiting for the lab reports to come back, not knowing how much it had spread—whether I had three months to live or fifty years.

I had to face my own death and overcome my fear of it in a few short days. That's something you rarely are called upon to face when you are thirty-five. I had to think through many things and it was a very, very intense experience. It wasn't very pleasant at the time, but it really brought out the best in me. It brought out the strength. Unfortunately, one never learns very much from happiness; one learns much more from pain. To lose a breast *has* to have a very big effect on your life, but for me it has had a very positive effect.

Looking back, I have always been grateful that it happened when I was thirty-five, and not when I was sixty-five, because it has given me a chance to apply what I learned to my life.

If I had the mastectomy at sixty-five, when most of my life had been lived, by then I might be insecure about my aging body and the operation might have turned me off men. But at thirty-five, I still had enough physical beauty in my body and a secure sense of self to counteract this feeling, so that now aging will bother me less than it would have otherwise.

Because of the mastectomy, I always cut myself off from emotion slightly when I meet a man until I know how he is going to react. I just casually in conversation bring out the fact that I had breast cancer—"I had a breast removed." If they are frightened, they have the option to veer off. It's very interesting because it has never made anybody shy away.

I have had many lovers since then, and I mean *lots!* It's made no difference in our relationships. If anything, it's caused men to love me more and with more tenderness because they feel that I have suffered, and that has been a revelation to me. It's even given me *more* self-confidence, because if a man can feel that way about me in spite of . . . well, he is obviously not just relating to me for my beautiful body, so I must be some special person.

●

In the summertime, I used to go with a group of my friends to the top of a mountain to a big lake where everyone swims in the nude. Six months after the operation it was summertime again and I was faced with this dilemma—what on earth was I going to do? After thrashing it around, I decided that I wasn't going to go through my life hiding, since I always loved to run around in the nude before.

So, I went up there with several friends and it was *very* difficult, but I took off my clothes and went swimming like I'd always done. It was really hard! None of my friends made any remarks, though I could see they were looking. I just braced myself. I realized that they had a very natural curiosity that I would have had also. Well, let them look, I thought.

Anyway, I don't think mine is so shocking because I have seen one other woman who's had a mastectomy. That's when I realized how lucky I am, because my scar is not at all disfiguring. Every time a doctor sees me, he says, "Wow, they did a really good job on you."

I'm the only woman in my entire health club —and there are hundreds and hundreds of women there—who has had a mastectomy. You know, I just walk around with nothing on and I don't pay any attention. It is really amazing.

You can control the way other people react by your own reactions, and since I am completely normal and natural and unselfconscious about my mastectomy, once people get over the shock, they respond that way, too. They see that I am not tense and so they feel there is no need for them to be. Another very interesting response has been that a couple of women with whom I have become friendly there have said to me that initially they didn't notice—standing right in front of me and talking to me—that I have a mastectomy! It's true because another time I mentioned it to a woman there and she looked at me in shock and exclaimed, "My God, I never noticed!" *That is a triumph of mind over matter!*

●

One thing that I wanted to mention is my brief experience with group sex which was quite something for me. At first I was pretty nervous about it, to put it mildly. Just to get into a room full of people and take off all your clothes when you have had a mastectomy is not easy, believe me, particularly when you are there basically for sexual purposes! (*Laughs.*)

The only bad reaction I ever had was with a guy who wasn't prepared for it—he was very young, early twenties. After a few minutes, when he realized, he was absolutely startled. He got up, went away, and didn't come back. I knew why and it didn't upset me very much at all. I felt sorrier for him and for the upset that he felt and the guilt he would probably feel afterward.

Every single person I talked to—male and female—said they were so turned on by my courage that they came over to meet me. The special attention didn't bother me at all, because they did it in such a nice way—like, "Wow, who are *you?* I think you are great!" How can you be embittered by that? Mind over matter again. I am probably one of the only women with a mastectomy who has done that, and it absolutely amazes people.

Before the mastectomy I was never particularly sexually oriented toward my breasts. In fact, if a man stroked my breasts thinking it turned me on, it sometimes annoyed me. Some men don't know when it's *enough!* But since I didn't have much for them to get hung up about, they usually turned to greener pastures! (*Laughs.*)

However, now, if a man strokes my breast, psychologically I appreciate it if he will stroke both sides. I am quite aware if he avoids the bony side and strokes only the other. I like being stroked—I think I'm half cat—and when it feels nice, I purr.

●

I have a friend who has quite large breasts and she *loves* them! Men have always responded to them and this and that, and she has often told me that if she found out she had cancer, she'd rather *die* than have her breast removed. To me that's ridiculous, but since then I have often wondered whether the mastectomy would have been more difficult for me psychologically if I had had larger breasts.

Another advantage of being small-breasted is that I am not too off balance with only one breast. I don't wear a prosthesis in the normal sense of the word. I simply use a pad—a falsie. For women who have heavy breasts, losing one often changes their posture and the whole weight tension of the body. Fortunately that has never been a problem for me.

Lately, I've been thinking about a silicone implant because my mother sent me an article about breast reconstruction. I've been seriously toying with the idea. I think I have strengthened my character enough, and if I could have the breast back it would just be nice. For one thing, I would love to go braless again. I mean—damn it!—all the years when I was brave enough to go without a bra when people weren't, and now that I could very easily, and I *love to*, it really is difficult. It's not that I would feel self-conscious, but I am afraid that *other* people will if I go braless with only one breast. My main reason for wearing a bra is that I don't want to make people uncomfortable.

If people see that you have lost an arm or a leg or that you're an albino or whatever, it makes them uncomfortable. As an anthropologist, I can say this is apparently just an innate trait in human nature. It is true all over the world, so I alone am not going to change it. There are some battles you can fight and some you can't. I don't think this is one that can be won because people just naturally recoil at abnormality.

Last summer, for the first time in my life I went to a nudist camp. There was another woman there who had had a mastectomy. When she saw me she came over to me and greeted me like a sister. I thought, Wow, somebody else has the courage to come out in public! Interestingly enough, I was a little *uncomfortable* looking at her. Strange. I'm used to my own body, but I wasn't used to hers. Just seeing someone mutilated. And her remaining breast was larger, too, so it was more noticeable. She was very warm and relaxed, which I thought was great, but I was so surprised at my own reaction. . . .

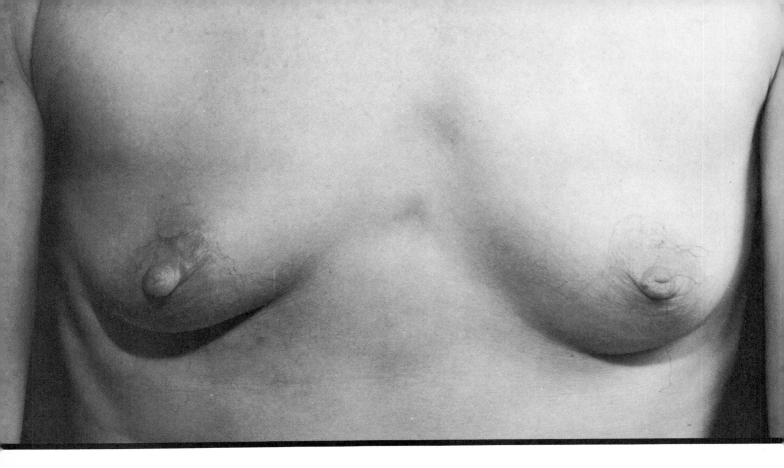

Vivian

Age 40 · Raised in New Orleans · Mother of one

I had one experience that really colored my attitude toward my breasts for most of my life. At the time that my breasts were developing, my godmother worked during the day and my godfather, who was a seaman, was at home. A couple of times, when I was dusting in the living room or something, he cornered me and started molesting me. He felt my breasts, which were really tiny little things then, and he kissed them and used his tongue, and my nipples got hard. That just scared the daylights out of me! I thought my nipples would never go back! Of course they did and I was very relieved, but the whole thing was really terrifying and disgusting to me. I didn't know what the hell to do about it, so I just tolerated it until I could get away.

I think that experience really affected how I felt about my breasts and particularly about anybody touching them. The first young woman that I ever fell in love with was more experienced sexually than I was, and when she touched and kissed my breasts, it produced such an anxiety in me that I wasn't able to enjoy it. It felt almost unbearable.

Later, when I was older, one advantage of my butch image [male role-playing] was that nobody could touch me, so I didn't have to deal with my breasts at all—it was as if I didn't have them. Even years later, after I dropped the butch role, I didn't really want anybody to touch my breasts.

I don't think I was breast-fed because I can remember being in a crib and having a bottle. My mother died when I was nine so I never got to ask her a lot of questions. After that I was in a bad situation emotionally.

I was very isolated, and even though I lived with a godmother who took me in, I was like a poor relation or something. I didn't feel wanted or even that I belonged. I was like a piece of baggage lying around. I mostly went unnoticed except whenever I did something that I was not supposed to. I spent a lot of time by myself, playing in the back shed with my chemistry set or carving wooden doll furniture.

I went "topless" until I was ten or eleven, and one day, long before I began to develop, putting on a shirt became a rule. I was outside in front of the house and my godmother said, "You shouldn't be out here without a top on, so you better go in and put one on." I was embarrassed and frustrated at the same time because it didn't make sense. I loved running around without a shirt and I resented the fact that I couldn't do that anymore. It was a hell of a lot to give up.

I was very angry and resentful that I was a girl. Whenever being a girl was called to my attention I hated it! So I never thought about when I was going to get breasts.

My first awareness of my breasts was when I was riding my bicycle. There was some movement on my chest that I had never noticed before. It was uncomfortable and I didn't like it. After that, I was aware of my breasts whenever I engaged in sports activities. I observed them developing with distaste and I just thought they were a hindrance and a nuisance.

My brother used to punch me in my breasts when we fought. I was always able to beat him up, but now he knew that it was a vulnerable place, so he deliberately aimed for my breasts. In my family it was believed that a blow or a bruise could develop into a cancer. That was one hell of a reason not to get hit in the breast! So I saw breasts as a liability, a vulnerable part of being a woman.

Even before I was an adolescent I had a thing about Amazons. They were communities of women where men took care of the babies and the Amazon women did the hunting and everything, and that really excited my imagination. I knew that Amazons had one of their breasts removed to make it easier to use a bow and arrow. I even used to fantasize that *I* would have a breast removed.

At thirteen, when I finally reached my mature breast development, I was glad that it wasn't worse. I don't think I've developed any more since. I always used to feel lucky that I didn't have large breasts because I didn't like them. I was happy that I had a very androgynous build and I was able to pass as a boy because I was slim-hipped and flat-chested. I've often thought that I controlled the way my body developed by my attitude—that's quite possible.

The only time I would have preferred to have larger breasts just like everybody else's was in school so that I would fit in. In fact, very often on the days we were going to have gym classes, I was so embarrassed that I skipped school. I was curious about how other girls developed but I didn't allow myself to look at them in the locker room because, since I felt more like a boy, I was afraid of how I might react. Looking made me feel like a peeping Tom, so I just kept my eyes glued to the ceiling!

●

In my early teens, a bus that I often rode went through the French Quarter down Bourbon Street, which is really just one long string of strip joints. I had a lot of fantasies about the strippers then—about seductive things that a woman might do and how exciting and beautiful it would be and she'd be doing it just for me. I used to sit in the bus and try to peek in the doors and see the strippers.

When I was about fourteen I tried to go through the motions of dating for a while. Mostly I was trying to fit in, but it was horrible and I never let boys touch my breasts or anything.

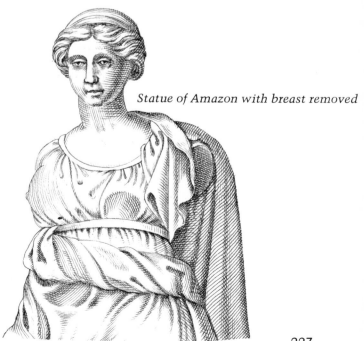

Statue of Amazon with breast removed

Once I decided I was a lesbian, I put pinups of nudes all over my room. I had Rita Hayworth and all those women, and at that time I definitely had an idea about the size of breasts I liked. I remember thinking that Jane Russell's breasts were bigger than I wanted to deal with—breasts that big were a little scary.

While I was living with my godparents, I had to live according to their expectations. Being a lesbian, I had to conceal a lot of things from them. I was terribly isolated. There was nobody in our community that I could talk to, so I started searching for people elsewhere.

I hung out at gay bars a lot. When I was fifteen, a bar I was in was raided by the police and the juveniles were arrested. The next day our names were on the front page of the local paper. I had a huge confrontation at home and had to leave, so I ended up living in the French Quarter.

It was quite a bizarre underworld. There were gay people and people into drugs, gambling, and prostitution. Many of the women in the bars made their living through prostitution, and because I had a Catholic upbringing I felt that wasn't right. But now I was a reject and outcast anyway, and there was an entirely different value system operating in the society I found myself in.

I got into a relationship with a woman who was a lot older than I. She had money and I had none, so I was very dependent on her. She was a little bit sadistic and, since I was just a teenager, she put me through a lot of emotional trips. If she got angry at me, she threw me out and I'd have no place to stay.

The only way for a butch to keep herself alive then was tending a gay bar or doing something illegal like selling drugs, theft, pimping, or prostitution. I kept finding myself broke with no place to stay so I got into a certain kind of prostitution—what they call "shows," where two women perform a sex act for a group of men to watch. I had to do whatever I could to make money.

I began to really bristle about the fact that I didn't have any control over my life. One day I had an argument with my lover and I found myself on the street and broke. Then some guy propositioned me; he offered me twenty dollars and I went. I thought that since I'd never been in bed with a man before, now I'd see what it was like. The man realized this and that just increased his sadistic pleasure. He was a very insensitive pig— really brutal. It was so fuckin' unpleasant, I never went with a man again!

I didn't realize I was pregnant for over three months. I was really a kid—seventeen—and I

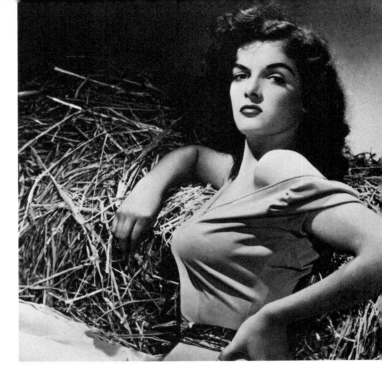

didn't even think ahead to the next week, so I wound up having a baby.

I often wonder if the police harassment of the French Quarter hadn't been so great at the time, just *what* would have happened to me? Fortunately, when I was still pregnant, a woman that I knew was found by her father through the Missing Persons Bureau because of a prostitution arrest. He took us both off to a wholesome life in Texas and my whole life changed. I discovered a few things that I didn't know anything about— books, music, everything! I didn't know about all those things and I started to find out.

●

After my daughter was born, I announced to the doctor that I didn't want to breast-feed. Somehow I couldn't envision myself having a baby nursing at my breast. I just couldn't see myself in that much of a woman's role.

From the time my daughter was five until quite recently, I held straight jobs and I wore padded bras. There were very few compromises in dress and appearance that I was willing to make, but that was one of them. It took me a long time to force myself to wear stockings and I *never* shaved my legs! I really looked funny! I had a short, masculine-looking haircut à la Tony Curtis, when there weren't any other women around like that, and I wore the most severely tailored clothes that I could get, and yeah (*laughs*) . . . padded bras.

I had a funny experience once, closing my padded bra—the one I was *wearing*—in the file cabinet without realizing it! Somebody was standing there and they just gawked! (*Laughs.*) Actually it was very embarrassing at the time.

As a butch, if I'd had larger breasts I don't know what I would have done, because butches don't like to admit they have breasts. I know that binding isn't good for your breasts, and I've only seen one woman whose breasts were bound. I was staying at this woman's house and she undressed in my presence. She took off her shirt and she had ace bandages wrapped tightly around her chest. When she unwrapped herself, her breasts just *fell* down to her stomach! They didn't relate to the rest of her body at all. I assumed that binding her large breasts so tightly on a regular basis had broken down all the tissues that would normally hold the breasts farther up. She was quite young. It was very horrifying to me.

●

For most of my life I never wanted anybody to see my breasts—particularly women. At one time I lived communally with many gay men around, and I would go into the shower with any of them, but never with the women. I thought the men would not view my body as a sex object, so I felt comfortable, but I was afraid the women might be critical of how my body looked.

When I was younger, reading all that garbage written by men about what lesbians were "supposed" to be and how they "behaved" gave me the whole idea about role-playing—being butch—and other ideas about lesbians being "sexual creatures." That's all a sexist perversion which I've since outgrown, but then, if you took your clothes off in front of a lesbian, it automatically meant something *sexual.* So my tendencies toward modesty were even more exaggerated.

I realized when I was raising my daughter that my supermodesty would be inhibiting to her, and I decided that I *had* to get over it. More than anything else, I did not want to transmit a lot of uptight feelings to my daughter. So if she walked into my room while I was dressing, it took all my nerve not to register that this was upsetting me. But by forcing myself I gradually got over my modesty.

●

For most of my life, I made love with my underwear on—my undershirt and pants—and that was a very strong message to my lovers that I had no intention of being touched in all those "female parts." They kidded me about that and sometimes, if I trusted them enough, I would take my undershirt off. But if they tried to touch my breasts I just said, "Don't!" and my undershirt went right back on.

I somehow felt that if I were sexually abandoned the other person would have control over me. I had tremendous anxiety about letting anybody have that much control, so I just didn't let myself go. I didn't get much real sexual satisfaction and I suppose that's the greatest sexual crime.

Recently, through consciousness raising, I've discovered sexual pleasure in my breasts and that amazes me! It's very related to a new feeling of surrender. It has been fantastic. Sometimes, when my breasts are gently sucked on, I experience a feeling of being gentle and tender and nurturing, which I guess you could call "maternal." It's a feeling of giving—giving your body—and it feels so good.

●

I think my breasts fit the rest of my body. Any other kind would look damned silly! They're soft and small, like a couple of fried eggs sunny-side up. I'm at the age where I am losing some skin tone and maybe my breasts sag a little bit more than they did, but even if they sagged forever they wouldn't get very far.

I've had hair on my breasts since I was an adolescent, and at the time I was confused about it. I liked it all right, and that might have had to do with my male-identified image—that "I have hair on my chest." But I also thought it was a sign that there was something *wrong* with me. I like my hair now!

It's been a struggle for many years, but I've finally come to feel good about my breasts. Until recently, every time spring came along and I could no longer wear a jacket to cover my breasts, I always felt vulnerable out on the street. I couldn't go out in a T-shirt because then my breasts would show and I couldn't pass as a boy. I wore sport shirts so that no one could detect I was a woman. But finally one summer I decided I was going to wear a T-shirt and I didn't care if my breasts showed. I wasn't going to be confined any longer and I wouldn't be ashamed either. It was a hard thing for me to do, but I *did* it!

I remember that day walking through the park and there was quite a breeze. The wind blew the shirt against my chest and I knew that my breasts were really showing, you know. I knew that somebody—*everybody*—could really see that I had *breasts!* I was elated! I had it all linked up with my new sense of being—discovering pride in being a woman—and I felt that my breasts are my badge that I am a woman and I'm proud of that. That was a joyful feeling.

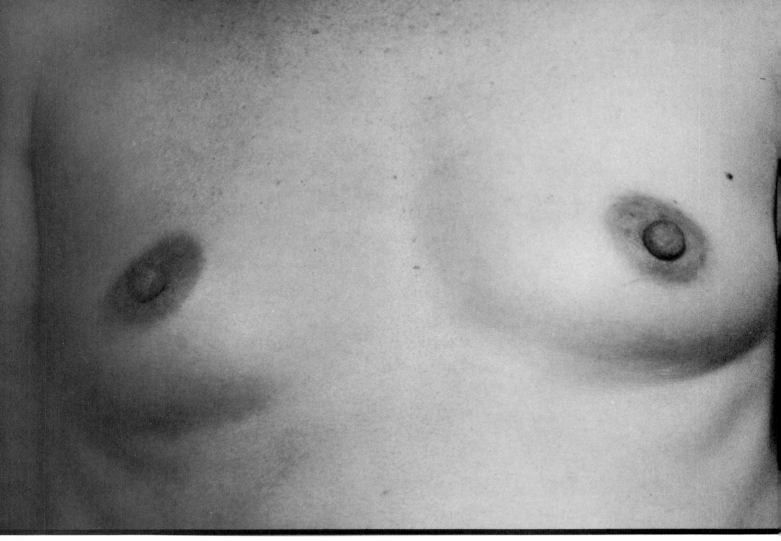

Christine *Age 41 · Raised in Appalachia (Ohio) · Medical Writer*

I think in a certain way my breasts probably saved my ass! Really! For all the self-consciousness that went along with adolescence, and for all the disappointment and inadequacy that I felt then, I think my breasts quite literally saved my life.

I recently attended the twenty-five-year reunion of my high-school graduating class. I saw what happened to those girls who had beautiful breasts. I know what became of their lives . . . and what their breasts and the emphasis placed on their breasts did to them. It made them small-minded, small-town housewives for a lifetime! If I had been a 34B, I'd probably be where they are now. It's peculiar—all the high-school cheerleaders, all the really busty girls . . . it was like a sentence to prison! That's what it really was! At sixteen I couldn't see it. . . . I can see it now.

I come from a *very* rural town on the West Virginia border. I'm an escaped hillbilly! My family goes back to pre-Revolutionary America, but I'm

hardly what you'd call a Daughter of the American Revolution, not by a long shot. My parents are Fundamentalists, and my father is the chair-

230

man of the Gideon Bible Society and teaches Sunday school and all that.

Mine was not a family that ever talked about any aspect of sexuality. My parents' way of dealing with the whole issue was to leave books lying around in conspicuous places. I was warned not to take candy from strangers and that men were all beasts at heart, but sex was never actually *talked* about. Even so, when you live in a rural area you are *surrounded* by the evidence of sexuality—cows, horses, cats, dogs—so you just automatically *know*.

My breasts began to grow at the same time I got my period, but it was *considerably* overshadowed by the *idea* of getting my period, which *infuriated* me! I was something of a tomboy—an absolutely wild-assed tomboy! It was *impossible* to get me down out of the trees or off the backs of horses. I was outdoors all the time. And what happened when I hit puberty was the most abrupt turnaround in everybody's attitude toward me. No more horseback riding, hiking in the woods, climbing trees and fences! No more fighting with kids! And I was a *notorious* fighter! I was also far and away the brightest student in the class, and my mother started saying subtle things to me like, "Don't contradict the boys in class or you won't be popular."

All of a sudden it was as if everybody who looked at me no longer saw a growing kid. They saw this potential woman—at twelve years old, no less—and they bombarded me with all this *woman* shit! But they were too late, because I wasn't buying it then and I've never bought it since. My mother has *very* feminine attitudes and when she looked at *me* she thought, What hath God wrought? and I looked back at her the same way.

I was very, *very* self-conscious about my breast development. When everybody else was developing, I earned the nickname of "Buttons" among my friends. You can imagine how much I loved that.

I went through a period where I did the round-shouldered bit, but my grandmother—may she rest in peace—was a feminist with an *arrest* record! When she saw me getting round-shouldered, she made me parade up and down the stairs and around the house with books on my head holding a yardstick stuck behind my back through my elbows! She *straightened* me out in no time. My grandmother was the great heroine of my life.

I read like a bandit—*everything* I could get my hands on—so I knew there was a normal varia-

tion in breasts and I just assumed that mine would develop later. But they *never* did! In all the reading I did, noboby ever mentioned that it was also *normal* not to get beyond a certain size. The Sears, Roebuck catalog listed A-cup bras as *small,* B-cup bras as *medium,* and C-cup bras as *average.* Now I never! Can you imagine a C cup as *average?* Well, that's what they said—I guess they were too used to *cows!* Since I never got anywhere near an A at all, I felt that I was quite far off the norm.

It got to the point where I was so neurotic about it that I used to quietly weep. My mother found me crying one day and I said to her, "You know, if I just was *sure* I was normal . . . if I just was *sure* that there wasn't something the matter with me!" And she said, "Of course, you're normal. I'm flat-chested and your grandmother was also flat-chested and we all nursed our children. It just runs in the family. As you get older I am sure they'll develop more."

I was so upset that she took me to the family doctor who was very understanding. He examined me and explained to me that I didn't have fatty deposits in that area as most women do. He said, "It doesn't run in your family. There is a lot of difference among ladies, and maybe when you're older your breasts will develop a little bit more, but you will never be a busty woman." I kept waiting and waiting. I'm forty-one and my breasts haven't *budged!* They never developed beyond the age of twelve.

I wanted to have a narrow waist and fairly narrow hips with little hipbones showing like the women in *Vogue* did. Most of all I wanted a pair of high breasts—not overdeveloped but about a 34B cup—you know, visible breasts. The kind that you could wear a horseshoe neckline with. As a matter of fact, I would have settled for cleavage! (*Laughs.*)

I knew that none of those miracle three-day developers or any of that shit worked. I've since met a lot of women who used them and got very frustrated while Mark Eden got very rich! But I did

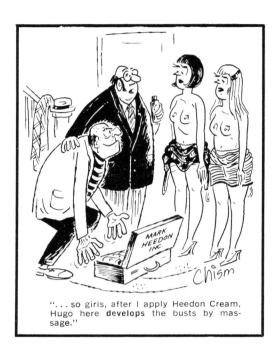

"... so girls, after I apply Heedon Cream, Hugo here **develops** the busts by massage."

exercises upon exercises upon exercises!! I went through life doing this exercise where you put your hands together and *pull*, you know ... but those exercises depend on moving weight around, and you can't move weight when you haven't got it. So I gave up on that.

Then I decided that my breasts were a reflection of my whole weight problem, because I was terrifically thin—at five feet ten and one hundred eighteen pounds. So in high school, I went through a period when I was consuming—and keeping track of my intake—about five thousand calories a day, including food supplement beaten up with eggs and whipping cream. I was downing it like crazy because I thought that if I put on weight I'd develop breasts. Nothing on earth could put weight on me! I never weighed more than a hundred twenty pounds until I was thirty-three years old.

Being flat-chested was, to put it mildly, a source of *real* aggravation. In the first place, I grew up during the Marilyn Monroe era when everyone wore bras with points. I wore Hidden Treasure bras which were as hard as *rocks!* The padded bras available in those days were very obviously padded, and were all the more obvious on

me because I was so skinny.

Of course, I never learned to dance because, you see, if I danced with anyone and they held me close, then they would feel those *goddamned* Hidden Treasures! They felt like cardboard!! I felt very inferior about it right through adolescence. I never went through the petting craze—and never dated at all in high school.

The town that I lived in is a coal mining town and a lot of Italian families settled there. I went to school with a lot of girls who were very early bloomers—the kind of girls who, at fifteen, are absolute *visions* of beauty.

Not only was I flat-chested, but I was also five feet ten; I was a *strange* sight. But I got along beautifully with the boys in high school because they considered me a *buddy.* I don't think any of them *ever* looked at me as a *girl,* which was just as well, you know. Otherwise I would have probably married a lineman for Ohio Power and Light and been sitting in a Sears, Roebuck housedress now, so ... As time goes by we see that our blessings are not always what we think they are.

Being flat-chested had a tremendous effect on every aspect of my life. I *never* dressed in a sexy, seductive way whatsoever. I put myself out of the sexual running entirely. This meant that I didn't play boy-girl games. I didn't act twice as stupid as the boys in class. I didn't attempt to reduce my grades. I concentrated strictly on intellectual development. I automatically assumed that I would go to college and I would earn my own living. I expected to marry eventually, but my primary orientation was not shuffling my feet, batting my eyelashes, pleasing boys, and doing the "let's play stupid and catch a man" ritual. Isn't that what *Seventeen* magazine tells you to do? Well, I had *better* things to do!

It was impossible to be both stylish and flat-chested in the fifties. The clothing was designed entirely different from the way it is now. The darts in the sides of dresses were so *deep!* They were made to accommodate these really big mammary glands. *Holy cow!* Even women of quite normal, adequate bust development very often wore padded bras. Sweaters were so tight they looked like they were *painted* on! Brassieres came to sharp points. Big breasts occasioned comments on the street and were literally the very *definition* of what was feminine. Women were feminine and sexy *directly* in proportion to the *size* of their breasts!

●

I was a virgin until I married my anthropology

instructor. Premarital sex wasn't too usual in those days. You just automatically said no. He did touch my breasts prior to our marriage, but *dressed.* I remember thinking afterward, Since he's aware that I'm quite thin and he finds it very elegant, it's logical to assume he won't expect me to be particularly busty. (*Laughs.*)

And yet, I went stark raving *crazy* trying to find a nightgown for my honeymoon—one that was sexy *without* revealing the breasts. Jesus! It involved about a two-month shopping expedition. I must have looked at five hundred nightgowns before I finally found one that fit the bill. It had an unusual amount of sheer material gathered onto the camisole top so it was somewhat three-dimensional and not transparent on top.

Luckily for me my husband turned out not to be the average *beast* of the fifties. He never mentioned my breasts one way or another in the two and a half years we were married.

It's interesting—I don't think that my lack of breast development has ever caused unpleasant comments, or had any effect on my sex life in either of my marriages or any of my affairs. One

To glorify the natural charm of your beauty zone*

Wear Life Bras

1954

of the men I had an affair with used to have an expression for my breasts which went something like, "A little is sufficient but more than a mouthful is too much." Obviously, a guy who is really a "tit man" wouldn't even glance twice at me.

Are your breasts sexually arousing?

Mmmmm—you betcha! . . . They *really* are! But during my first couple of years of sexual activity, they weren't. In fact, I did not particularly like having my first husband fool around with my breasts—I would move his hand away. But that was really a reflection of the self-consciousness I felt. As time went by, my breasts became very erogenous and they still are.

●

In 1963 I worked in a plastic surgeon's office and part of my job was to read all of his journals, so I had plenty of opportunity to read up on breast enlargement. Basically there have been three procedures. In the original procedure, they inserted a mold made of foam. Unfortunately, the flesh grew into the foam and the breasts became as hard as baseballs!! That was twenty years ago. After that, they tried silicone injections—no good whatsoever! The silicone not only shifted into the wrong places, but if it accidentally got into the bloodstream, it *killed* you. There were many fatalities, so they were stopped. The third procedure, which is still used today, had just been developed then.

It was a breast form made out of a pliable plastic material filled with a silicone gel. They made a half-moon incision in the crease underneath the breast and separated the breast tissue away from the musculature of the chest wall. They inserted the breast form and attached it to the muscles on the chest wall with stitches so that it couldn't shift. Then they replaced the breast tissue over the form, and closed it with a single filament nylon suture, which is finer than a hair and leaves absolutely no scar.

From what I heard they're completely safe. The only danger was if you were accidentally stabbed in the breast or, God forbid, had an accident in which you were thrown through a windshield and perforated the silicone sac.

When I inquired about the operation, I saw a patient who had the implants and I had the opportunity to examine her. Those breasts were normal in appearance in every way—they had normal motion, weight, everything about them. They were just absolutely flawless, and of course they will still be flawless when she is sixty!

At any rate, it would have cost thousands of

dollars then and it just simply wasn't that important to me, not anymore. Had I been able to at age eighteen, I would have done it at the drop of a hat. Over the years I changed enough so that it didn't matter anymore.

What changed my attitude was the discovery that it wasn't as important to the rest of the world as I had thought it would be when I was still growing up. You see, I wasn't a hick from Ohio anymore! I was in a world where women were not judged primarily by the size of their breasts. I had discovered that I was attractive and that men didn't drop *dead* at the sight of me without clothes on. After my divorce, I had several happy affairs in the ten years before my second marriage, each lasting a couple of years. So I just didn't feel that I had a desperate need to prove any points. To hop from bed to bed or go through plastic surgery or anything like that.

To this day, I still wear padded bras and I don't mean fiberfill. I mean real, honest-to-God padded bras! Now they're seamless and unobtrusive and much more in line with what my figure would "normally" be. If anything would ever motivate me to have that plastic surgery, bras would. Bras are just plain uncomfortable and padded bras are *twice* as uncomfortable. In the summertime padded bras are hot, and when you sweat, Goddamn it, they soak up the sweat and there's just nothing like a cold, clammy padded bra. But I wear a bra because I really *need* to.

Aside from the fact that my clothes fit better, the main reason I wear bras is as a conscious preventive measure. For example, if I were to go out on the street without a breast . . . er . . . a bra (that was an interesting Freudian slip!!) I would probably attract some comments. If the comments were unpleasant enough, they would result in assault and battery, because mine is a sharp temper to say the least. I don't go around beating people into the ground, but I'll tell you right now that I've put two grown men in the hospital, being sufficiently motivated. At five feet ten, I can damn well do it!! All I need is for some asshole to make a comment like, "Geez, you don't have any tits at all!" and I *promise* you, they would carry that bastard off on a stretcher!! (*Laughs.*)

So when I walk down a street I want to be as unobtrusive as possible. Without a bra, flat-chested as I am, it would only be a matter of *time!*

●

In the last year or two I have thought my breasts are beautiful—I think that's a part of being over forty. At my age, I'm very glad they've stayed where they belong! They don't droop, sag, or get in my way. I saw what happened to those big, beautiful breasts the girls in my high school *used* to have.

For a long time I was very self-conscious about trying on clothing in open fitting rooms, but lately, after looking around at the other ladies present, I felt that their problems were at *least* equal to mine and I've stopped being self-conscious about it.

On the street last summer, I passed a girl who must have been nineteen or so, and in *every* way she had one of those really beautiful adolescent figures, but I can't say I'd have traded spots with her. It's taken awhile, but now my breasts are something I'm very comfortable with.

I'm sure that this world is absolutely full of beautiful breasts on lots of beautiful people, but as far as an "ideal" breast, that's like saying there is a great American novel . . . or a perfect rose. As I have gotten older, I've come to love and appreciate the varieties of life. In this, I'm with Mao Tse-tung—"Let a thousand flowers bloom."

●

It occurred to me this morning before the interview that in the past eight or nine months that I've been in therapy, the subject of my breasts has *never* come up, though did it *ever* in past therapies years ago. It's as if concern about my breasts has passed into the irrelevant in my life now.

I would *never* have done this interview . . . let's say six years ago. I wouldn't have immediately faded into a shy, "No, no . . . no" sort of thing, I wouldn't have admitted to that, but I would have said, "Nahh . . . what difference does it make?" or "That's *counterproductive*," or whatever. I might have said, "You know, there's been too much emphasis on breasts already and what difference can it possibly make?" I would have found *some* excuse not to do this interview.

I don't think that I had enough awareness six years ago to realize the value of sharing, because *sharing* is precisely one of the things that women have been deprived of. Divide and conquer! Each one has been tucked into her own little kitchen and isolated from other women, and taught that we are *rivals* and *enemies* for no other purpose than to prevent us from sharing and comparing and learning . . . and maybe even rebelling!

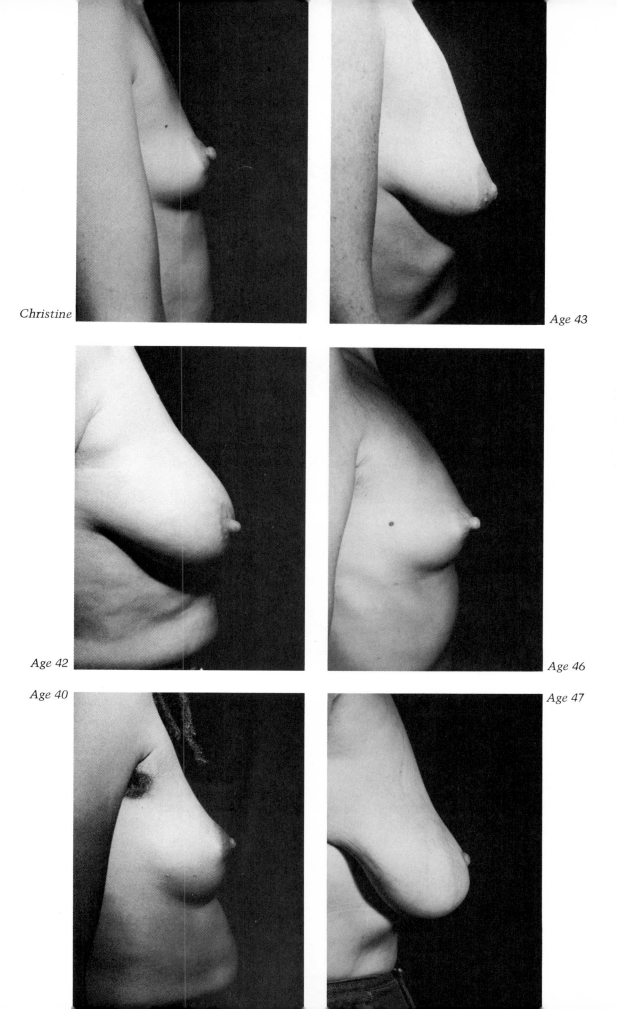

Christine

Age 43

Age 42

Age 46

Age 40

Age 47

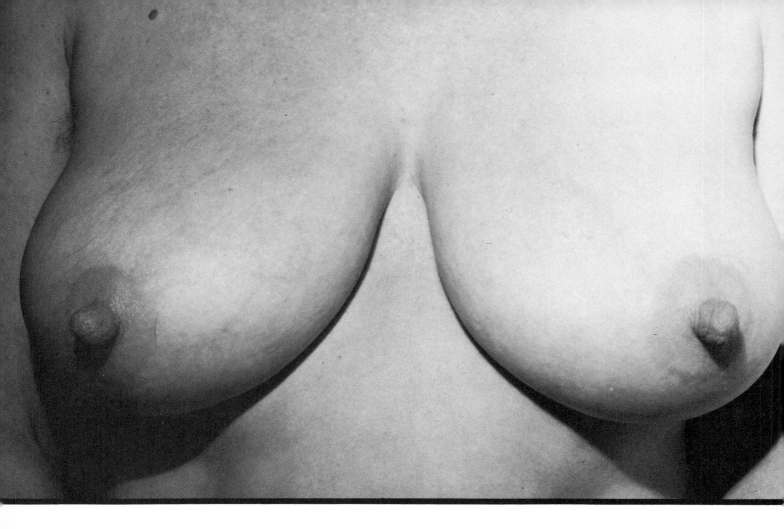

Simone

Age 50 • Raised in Europe • Painter • Mother of one

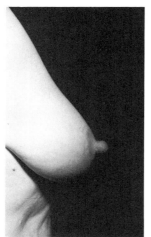

I am the only one in my family with breasts like my mother's—big with large nipples. My sisters don't have much of a bosom so I am better off, you see.

My nipples are practically the most erogenous part of my body. I can have an orgasm simply by having them fondled—if they're manipulated long enough, I come. Men tell me that some women are just not sensitive in the breast area and they couldn't care less about being touched or sucked there. They say that some women dislike it so much they just don't allow it. I cannot imagine it.

Every man I've ever been with is crazy about my bosom—this is one of my great attributes. Men are particularly crazy about my large nipples. They say they have never seen anything like them before, ever, and they are completely astounded!

When my breasts were just beginning to grow, they were teeny-weeny pointy things. The nipples were there before the breasts, hard and protruding through my sweaters. I noticed my child-hood boyfriends suddenly eyeing me—looking at them—and that was the first manly, masculine look I ever got. It made me feel really happy. Finally, I had something to *show!* Until then I had

236

the feeling that I was absolutely ugly and repulsive.

Then I had my tonsils taken out and suddenly everything shot out! This is perhaps the first time in history that there is a connection between tonsils and breasts! (*Laughs.*) When my breasts finally started growing, they *really* grew—out and up, forty-five degrees northwest so to speak. And my mother said, "Well, they're swinging around now, so you'd better wear a brassiere."

Years later people told me, "Don't you know that you were famous for your bosom? You had a beautiful figure." It surprised me—that's not what *I* remember. I had a figure like a boy, thin and flat, for much too long.

I'm not conscious of it, but I have been told that I must be proud of my breasts because I carry myself very straight, as if to show them off. I have a very upright way of walking. If I walk in the street without a coat, no matter where I am—and I've traveled all over the world—every man's eyes turn to look at my breasts. It is the first thing they look at, and sometimes men have even followed me! My breasts are a great success! They're even a conversation subject. It's almost like taking puppies out for a walk and having strangers stop and pat them. (*Laughs.*)

The other day I was waiting for a bus late at night and some man who was not in the least obnoxious or drunk walked past me. Suddenly he turned his head around, walked back toward me, and politely said, "Please don't misunderstand me, but I want to compliment you on your bosom—it is beautiful." So I said, "Thank you very much. It is very kind of you." And he walked off. It was done in good taste and I felt like I'd been paid a compliment. It was the most extraordinary thing, no? I think it was homage really.

I am quite capable of meeting a man who really fascinates me, whom I find attractive, intelligent, and interesting, but if at any time in the conversation he uses the word "tits" I will not see him again. The word I use for breasts depends on what language I am speaking. "Breasts" is a lovely word. In French the word for breast is "sein," but they also say "teton," which is used like "tits" although it actually means nipples. I *loathe* these words! There is something terribly vulgar about them.

●

Something terribly funny happened to me many years ago when I was living in Paris. The studio I had then was very large and the whole northern wall was glass, facing a fairly wide boulevard. I used to rush naked from my bathroom at one end of the studio, upstairs to a dressing area. And though the entire wall was glass, it never occurred to me that anyone could witness this. There were trees there, and then houses far, far away.

Well, one day I started getting what they call "obscene" phone calls. The caller said, "Why don't you come and have coffee with me," and I said, "Why? What for?" So he said, "Because you have the most beautiful breasts that I have ever seen," and he started describing my breasts. That shocked me. Every time he called I put the phone down but he would call again. At first I thought it was one of my friends just kidding me or something, but it went on for two weeks.

One day he gave me a very accurate description—some real details—and I figured out that he must live across the boulevard and must actually be watching me with binoculars because he said, "You go naked upstairs and then get dressed." It upset me terribly because, for all I knew, I was going to have him there for all *eternity*.

Finally, he said to me, "You know, I pass you several times a day. We go to the same café down the road." Suddenly I realized *who* it was, so I said very coolly. "Oh, if you saw my breasts so well, I am astonished that you didn't realize I'm wearing falsies." There was a stunned silence at the other end and he said, "No, madame. It's impossible! You're not serious." I said, "Can you imagine any woman crazy enough to tell you she wears falsies if she doesn't? Of course I'm serious—they're falsies! Your eyesight is wrong!" And I hung up.

This man obviously had the shock of his life. I went and bought—at great expense I might add—a pair of falsies, wrapped them up, and sent them to him. I put a note inside saying, "Here they are since you like them so much," and from then on whenever I passed him on the street, he turned his head away. He was so embarrassed.

For all I know he really believed it. He must have said to all of his friends in the café, "Look at her. You think she has a nice bosom? Well, it's just falsies!" By now half of Paris must think I wear falsies. But I got rid of him.

●

I think that the excitement my nipples cause for men is that there is something to really touch, to hold and to suck. I suppose it is very satisfying for a man to put a nipple in his mouth—it must be very erotic. The penis must be erotic to women for the same reason—because it is something to grasp, to hold or to suck. And sucking is primal, of course. I like to put a man's finger in my mouth and suck it. It's very sensual to suck whatever is

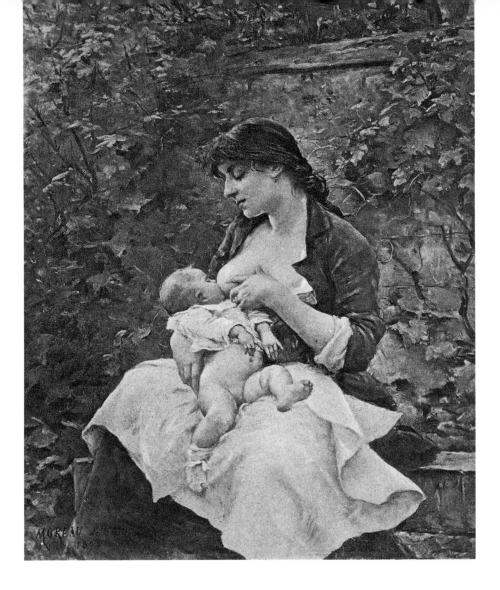

protruding, but why make such a tremendous distinction between a nipple and an earlobe? If a man is really a sensual person, he sucks every finger you have and even toes sometimes.

But also I think that when a man sucks a woman's nipple, part of what's involved is the fact that he did that as a child. Once I was in bed with a man who was about sixty or so, but he probably had the emotional development of an eight-year-old because he just driveled and drooled all over my breasts and he didn't seem to care at all about the other end. Some men go for breasts much more than any other part of the body, and that is obviously a mother fixation. There are all types. (Your readers are going to think that this woman is talking about "some men" as if she has taken on the whole world and is now making statistics!) (*Laughs.*)

●

When I was in my early thirties, I became pregnant. I remember how beautiful my breasts were. They got swollen and more swollen, and bigger and bigger. My God, I wore such enormous brassieres! How I loved to look at myself in the mirror. I made lots of drawings of myself at the time. Since then, whenever I get a chance, I like to sketch pregnant women. There is nothing in the world more beautiful!

One of the main reasons I became pregnant was that I wanted to breast-feed. I was looking forward to it because I felt a tremendous need to have a baby suck on my breasts—after all, that was why they were there, why I had them!

At the time I was pregnant I lived in Paris among a group of highly intellectual people. One of the women whom I knew casually was expecting her child at the same time as I was. After our children were born, we met and talked a bit, and I said, ". . . and isn't it absolutely wonderful when the baby sucks?" Because when my baby sucked my breast I actually had orgasms. After all, the sucking of the breasts, especially by infants, is very intense, so I got all the tingling in my lower belly and pleasure all over my body.

Well, she looked at me askance and said, "Do

238

you mean to tell me that you are *breast-feeding?*" I said, "Of course! *That* is one of the reasons I had a baby." So she haughtily said, "Obviously, Simone, there is a tremendous difference between us. I am so much more mental than you." I burst out laughing. "Intellectual" is what she meant—that she's a superior "mental" woman and I am a peasant and an animal. Everybody we knew thought I was more of an intellectual, so it was terribly funny. (*Laughs.*)

To my amazement, a number of times people were shocked about my breast-feeding. I once sat in a park and breast-fed, and all these bloody women looked at me as if I was *demented.* But I was proud and felt part of nature. I think it's horrendous to cut yourself off from nature, as if human beings are self-made.

In a way, it is the same as the cheapening of sexuality. I have always had the Tantric sentiment about sex—that it is sacred and orgasm is reaching out to God. The moment of penetration of man into woman is the grace of God. You are penetrating into the rhythms of the universe—it's cosmic! And you are potentially creating life. I cannot understand how the creating and nurturing of life could have been dirtied, cheapened, and degraded. It upsets me.

●

There is something I once did which is interesting because I suspect that it was more deliberate than I pretended. I've been divorced for many years and my son lives most of the time with his father. Two summers ago, when he was fifteen, he came to visit me while there was a terrible heat wave. My house was not completely built yet, so he and his friend and I all slept in one room. We had no air conditioning. . . .

I lay in my bed across from them and at one point I said, "It's so hot in here, I hope you don't mind but I just have to take my top off," and with just knickers on I wandered around the house.

I don't know what effect it had on my son and his friend. At the time, I really believed that I was so hot that I didn't care, but I'm sure there was more to it than that—some kind of provocation. Everybody talks about the Oedipus complex but no one ever bothers to mention the Jocasta complex. After all, if Oedipus slept with his mother, Jocasta, then she obviously slept with her son . . . and I do imagine that every mother subconsciously wants to do that. But nobody will admit it!

Every year I go for younger men and I am well aware that when I put my hand on the body of a young man, in some way this is a substitute for my son. So I imagine that subconsciously I was playing the coquettish female with my son and that I was well aware of what my bosom might be doing.

●

I am always absolutely aware of my breasts because they predominate my body. I can't turn without feeling my breasts jump and I can't even *walk* without a bra. But I also wear bras for aesthetics. I look at my silhouette and, according to my build, my bosom should be high up on my chest, not down there. The kind of bras I wear are stiff on the underside to pick me up and separate the breasts. They must have a good, strong uplift.

I would love to be able to go braless. The other day I went to a party and a friend of mine was there braless, and she is fifty-five, for God's sake! She has small, beautiful, firm breasts. I was so envious.

There are all kinds of clothing which I can't close over my breasts without feeling uncomfortable, and I hate tight sweaters. I hate it when my breasts look too obvious because there is something vulgar about it. Also, I can't wear anything too low-cut. I don't like to show too much of the actual flesh of my breasts because the skin is getting wrinkly. I have a complex that if my cleavage showed too much it would make me look like an old woman. Twenty-five years ago, when I was a young woman and the low-cut look was fashionable, I wasn't liberated enough to wear it. And now that I am liberated enough, I don't dare! I'm vain. . . . (*Laughs.*)

In a way I am proud of my breasts because they are large and still full with strong, hard nipples, but I am also ashamed because they are drooping. I am afraid that they may be considered a bit passé. I am becoming self-conscious about my breasts when I am in bed with a man. If I get up naked to walk across the room and there is a light on, I try to hold my breasts up because I think they are sagging. My lovers tell me, "It's perfectly all right—they're big so they sag." Men don't seem to think my breasts are too old-looking, but I still worry about it.

I have many friends who are younger than I so, by God, I am really aware that their bodies are more youthful-looking, and it upsets me. Naturally, I would like to be as youthful and firm-looking as ever. From year to year I ask my friends, "How do I look? Is it all right to walk around? Dare I show myself in a bikini?" They say, "Of course! How do you do it?" I must say that even though I'm self-conscious, I am proud of my body when I compare myself to other women my age.

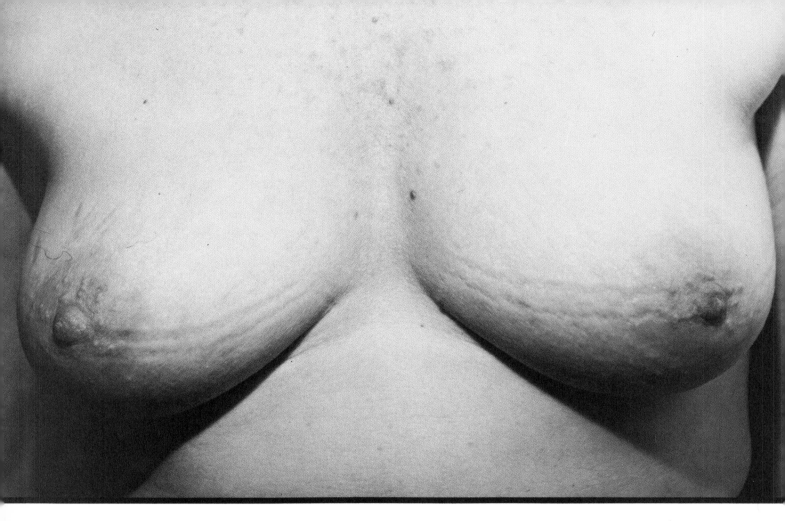

Ellen

Age 49 • Raised in Brooklyn, N.Y. • Nurse • Mother of two

Breasts should be accepted as more than just an implement of sex but they're not. Women's breasts have been exploited in movies, in television, in magazines, in advertising—everywhere—and it's very damaging!

I'm sure that the feelings I had when I was nursing are probably the same feelings that many women have—that breasts are just a sexual implement and thus breast-feeding is an animal thing to do and in some way disgusting! You know, calves nurse on cows, but babies should not nurse on mothers. Now twenty-seven years later, I realize that feeling is disgusting and that I could have saved myself a lot of troubles.

The only thing that has ever embarrassed me about myself, that is constantly with me, is my small breasts. To be honest, if I were single, I would feel very self-conscious about exposing my breasts to a man. I would probably prefer undressing in the dark. And the first time a man put his hands on my breasts, I would probably think to myself that he didn't get as much as he bargained for.

My husband has affectionately referred to my breasts as "cupcakes" and other things that are small. He always says that everything over a handful is wasted. He doesn't seem to mind my being small, although when we were dating and planning to get married, one of his pet comments was, "You know, I always wanted to marry a blonde with big tits." Of course, he married a little brunette with small ones. . . . So it has been a joke over the years. But when he said that, it always made me feel inadequate. I'd always find myself wishing that my breasts were bigger. I imagine if he ever had a lover, she would be a blonde with big boobs—for what he missed!

When I was pregnant my breasts were bigger and that was the one time I enjoyed having large breasts, and so did my husband. He *loved* it! He thought it was great! He certainly liked to hold them a lot more than usual.

●

After I gave birth to my oldest daughter, I really did not want to breast-feed, but my obstetrician was a firm believer in breast-feeding, which was unusual at the time. I was not really strong enough to say, "Look, I don't want to breast-feed and that's it." So I nursed her in the hospital under duress.

I didn't like the feeling. First, it hurt because my nipples had not been toughened, and she really got hold and *pulled.* Then, when the milk came in and she burped some up, I realized that the milk came out of *me!* It gave me an absolutely *horrible* feeling! I felt like a *cow!* I got very upset. I cried and got hysterical and I *refused* to nurse her!

The doctor gave me an injection to dry up the milk, but by this time I had a lot of it so when I got home from the hospital I was terribly ill. I developed a very high fever because of my breasts and they were very hard and tremendous and red. It was terrible! My mother-in-law had to take care of the baby. I couldn't even lift her! I was quite ill for about three weeks. My breasts weren't being relieved of the milk so it just got all caked up, and I remained with lumps in my breasts for years afterward.

Since then, my breasts have been a continual source of worry and anxiety. I've been *terrified* of getting breast cancer. I've had cystic mastitis over the years and I've even had to have the fluid taken out of some of the cysts. There is still one big cyst in my left breast which has been there all this time—for twenty years or more. Of course, I've had many mammographies—too many. So I feel more frightened and panicky about developing breast cancer than I think is normal.

●

I walked into a brassiere store about a year ago. There was a box of bras on the table and they were absolutely *gigantic!* I never saw such huge cups before. I picked one up and looked at the size and said out loud, "Forty D!? Who on earth wears a forty D?!" Naturally, the woman who had been trying one on was standing right behind me! I was very embarrassed. She was good-natured about it and started to laugh, but meanwhile I just slunk away.

The reason I wear a bra is habit. I feel more comfortable with one on because I've become accustomed to wearing it. But at times I've said to myself, What the hell am I wearing this thing for? because I really don't *need* it. I could get along very nicely without a bra—nobody would ever notice. Why haven't I done it? Because I look better with a bra according to the standards of my peers, according to the standards I was taught, and *not* according to young people's standards today. So it's a cultural motivation.

Neither of my daughters wears a bra, and it used to disturb me but I've become accustomed to it. When they walk and their breasts bounce around, or when they get cold and the nipples stand up, I don't think it looks nice. It looks *sloppy!* And nipples protruding from a cotton T-shirt are not pretty at all.

I'm sure my daughters' bralessness disturbs my husband. I find it a little embarrassing, too, depending on who the company is. If just my husband and I are home and the girls walk around with their nipples sticking out of their T-shirts, that's one thing. But if other people come into the house, I have to admit it makes me uncomfortable.

Lately I'm finding that in some ways I'm better off that my breasts are small. I can wear clothing that big-breasted women can't, like dresses that have a very long, low-cut V in the middle. If a big-breasted woman wears one, half her breast comes out, and with me it doesn't. So it's rather advantageous to have small breasts with today's kind of clothing. Fashions are kinder to me now than when I was younger.

I used to get tremendous sexual feelings in my breasts, but I really don't anymore. I don't know why that's happened—whether it's physical or whether it's mental—but the feeling certainly has decreased. It's a gradual change that came about over the last ten years. It doesn't upset me though.

When I was younger, aging bothered me a lot. Because of the milk problem I had at twenty-five my breasts drooped a lot for that age . . . and it upset me! I read articles about keeping the breast tissue firm with exercise and I tried it over the years, but I always got tired and gave up. Ten years ago I completely gave up. I certainly would have liked my breasts to remain fuller—to stay young-looking. I think it's very normal to feel that way, and not just about breasts—I'd have liked my skin and *everything* to remain young, but that's not possible.

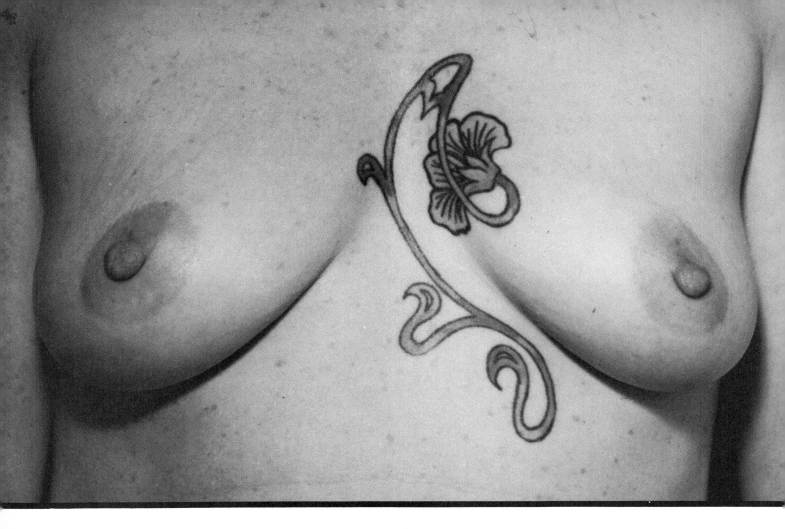

Harriet   *Age 41 · Homemaker · Mother of three*

Awhile ago my husband and I were making love and he felt a lump in my breast. I panicked! It was just after we heard about Betty Ford and Happy Rockefeller—I was terrified! I ran to my doctor immediately.

After having a mammograph, I went to see a terrific surgeon. Both he and the doctor who gave me the mammograph told me that because I had had a baby before I was twenty, unless every female member of my family had breast cancer, I could not possibly have it. What I had were cysts, which are very common, so there was nothing to worry about.

For years I had wanted a tattoo on my breast and after that scare, I finally had it done. I was at a party and a woman was there wearing a dress that showed a tattoo on her arm. I talked to her and she turned out to be a tattooist. I liked what I saw, so I went to her.

I'd always wanted a very tiny rose on my breast, but when I looked through the dozens of books

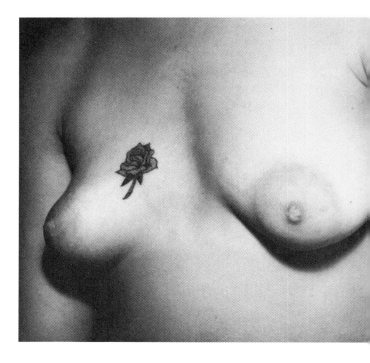

242

that the tattooist had and found this flower, I fell in love with it. It's an art nouveau design. I didn't tell my husband what it was going to be, so he just expected the small rose I'd been talking about. In fact, until I convinced him, he didn't want me to have a tattoo on my breasts at all. (*Laughs.*) His feeling was that they're *his* breasts. He always says, "They're *mine!*" He really loves them. He thinks my breasts are terrific—the best!

When I came home with my tattoo, my husband was in the tub. (*Laughs.*) I thought he would *drown* when I took my shirt off. He was not prepared for it at all. In fact, I wasn't either really—I just went in and trusted the tattooist. It didn't take long to get used to it. I *love* it! It's a very sensuous design. I've always loved flowers and I can't get anything to grow in my house, so it makes me feel as if I'm growing a flower on my body. Eventually my husband got used to it and now he loves it, too. He *loves* it!

I like wearing low-cut things to show off my cleavage which is why I thought it would be so pretty to have a tattoo there. It's like permanent jewelry. It's something to make me feel and look better than I do.

Living in the city with all the nuts around, I have to wear clothes to cover it up during the day. But when we go out at night, I wear something that shows it all off. Now all my good clothes are very low-cut and open so you can see my tattoo. I love the attention. I also have a lot of see-through shirts. And by the way, I *never* try to cover up my nipples. (*Laughs.*) I love them!

People are always shocked about my tattoo—they don't know what to say. They stare at me and just don't know what to make of it. (*Laughs.*) Everybody else is concerned about how permanent it is, but I'm not. I feel that everything we do is permanent in some way. The tattoo is totally part of my body.

It always comes up in conversation that I have a tattoo. In fact with one woman, while I was bending over the stairs to let her son out of the door, she said suddenly, "Were you *drunk!*" I said, "I don't drink. What the hell are you talking about?" And she says, "That *thing!*" "Oh, my tattoo!" She didn't approve of it. Many people don't approve. They think it's very weird . . . and *permanent*, but I don't care. I've always wanted a tattoo and I have a group of very positive friends who just love it.

I really like my breasts. They're saggy—I've had three children. Gravity has taken its toll, but I like the way they look. I have some freckles in the middle and one is bigger than the other and they're not spectacular, but I'm very happy with them.

When I was nursing my middle child, we were going out to a concert one evening and a friend walked in, looked at my chest, and said, "Why don't you use some tape and pull 'em up!" She wanted me to put transparent tape on my breasts like the *Cosmopolitan* models do so they wouldn't hang. I said, "What for? My breasts hang down a little bit. I'm a grown woman. I have two children and I'm a nursing mother . . . I'm not eighteen years old anymore!" She said, "How can you feel that way?" And I said, "Well, I *do.*" She was very surprised. But after she had children she realized what I was talking about. It upsets me that people think like that, but we each deal with it in our own way.

●

I guess by having this tattoo I'm making a statement which I really wasn't conscious of at the time. What I am saying is, "I like me. I like who I am. I like the way I look." I'm proud of that. I didn't *always* like the way I looked. It takes time to accept the fact that you're not going to be eight feet tall and weigh ninety-six pounds and have an enormous bosom and a tiny waist and look the way everybody thinks you should.

For years I was not happy. I thought my body was ugly and that I was ugly! It took me a long time to realize that I wasn't, and that realization was very liberating. I have finally accepted who I am and what I look like and I guess I'm decorating myself because of it!

Solomon Islands

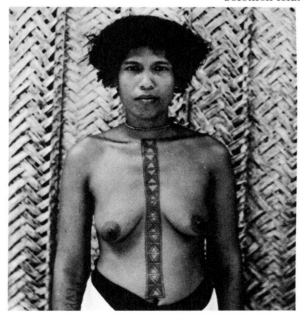

243

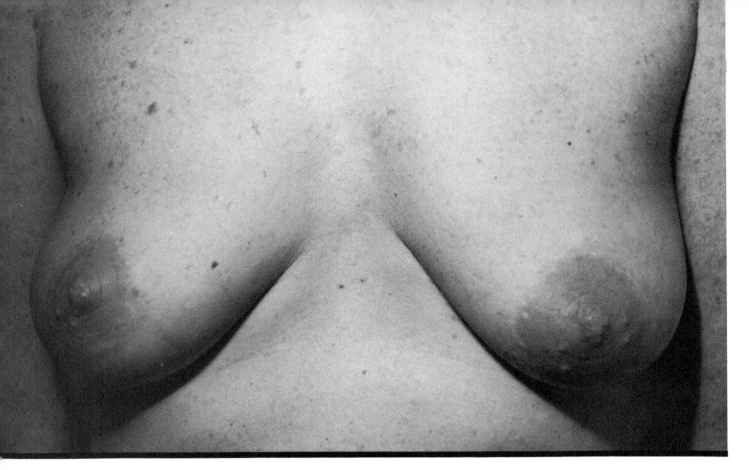

Age 43

Age 40

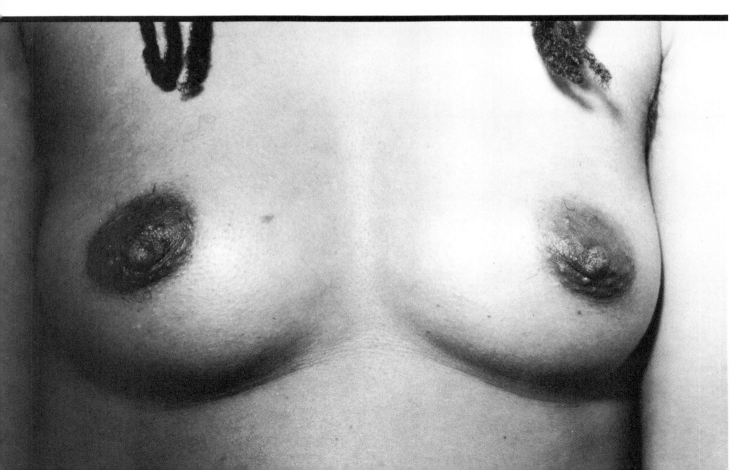

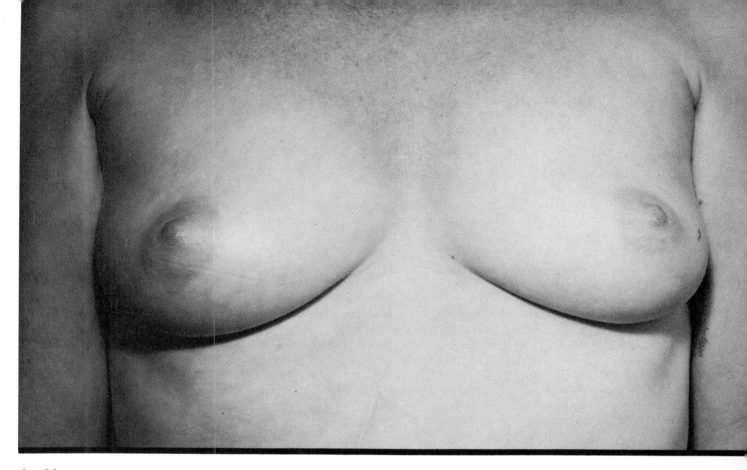

Age 54

Age 51

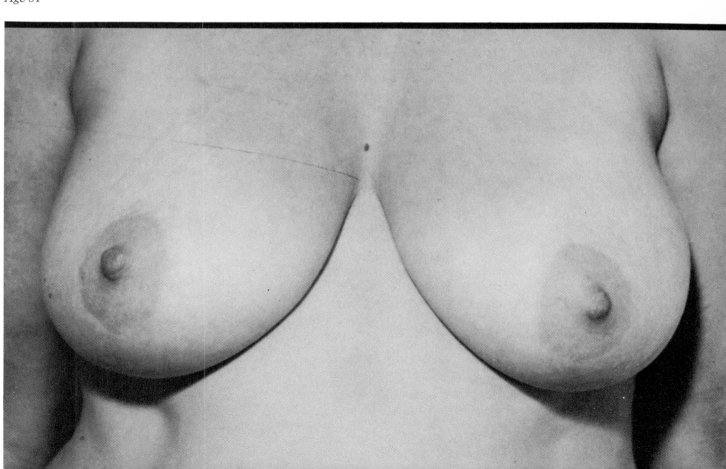

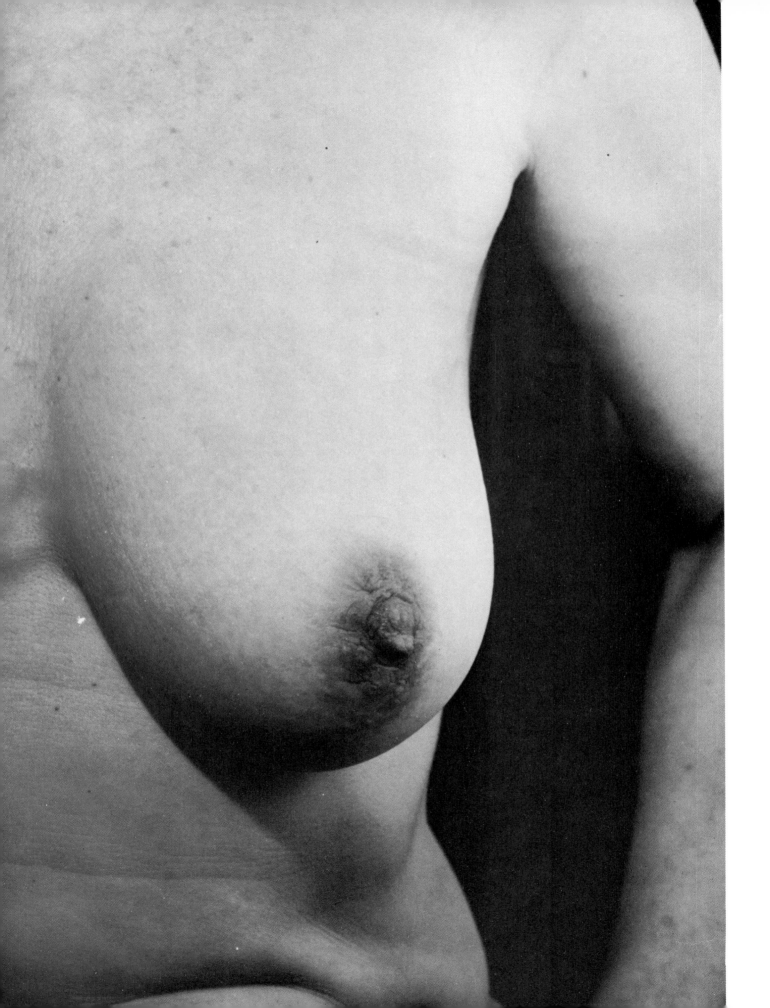

Ruth

Age 50 • Designer • Mother of one

My breasts were always very important to me, particularly the way I looked in clothing. And having my breasts fondled during sex was so very important. My husband and I used to have names for my breasts—we thought it was very funny. We finally settled on "Mutt" and "Jeff." Whenever he was away, he sent me a postcard saying, "How are Mutt and Jeff?" And I always signed my postcards to him with those names in the middle of two breasts . . . which I haven't done, I'll admit, since I had my mastectomy.

I was born in 1928 and I don't think my mother thought one way or the other about nursing me. In those days, women normally did it unless they were sick or the child was sick. So I was breast-fed.

I don't really think breast-feeding is very important. In fact, I was against it. I didn't breast-feed my own child because it was more important for me to go on working than to be involved in that. I didn't want to get hung up on the idea that my child was causing problems in my life-style. I wanted her to be a joy, so I didn't want anything about her to interfere with my work which I am devoted to.

I really felt that giving her concentrated attention when I was home was more important than being there all day to breast-feed her. I told my doctor, "I'm not going to do it because I'm working." He didn't seem to mind—doctors weren't supporting breast-feeding in 1960. Maybe I could have fit breast-feeding into my busy schedule, but I didn't want to, so I bottle-fed her.

●

Long before my breasts ever made an appearance, I knew that they were somehow important and that women had to have breasts in order to be attractive. It was just knowledge I absorbed from the environment. We all saw movies and ads, and Petty Girls . . . all of that!

Illustration: George Petty

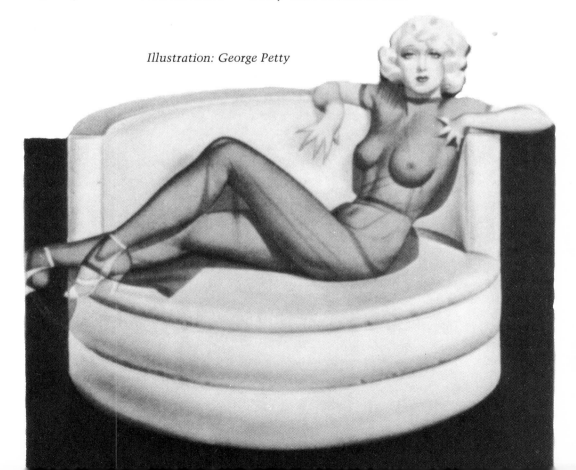

I got my period very late, when I was around fourteen, and I had the tiniest breasts and I thought it was the biggest *disaster!* Just awful! And that wasn't my only problem. All through my teens I had terrible acne—the worst!—and my mother would rush me from doctor to doctor. She tried everything and nothing worked.

All through my teenage years I hated being flat-chested and one of the biggest reasons was that I was mistaken for a boy. Finally, in my second year of college when I was eighteen, I met an incredible doctor who was experimenting with an estrogen pill. He put me on the pill to cure my acne, and I had some side effects. I didn't have my period for a whole year *but* I developed real breasts! It was actually one of the estrogens which is now known to be dangerous to take if you are pregnant. If we knew then what we know today about cancer, he might not have given it to me.

So the major part of my breast growth was during that year. They might have gotten bigger by themselves, but I doubt it. I think I would always have had small breasts. So I was very pleased. I got rid of my acne and got breasts all at once! It was fabulous!

At that point my body was very attractive. When I walked on the beach in a bathing suit I looked terrific. But it embarrassed me because I thought that if I looked so terrific, what was I going to do if a man approached me and I actually had to talk to him? It was very slow with me—I grew up *very* late.

Right through my twenties I was very shy about my body. I don't know whether I was really "growing up" or whether I was influenced by the changes happening in the outside world in the sixties, but in my thirties, for the first time, I started to wear much sexier clothes. I wore very low-cut things that I never would have worn in my twenties. I felt more secure about myself as a woman and more sexy. And I had pretty damned good breasts!

There were a few times in the late sixties when I didn't wear a bra, on and off, for certain kinds of clothes. I was proud of the way I looked and getting prouder and prouder because I kept getting older and older and nothing was happening to this great body, and I loved that! The outside world became more tolerant and I grew up with that. The sixties certainly affected all of us—even the older generation. We all became much freer about our bodies, and that's why I was so *furious* when all the trouble started.

How did you first discover that you had breast cancer?

It was completely accidental! Five years ago I went to the doctor for a checkup and he was going through my records. He said, "My God, you're over forty—why haven't I ever sent you for a mammogram?" I had always had Pap tests and breast checks regularly and there was never anything wrong.

Well, my doctor sent me to a very famous man, the one who developed the breast X-ray technique. I went very casually, not really concerned about it at all, and about a week later my doctor called and asked me to come over. He told me they had seen a shadow on the X-ray, so I said, "Well, what does that mean?" And he said, "We don't really know enough, but I think you should go and have a biopsy." I said, "What if they find something?" He said, "Well then you might have to have your breast removed," and I burst out crying.

He sent me to a famous surgeon who shall also be nameless. Actually, he shouldn't be, because I think he is the *worst* doctor in the world! He showed me something on the X-ray that looked no bigger than a pencil mark! It was like a dot and I said, "A dot can't be *that* important." I was scared really, but I tried not to show it too much. The surgeon, whom I didn't know but went to *because* he's famous—"the best"—booked me into the hospital.

When I arrived at the hospital, he asked me to sign papers giving him permission to perform a mastectomy and I said, "Not me! I'm not going to sign any papers! If you find something, I'll decide later whether I am going to do it." He said, "No way!" He got furious, but I mean *furious!* He thought he was being challenged, that I was presuming to know more than he did. I didn't, but I wasn't going to wake up and find that I had cancer and *no breast* . . . and be traumatized! I wanted to wake up and find out that *maybe* I had cancer, and then I would look into it.

Well, I had a big argument with the surgeon about those release papers and he finally stormed out of the room. My husband went after him and he finally agreed to perform a biopsy.

When I woke up after surgery, he told me that I had cancer. I said, "What does that mean . . . *cancer?*" And he vaguely explained what it was. I didn't learn very much, so I told him, "Well, I don't know what I am going to do."

Then my doctor came to the hospital absolutely hysterical, saying, "You've just got to cooperate!" Obviously the surgeon had spoken to him. I said, "No, you haven't even told me what *kind* of cancer it is. You haven't told me what it's all about! I am going home and I am going to find out for myself." Which is exactly what I did. It was my way of getting ready for whatever had to be done.

When a doctor says something, most people believe him *because* he is a doctor. I never do because I know too many people who've had very bad experiences with doctors. I'm really very sour on them. Most people think doctors know *everything.* They don't, and most people don't want to take responsibility for finding out the truth, either. Women are too scared to question their doctors' procedures. But we should know as much about them as possible. Women shouldn't accept answers from anybody—information, yes, but not answers. We shouldn't be snowballed or railroaded into *anything!*

I decided I was going to find out *everything* I could about my tumor. Even while I was still in the hospital, about an hour after the doctors left, I called people I knew all over the country to find out what it all meant. I knew that it was an "encapsulated tumor," and suddenly there I was talking to people about something I had never discussed before—cancer.

I refused to go back to my old doctor, so finally I got in touch with a marvelous woman—a pathologist—who in turn recommended me to a fantastic doctor. I called him up and he said, "I'd like to see your records." So I went to my previous doctor's office to get the records, and there was a *scene.* The nurses didn't want to give them to me. They were hysterical and they practically told me I was going to drop dead if I didn't have a radical. "Do it!" they insisted, but I refused to just "do it." Reluctantly, they finally gave me my medical records.

With the records in hand, I went to see the new doctor, who turned out to be incredible. He sat down and really explained my situation to me. His attitude was that it was my decision to make. And it was a hard decision because I had an encapsulated cancer—it was totally confined to the tumor so it had already been taken out in the biopsy. The problem is that seventy-five percent of the women who have encapsulated cancers removed may eventually develop a more severe cancer. They just don't know for sure, so the only thing they can recommend is removal of the breast. Then there is a hundred percent chance of recovery.

I had to make up my mind. I could have said, "No. I don't want to do it. No one is saying I have cancer. I want to take the chance." But I thought that was not a good idea. Seventy-five percent is

a very high percentage, and they can't X-ray you over and over again because it's too dangerous. So it was a very *difficult* decision to make.

At this point I decided that if I was going to have it done, I was going to have it done right. At the first hospital, even though I had an encapsulated cancer, I would have been forced to have a radical. There is no choice there with that particular doctor. From what I've heard, at that hospital, even if you manage to have a "simple mastectomy," it is done differently from the one that was eventually done on me. The scar usually ends up being far down below the breast.

Once I felt sure that I had all the information I needed, I called back my pathologist friend and asked her who the best surgeon was. She sent me to a fabulous man who had been doing breast surgery for years. He really seemed to know his stuff. He was even furious about my biopsy scar because it was done wrong. He also explained my situation to me in very complete detail. He thought I should have the breast removed—in his experience women with encapsulated tumors who didn't have their breasts removed had a recurrence of cancer.

He also told me something that is not generally known, that there are tremendous differences in the procedures depending on the type of cancer. There is no one solution because everyone's case is different—*everyone's!* He was somebody I believed and trusted, so together we made plans for my operation.

●

Right after the operation, a Reach to Recovery [see page 214] woman came by and said, "You are in such good shape, I don't need to talk to you." I

Reach to Recovery volunteer instructing mastectomy patient in therapeutic exercises.

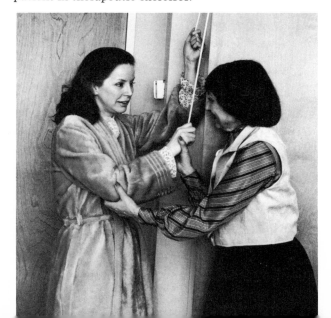

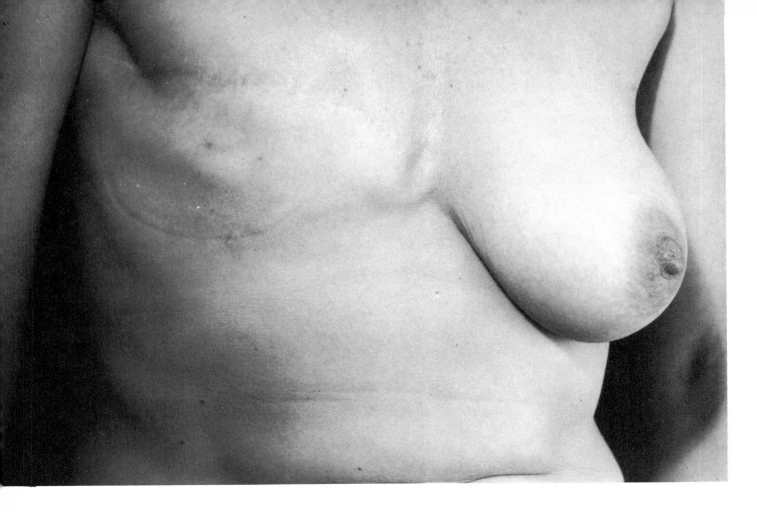

was! Once I made up my mind to have the operation, I was going to do it better than anybody. It was a challenge to me to get the best possible treatment.

I had a simple mastectomy. My whole breast was removed but it was very well done—the scar is extremely good. I have all my muscles and the only thing that was removed was the breast itself—the mammary glands and the fat. One lymph node was also removed but I have everything else, so I was lucky in that sense.

The second day that I was home, I went out looking for a bra and a prosthesis—I couldn't wait! I don't know what happens with women who have muscles removed. I am sure it is a much harder adjustment. I had very few physical problems because so little was removed from me. I was back at work and doing everything in no time.

It's very funny but losing a breast made me feel less threatened *sexually* than about other things. I was more nervous about dressing and wearing bathing suits and the world out there, because my husband made me feel very comfortable about sex. Before I'd been very proud that I was in my forties and still had a good figure. When I walked

on the beach I still looked terrific, so that's where the mastectomy really challenged me. I didn't know how I was going to handle it. I was terrified that everybody could see it and everybody would know! What was I going to do about all those low-cut dresses? How was I going to wear a bathing suit?

The first six months I changed bras endlessly! I would put on a dress and be absolutely *convinced* that it wasn't going to work, that it would be too low and everybody was going to see. If I wanted to wear a tight sweater, I was afraid only one nipple would show!

Why does it matter that anyone knows? It may simply be pride. I am sure it has to do with my own sexuality, that I felt slightly damaged. But I would feel that way about *anything* that came off my body—the feeling of being "less." It's an embarrassment that you are "not all there."

It doesn't bother me as much today. I am not as conscious of it as I was at first, and it never occurs to me that someone is looking at me. It took me six to eight months to learn to handle myself.

Before the mastectomy I always wore one-piece bathing suits because I never liked bikinis. I liked the ones that are cut really low and go down in the back. I can't wear them now. Ironically, I now wear bikinis because the tops are built like bras and they hold you. My method is to put a little piece of material across the center where the cleavage is, like in a sailor suit, so it isn't too low. I wear the prosthesis in the cup and it stays. I mean, if I really lean over you can see it, but that doesn't bother me much. You see, I have no other scars, so it's okay. But if you have a radical, you can't do that.

•

There is one thing that I did because I'm a very pragmatic person. About a year after I had the mastectomy, I went to bed with someone whom I had a very brief affair with some years before, at a time when my marriage was going through a difficult period. The occasion presented itself—I mean, I didn't go looking—and I did it as an experiment to see if this whole thing would turn him off. I was fascinated to know how somebody who is single would handle it . . . and could *I* handle it if I wasn't married? That's the big question, right? It immediately occurred to me, and I wondered and wondered. . . .

And I still don't know! It was a very little experiment and it wasn't very conclusive—I didn't take off my bra! I never got to that point because I was too afraid. So I still don't know how I would deal with it. I *think* I could handle it.

Yet I imagine a mastectomy is more difficult for single women. Jack, my husband, reacted fabulously! He couldn't care less, but he is a very unusual man. He's been terrific.

Jack and I have a very good sense of humor about the prosthesis. If I'm getting undressed, for instance, I'll take it out and begin to jiggle it around and play with it, and we both have a good laugh. Or if I throw my clothes down next to my bed and Jack comes over to that side, I squeal in a funny voice, "Oooh! Don't step on it!"

There definitely has been some change in my sexual relationship with my husband. The breast is not quite as important as it used to be. For the first year I always wore a bra to cover the scar when Jack and I had sex. I hated that because I wasn't getting enough . . . I mean Jack would sort of avoid my breast altogether and I didn't like that. I could at least have *one* breast fondled! I finally took the bra off and then it was like before. It doesn't bother Jack and it doesn't bother me.

Sometimes my husband accidentally touches the area where my breast was removed. . . . I mean he won't touch it on purpose, but he doesn't avoid it either. It's certainly not a turn-on. The sensitivity in my remaining breast is exactly the same as before. The mastectomy really doesn't affect my capacity for arousal. That sensation is there, so it doesn't matter if I have one breast or two.

Occasionally, I've thought about the possibility of having the other breast removed. At this point, I don't think it would affect me, but I really don't know. What kind of bra would I wear? Specially designed with two prostheses? (*Laughs.*) The thing about that which really worries me is that I do find breast fondling very exciting. What would happen if I didn't have that other breast? I know there are millions of other parts of me that get me excited, but the breast is one of my favorites and I would miss that more than anything. My breasts have always been a part of my sexual fantasies.

One thing I've noticed since the mastectomy is that any fantasies about breasts I once had no longer exist. Why can't someone have a fantasy about one breast? (*Laughs.*) Maybe . . . I don't, though.

The thing that scared me before the mastectomy was that somehow I would be changed and people's relationships with me would change. That something would be taken away—like the breast—everywhere in my personality! I've learned that I am who I am, and it doesn't matter—it didn't really change me. But I consider myself lucky because it was fairly easy for me to adjust to something that, to most people, doesn't sound so simple.

None of my friends has ever asked to see the mastectomy. No one at all. I think people really don't want to know. . . .

How does your daughter feel about your mastectomy?

It was difficult when the scar was still bad, but now I walk around the house naked all the time. My daughter has very mixed feelings about it. She'll talk to me about the mastectomy and she is aware of it. She'll look at me naked, but she's not really comfortable doing that. I may be projecting this, but I think it is less looking at *me* that bothers her than a slight terror about herself. That's the reason I don't force it on her, because every child of a parent who has had cancer must have it in the back of her head that she may get it. She's a teenager and I just hope that by the time she is my age they will solve this.

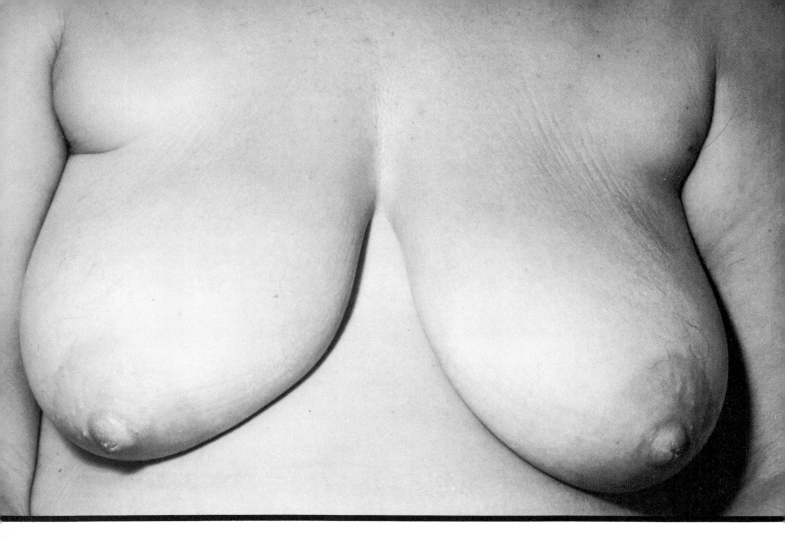

Irene

Age 54 • New England • Writer • Mother of three

I've been extraordinarily conscious of my breasts for the past few years. Since I am in my menopause and my breasts have significant symptoms of it, I probably watch my breasts more than most women. My breasts are much more important and interesting to me in my menopause than they were in my early development, which was very pedestrian.

I am very interested in listening to my body—I think our bodies tell us a lot, but we don't pay attention. As I listen to what my breasts tell me in my menopause, I know from the way they feel some days that I should be quiet. My breasts tell me a lot about my hormonal changes, and if they are sore it means that I'm going to be more sensitive and fragile that day. And so that knowledge is very helpful to me.

I was born when the flapper era was just beginning, but my mother, being an immigrant woman, was certainly not a flapper. She wore those strong brassieres that seemed to be shapeless and flat. They were very elaborate and long, with a lot of snaps. She also used to wear a corselette, which was a big engineered thing with stays, a heavy-duty number. Since she was a woman in business, always meeting the public behind the counter of a store, she had to be "together" looking and was always very locked up in those corsets. Even at home she never wore a housedress.

When I was a little girl I slept with her in the same bed. I always felt that my mother's breasts were a positive part of her, representing warmth and cuddling. I think breasts symbolize the most positive elements—nurturing and protection and love. There's nothing as sweet as being comforted at your mother's breast and I'm sure that was the source of attraction to my mother's breasts. I remember wanting to touch her breasts but that would have been taboo so I didn't.

My mother's breasts were pendulous and so were all my older sisters', so I expected the same. And from the minute they started to grow, when I was twelve years old, my breasts have *always* been pendulous. I took it very naturally. My pendulous breasts never bothered me because that was the time of uplift bras.

I've always worn brassieres for support, so they are usually the sturdy type. Sometimes I go without a bra around the house and I have a very different feeling of myself. I have a different configuration then because of the way I am built. Since I'm short-waisted with pendulous breasts, when I don't wear a bra there's a whole area of me that

Advertisement, 1920

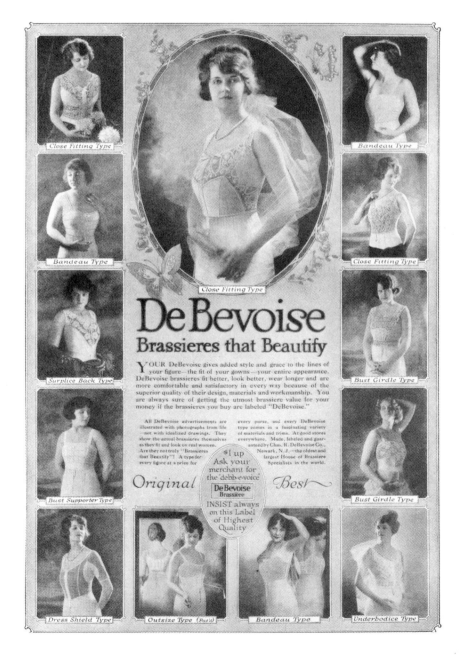

253

gets lost. When I do wear one, my body seems elongated because my waist is differentiated—I have a feeling of being more defined.

I've been very conscious of my breasts and the clothes that I wear. I've never had to draw attention to my breasts with particular clothing because they are such an obvious part of me that I could hardly keep them hidden if I tried.

I've always liked having large, opulent breasts, and I consider them one of my positive points. I always liked the attention given them and just took it for granted that I was admired *because* I had generous breasts. And by the way, I like my cleavage! I remember that in the 1950s, when cleavage was in, I was admired by many of my friends. There was one woman, a poet, who told me, "Oh, I would give *anything* to have a cleavage like yours."

How has your menopause affected your breasts?

Throughout menopause, my breasts have often been very engorged. This is a phenomenon that frequently happens to menopausal women. I get the swelling and soreness and engorging as though I were premenstrual, but the symptoms last throughout the whole month. Sometimes my breasts are so sore I have to wear a brassiere to sleep. It hurts if I lie on them, they get *that* sore. They have also been heavier a lot of the time in the past couple of years. My breasts change enormously and I am sure they are manifesting the hormonal changes that are going on in my body.

It is important for me to understand and keep track of these hormonal changes because they also affect the way I feel emotionally. I have four points on my body that I chart, but my breasts are the number one point since they are the *most* changeable.

Since this knowledge is so important to me, I keep a detailed daily record on the calendar of my breast condition during my menopause. The notations on my calendar are: "sore," "very sore," or "very, very sore," "tender," "heavy without soreness," "swollen without soreness," "swollen with soreness," or "swollen, heavy, very tender," etc. They sometimes change daily, but they can also go for three or four days in the same condition.

I'm consciously aware of my breasts—I know from the degree of their sensitivity whether I should be active or whether I should rest on a particular day. The degree to which my breasts are sore on a particular day is often a sign that I'm going to be more emotionally sensitive and fragile that day.

As far as the sexual feelings in my breasts, that really didn't change with menopause except that, of course, when they're very tender I'd rather not have them touched. My breasts have always given me sexual pleasure.

I expect the changes in my breasts to continue for another couple of years. Menopause generally takes five years. Not everybody has these symptoms—I just happen to. I don't have hot flashes and some women do, while others don't have anything.

Menopause has become my specialty and, in fact, I run menopause workshops for other women. There are an enormous number of myths that exist about women and their breasts as they age. The books that are written about women aging tell about women's breasts getting smaller and that's the largest myth. The books imply that *all* women do and that's not true. Many women that I know have not gotten smaller breasts. My neighbor across the hall is eighty years old and she is as well endowed now as she ever was.

●

I think my breasts are cuddly and soft. I think they're . . . Well, there are such distortions about what beauty is, and I am affected by that, too. Since I'm fifty-four now, I wouldn't use the word "beautiful" to describe my breasts.

When I was younger I was uncomfortable about having new lovers initially see my breasts. I was shy because of my fear of being judged. But I've recently learned that the more a woman accepts herself, the more that people around her accept her.

It is only recently, being involved in the women's movement and in workshops, that I have seen other women's breasts. And because of that I am less self-conscious about other people viewing my breasts—other women, that is. Last winter, I was in an older women's "female sexuality" workshop, and in one meeting we all exposed our breasts to each other. It wasn't easy at first—I really had to warm up to it. The woman who ran the group is a very sensitive person and we just progressed to it through a series of sessions so it wasn't too bad.

I don't usually have much opportunity to see other women's breasts, but when I do I always find it very interesting. This summer, in another workshop held in the country, we sat in the sun on the grass and it was very hot. I was delighted that some women took their shirts off—it was a very natural thing to do. I admired them and I would have liked to be so free, but I can't be. Perhaps someday.

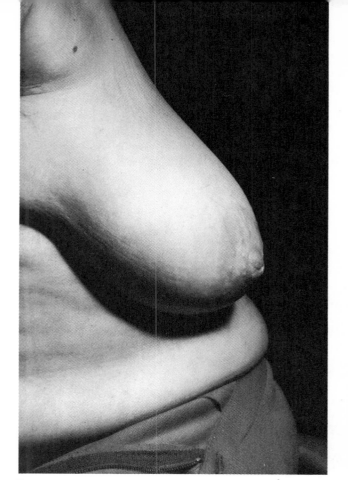

Irene

Age 54

Age 51

Age 55

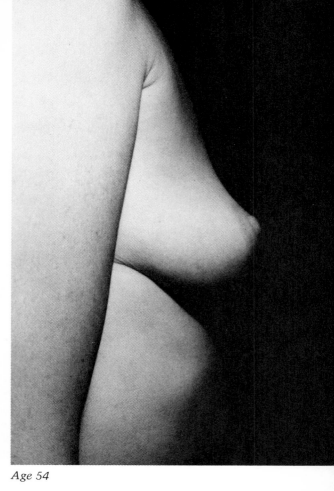

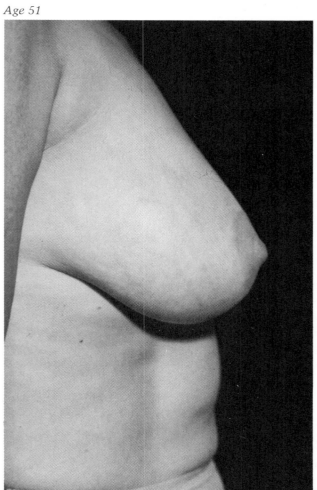

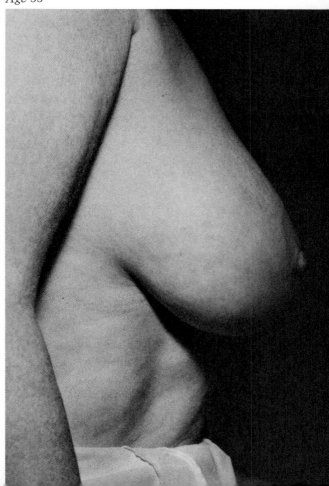

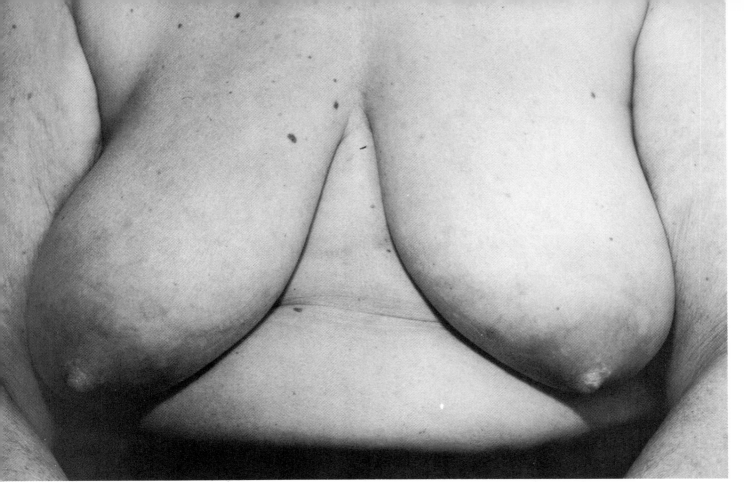

Age 71

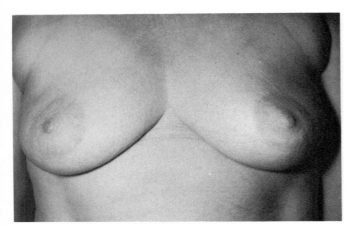

Age 60

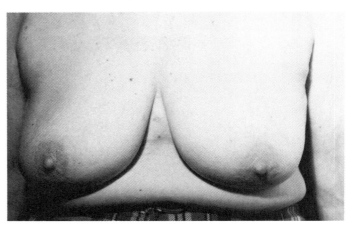

Age 72

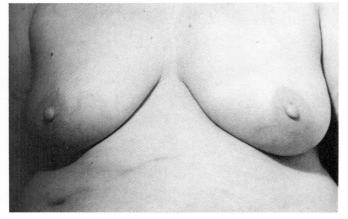

Age 76

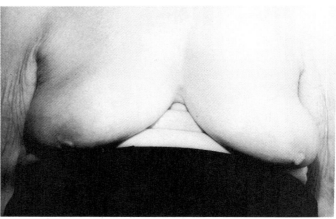

Age 85

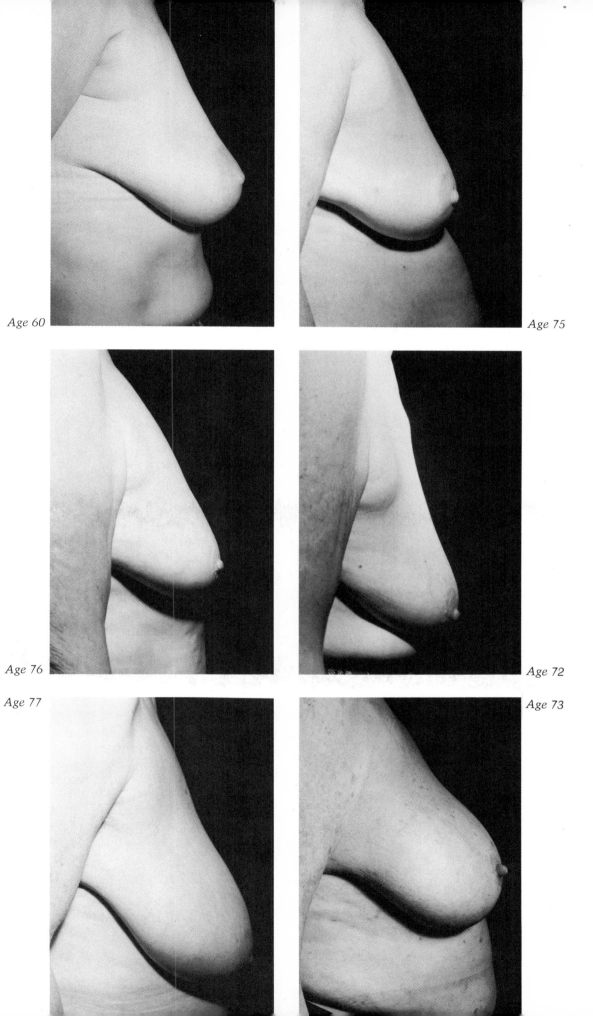

Age 60

Age 75

Age 76

Age 72

Age 77

Age 73

Laura   *Age 73 • Born in Russia • Former Dancer*

I used to dance and I was always conscious of the shape of the body—always hoping that my body would be nice. It meant so very much because I always wanted to do one thing—I wanted to *dance!* So I wanted to be *perfectly* proportioned. I hoped that my breasts would be the right size, not too small and not too big.

I almost *worshiped* a beautiful body. When I looked at classical sculpture, I especially admired the breasts. To me, the ideal breasts were ones that didn't hang down too much—they stood up and out. I admired that kind of sculpture because I thought that's how breasts *should* be. Yet few women have breasts like that. I guess that is what makes it great sculpture.

It was a tremendously painful experience for Laura to recount the trauma of her mastectomy, and during the interview she broke down crying a number of times. Yet she continued telling her story, believing that it was important for other women to know about her bizarre experience.

Almost twenty years have passed since her mastectomy. . . .

It was 1959. I was spending the summer in Atlantic City as I had many times before. One evening as I lay in bed and adjusted the pillows, I touched my breasts. I felt something strange there, something unnatural. I couldn't believe it. There was a hard thing inside. I tried to forget it, but I couldn't. I was immediately worried. I couldn't relax for one single minute from the time I discovered it.

I went to a doctor almost instantly. He told me there was something in the breast—a lump—and without further hesitation he said that the lump should be removed. I got very frightened. I went to see three other doctors before making any decision, but that only confused me more.

I thought there must be another solution. I needed time to think. But the doctors frightened me so. I wanted to wait and chance it for a while, but the doctors were opposed to that. "Quickly! We must act quickly," they kept saying. They felt it was their duty to frighten me and to tell me there was only one way out—surgery! They also told me a terrible thing, that if the surgeon finds it necessary to remove the breast during the biopsy, I must allow it. They said, "You must give

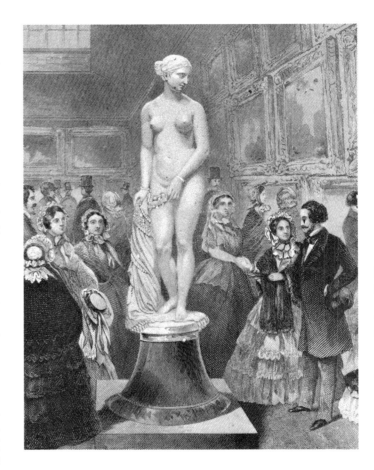

the privilege of making the decision to the surgeon while you are under anesthesia."

All the while I felt I should wait, but I had no one to turn to. The indecision was *torture* . . . and the unhappiness and this . . . Oh! . . . this terrible depression came over me. I didn't want to eat, I didn't want to sleep, I couldn't take an interest in life anymore until *some* decision was made.

I knew that if I was going to have the operation, I had to do it soon, because after discovering the lump, my mental and physical condition rapidly worsened. Not much time had passed, but to me it seemed like an eternity! I grew desperate and afraid. I was losing a grip on myself with it *constantly* on my mind. I was in a muddle. I desperately wanted to make up my mind, but I couldn't even decide which doctor was good enough.

Everybody left Atlantic City on Labor Day, but I stayed on . . . and on and on and on. . . . The village was empty, the beach was empty, and I was the only one on it—I *clung* to it. I asked myself over and over again, What am I staying here for? I was paralyzed with terrible fears of the operation itself, of the surgery.

One day on the boardwalk, I was sitting on my bench, desolate, when a woman sat down next to me. She saw that I was very depressed. We talked for a while and finally I unburdened myself to her. She said not to worry because she knew a great surgeon who had operated on her and had saved her life.

When she introduced me to him, I was able to cover up my nervousness so well that he didn't realize how depressed and weak I really was. He apparently didn't see any outward signs. He felt there was no time to waste, so arrangements for the operation were quickly made.

I was so frightened about the operation that I arranged to have a nurse with me in the hospital the day before. On the day of the operation, she came in at six in the morning to get me ready, but she didn't give me any sedatives. I was so nervous that I hardly knew what to do with myself, so in desperation I began to draw. I drew the nurse's face and I made a beautiful picture. Then I began to draw face after face after face. You have to concentrate to draw faces, so it helped calm me down.

Outwardly I seemed to be quite relaxed, but inwardly I must have been in terrible turbulence. It was the prospect of "not knowing" when I went under. . . . This awful, *awful* feeling. The surgeon later told me, "You gave us a hard time—you didn't let us operate." It seems that the subconscious is always working for us. We don't know it, but a very deep, deep consciousness within the body, a survival instinct, acts to protect us.

Perhaps I should have waited. By that time, I don't think I was strong enough to undergo major surgery. As it turned out, I had an extremely difficult time recovering from the operation—I nearly died!

I was *mortified* when I woke up and found myself all bandaged. The shock was so great because *that* was the *only* thing on my mind when I went under the anesthetic, and it was *exactly* how I was afraid I would find myself when I awoke!

The last thoughts I had as I went under were the same thoughts that brought me to consciousness again. When I awoke, the first thing I did in my stupor was to feel for the breast, and I knew immediately that it was gone.

Strangely, I was too sick to care. At first you are so ill from the operation that you really don't know how to react to the loss of the breast. All I wanted to do was to be able to feel better again—to live. I didn't want to die! And then slowly I realized that I might not be so lucky as to die, but I might just have years of incapacitated life!

When I began to recover it hit me. I hadn't eaten for weeks prior to the operation because of my depressed state of mind and not knowing what was going to happen. I couldn't swallow much food, so I lost a lot of weight and a lot of strength. And I went to pieces!

It was the surgeon's fault. I wanted a nurse during the first three crucial days after the operation, but the doctor thought I was doing so well that he allowed her to go. If the nurse had been there, I think I might not have had the nervous breakdown. I just cracked up in the hospital and I couldn't get myself together. I went down and down and down, down, down. . . . (*Cries.*)

They should have treated me very tenderly and very carefully, but the new rules were to get them off the beds, get them circulating. I spent more time in the hospital than any of their other patients. They tried everything, but nothing could help me.

The surgeon said that I had an infection and he had to drain it, but I didn't feel any pain because I was so numb. I could have been operated on again without the anesthetic and I wouldn't have felt it. They cut off all the nerves . . . the *numbness!* . . . Even right *now* I feel it, it's so deep in me!

All right, my breast is gone, I thought, but will that feeling *ever* go away? The feeling that you are bound by steel, as if you are wearing a steel corset where they operated? The stiffness is so dreadful! When I asked the surgeon, he said it would ease up. But it never did.

It's funny, but I didn't think of cancer. Even after the operation I never actually connected cancer with *my* body. It was a long time before I could ask my surgeon about it. Finally I said, "Why the mastectomy? Why? Did I have cancer?" He said, "No. It was just a cyst and it was benign, and I was getting ready to sew you up when I looked into the breast and I saw a whole line of little, not yet mature cysts. You would have had to come to the hospital perhaps every six months to have them removed, and by the time I was through with you, you wouldn't have had much of a breast left." He thought he would *save* me all that trouble, so he took off the breast! He said, "I

WHOSE "LIABILITY"?

A Rhode Island doctor, Karlis Adamsons, chief of obstetrics and gynecology at Women and Infants Hospital, was quoted in the Providence Sunday Journal about some women's fears that hysterectomies will induce depression. He insists the uterus "is just a piece of muscle." In fact, he maintains, "it's a liability after the children are born because it's a cancer site. If there were no risks and the costs weren't so high, then, ideally, it would be best to remove the uterus." Dr. Adamsons added that "ideally," his theory would apply to breasts, though this would be "a hard concept to sell in this society."

Ms. Magazine, Nov. '77

made a very quick decision." Oh, what a feeling of *regret* I had! My God! . . . (*Cries.*)

●

The real shock comes after you begin to feel better from the actual surgery. Losing a breast meant the *end* of all things to me! Because of the terrible feeling and the stiffness, I thought I would never, *never* be able to relax again. I would never be able to dance or even to just exercise. Dancing is the thing I love the most. To me, to live was to dance! If I couldn't move my body anymore, then what was the use?

Physically and emotionally I was completely lost. And I didn't know *how* to come back to life. When I went home, I lost an incredible amount of weight. I wasn't able to *stand up!* I had a fear of standing up and going out . . . *anywhere!* I didn't know *how* to get well. I wasn't doing *anything*—just lying around and getting weaker from lack of living. I didn't know anything about Yoga at the time. If I had known about Yoga, it might not have been so bad—I wouldn't have allowed myself to get so down. As it was, I just didn't know *how* to turn the tide.

A woman of great moral strength had heard that I was ill, and she came to see me and nurse me. She was a retired nurse and a follower of Meher Baba.* She took me . . . (*cries*) . . . she ac-

* An Indian spiritual leader.

260

tually took me physically, held me, and made me eat and drink and walk, mostly walk and *use* my body. I hadn't been using it at all.

She gave me a lot of courage. She would get me into the elevator and we'd go downstairs. I hadn't done that since I got home, but with her I did. But I wouldn't stay downstairs more than a minute. As soon as I got down there, just the thought of being outside was too overpowering! I felt *terrible!* I said, "Take me right back. I feel as though I am going to die." "The next time," she told me, "just keep repeating 'Baba' all the time and the terrible feeling won't be so bad. When you feel badly, just repeat his name again and again."

The next time, while holding onto her, I had the terrible fear again—that I would *die* if I stood up and walked. But at that moment, I diverted my mind for a few seconds, or a minute, or a half minute, to thinking about Baba and calling him. And while I repeated "Baba" over and over, I didn't think of my own self, and that strengthened my will. From that point on I began to recover. I broke that crisis and there was no direction to go except up. From then on I began to get hold of myself. I decided to like myself again and build up my body.

I remember it was on Election Day, November sixth, one of the coldest days with a terrible wind, that I walked alone outside for the first time since the operation. I walked to the voting station to cast my vote.

A few weeks after that, my boss called and said, "When are you coming back to work?" I said, "What?" I thought all I could hope for was to go down in the elevator and walk a block. He said, "Come on, you'll be all right." We can, if we allow ourselves, survive temporarily on the energies of other people, so when he said, "Come," I couldn't resist. I was ashamed to say, "I can't," and then I just went back to work.

●

When I first came home from the hospital, I couldn't bear to look at my body. I *still* can't. The lymph glands which are directly under the arm have all been removed, so there is a deep cavity there. The bones have no flesh around them—no more flesh ever grows around there.

I think the main thing women are afraid of is that their husbands won't like them anymore. It hurt my husband very badly. He felt that he could never touch me, that he wasn't *allowed* to touch me anymore. The doctor tried to reassure him that sex was still possible, but it didn't help. Our sex life stopped! It was my husband's fault. I was devastated that he felt *that way* because I didn't. He never *looked* at me, he just couldn't. So I was very careful. I always wore a bra because it seemed a horrible thing to confront a man with.

Since my husband died, I have made many new friends and I never tell them I have only one breast. If I ever have anything to do with a man, he would soon . . . Well, having one breast holds me back from any personal relations or lovemaking because I don't want to be found out.

Is it necessary to inform a man ahead of time? That question is forever in my mind. I've gone over it so many times. What would I do? Finally it would *have* to come out! But I've made a personal decision that I wouldn't inform the person ahead of time. I would let him discover it himself, and hopefully by that time it wouldn't make any difference. After all, I am an older woman and I don't know if there are any possibilities. But should anything come up . . .

My mind was almost changed by a woman whom I met this past summer. We discovered that we each had a breast removed. I have never met a more wonderfully adjusted, happier, or more successful person with men. She's a man's woman. Men just can't *resist* her! She is fifty-two and she is just great.

The thing that really intrigued me about her was her successful relationships with men. And it wasn't just one man who said, "I love you whether you have one breast or two. I love you." She's had experiences with *several* men! I don't know *how* she does it! Funny, I never had the courage to ask her that one question that was foremost in my mind—"Do you tell a man ahead of time?"

●

Many years after it happened, I learned of a woman who refused to have her breast removed though she was warned repeatedly by many doctors that she was being childish and risking her life. She had a terribly strong feeling that there were other ways of healing.

Well, she refused to have her biopsy unless she could find a surgeon who would promise not to remove the breast, *even* if she had cancer. She was a writer and a wonderfully strong woman, a very independent type. She finally found a doctor who agreed to perform only a lumpectomy. She and the doctor believed that having caught it at such an early stage, statistically she had the same chance of surviving that she would if a mastectomy had been performed. That took a lot of courage. She got well and never had her breast removed. In fact, she wrote a book about it.

I always intuitively believed in natural healing. Since my operation I have become deeply involved in nutrition and healing, and I have discovered something which I believe works.

It is a very special honey, full of enzymes, made by bees that live on only certain foods and flowers. An old and very wise and healthy man has spent most of his life perfecting this honey. It isn't advertised—the people who use it only know about it through word of mouth and personal recommendation. I was advised to take it to help me regain my strength, by the nurse who helped me recover from the mastectomy, and I have used it ever since.

Quite some time ago, I was told by a doctor that I might have cancer of the cervix, but he wasn't ready to operate. "Let's wait a month," he advised, "and if it doesn't get better, I will have to operate." I took the honey furiously! I gave myself completely to it. As I said, that was quite a few years ago. . . . I never needed the operation.

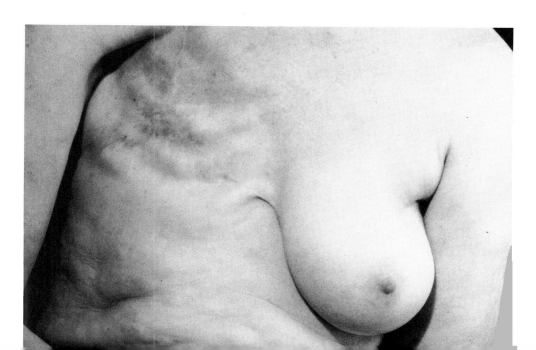

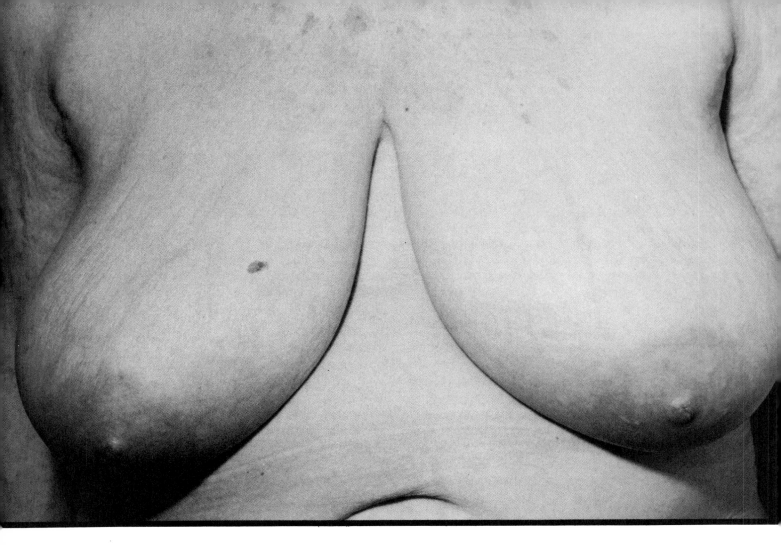

Sybil   *Age 79 • Raised on the French-German border (Alsace-Lorraine) • Journalist*

As a child, every summer I was sent to Bavaria in southern Germany to stay with Grandmother. Hers were the first adult breasts I ever saw. She had big ones and I noticed them. In fact, I inherited them! I loved to watch her take a bath. Even before I started school at five, I would admire her breasts and ask, "How do you get that?" She'd say, "You take cold showers and you rub your chest with cold water," which I did.

Unfortunately, I got much too heavy breasts, and that is my big inferiority complex as long as I live! I was ashamed of them! I hated them! I still hate them today!!! They're too big for my small body, like a cow's udders. I think they're absolutely ugly. I hate myself! I hate my breasts and I hate myself! In a way, they're the same thing.

Are you saying that you are your breasts?

Maybe? . . . Yes! There is something to it. I think my breasts affected my life a lot and that should not have happened—this stigma, this self-hate. My breasts bother me physically and mentally, in every way!

In 1899 when I was born, there was a kind of bottle used in Germany which was very similar to what we have today. Bottle-feeding was the fashion and my mother, being a very elegant, bourgeois lady, wanted to have beautiful breasts and not spoil them by giving me milk.

From what I hear now, breast-feeding is better in every respect—for your relationship with people and your physical health and development—so I regret not being breast-fed. If I would have been nourished better, maybe I would have been taller—I'm so little!—and my relationship to my mother might have been better. In fact, it was very bad.

I was an unhealthy child, and even later sickness was always a terrible part of my life. I have a history of female sickness, and somehow I think it all has to do with my not being breast-fed.

My mother had beautiful breasts. They were tiny and pretty with very nice pink nipples which stood up in the air. And I absolutely *envied* her because I had not inherited her breasts but my grandmother's!

My mother was a very erotic woman and she had a lot of lovers. I had a lot of so-called "uncles." She would have "afternoon affairs" with officers of the several armies that went through Strasbourg where I grew up. Strasbourg was a fort on the frontier and was full of French and German officers before and after the First World War. Meanwhile, my father was busy making money in the office, and when he wasn't working he played cards. He only came home for dinner. I was raised by governesses and maids. Nobody seemed to care about me very much. I was such a lost child.

My mother neglected me. I was taught absolutely *nothing* about why women had breasts or what they were for! Besides the advice my grandmother gave me about rubbing my chest with cold water, I wasn't prepared in any way. My sex education came out of the gutter.

My mother used to go to a French dressmaker and I went with her and sat in the waiting room while she had her fittings. Sitting in a glass case was a row of green leatherbound encyclopedias, *The History of Sex.* There were many pictures and they were quite pornographic actually. I learned *everything* there! As soon as Mother went inside, I would go to the case and pull out a book. I remember vividly some pictures of the French Revolution where the women spectators at the guillotine were leaning out of windows with their heavy breasts. I was fascinated! How I *loved* to go with mother to the dressmaker! (*Laughs.*)

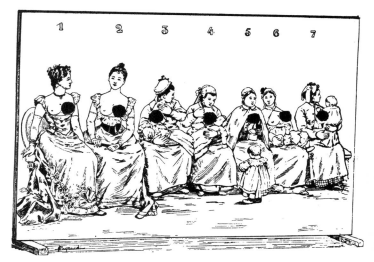

Perforated breast screen used in Paris in 1896 for the judging of women's breasts

When I reached puberty at about twelve, I had a cousin who tried little sex games with me. He told me to massage my breasts so that they'd develop and become beautiful Venus de Milo breasts. He gave me special lessons on massaging them, and of course he wanted to massage them for me!

One summer day I was taking a lonely walk through the woods and a man came from behind and just *grabbed* my breasts. That made me very conscious of them, and that I had something which made men do *that.* I got so scared! If that wasn't bad enough, soon after I had another bad experience at the dentist's.

While he was working on my teeth, the dentist put his hand inside my blouse on my breast. I became enraged! His response was, "Oh, you are acting like a little goose. You don't want to be a silly goose, do you? I'm not hurting you. Why don't you let me fondle your breast?" I shouted "No!" and I jumped out of the chair and stormed out of his office. I was thirteen, but I had already developed quite substantially.

As a girl, I wore an undergarment called a "liebchen" in German. It functioned as an undershirt, but it was more fitted, with buttons down the front and thin straps. While I was developing I continued to wear the "liebchen." I would pull it down tight, and fasten it with safety pins to my garter belt, in order to flatten and conceal my breasts. There was no reason not to conceal them. From the little experience I'd had my breasts only seemed to bring out the "beast" in men.

I began to carry myself so that my breasts couldn't be seen. As a result, I developed a round spine and I still have it to this day. Only when I got older and wiser did I try to straighten myself out. But then I always walked hunched over, and my father once said to me, "Don't go like the hunchback of Notre Dame! Go straight!" And I answered, "No, I can't! Look—then *this* sticks out!" So he said, "But that's beautiful!" And *that* I detested, that my own father would say something like that.

I only began to appreciate my breasts later on when I was a little older. I enjoyed touching my breasts for the sensation of it—experimenting with sexual feelings.

As a young lady, there was a fellow whom I saw for a while. In the beginning there was never any petting, just kissing and holding hands. Soon after, he joined the army and went to war. He sent me love letters constantly and then one day he came back on furlough and declared, "I want to marry you." Then he went and asked my father for "the hand of your daughter." I was holding my ear to the wall and listening in from the next room. And I could hear my father say, "You're ridiculous! How could you marry her? How could she live? She's only a child!" I was fifteen.

Every afternoon I said that I had to do some shopping or go buy bread or whatever, to get away from home and meet this boy at the *Konditorei*. In the front they sold bread and cake, but in the back you could sit and eat and drink, and there were red plush chairs where we had "love scenes" every day. He would get down on his knees pleading to be permitted to touch my knee . . . and then above the knee. (*Laughs.*) And though we were alone there, I would resist that. Instead I always allowed to him to put his hand inside my blouse on my breast—*that* I allowed! And that was how we carried on every afternoon.

Once after a breast-fondling session a remarkable thing happened. We were walking along the street and suddenly I couldn't go on. It became very hot between my legs and I thought I was *sick*. I suddenly had an orgasm, a delayed reaction. It was my first orgasm, and of course it was from him fondling my breasts for *hours* in the café! I couldn't bring myself to tell him—that was a lonely aftermath. (*Laughs.*) It's so vivid in my memory that still today I remember that feeling.

I was born at a time when sex was taboo and everything connected with it was never talked about . . . we were *afraid* to talk about it. I only understood what it was all about when I began reading certain books on my own initiative. When I was seventeen years old, I read Freud's *Three Theories on Sex* and other books. These books were the greatest revelation to me, but my parents thought they were dirty and tried to punish me for reading them. They even threw the books out the window. My parents were old-fashioned people who didn't understand the changing world. They didn't understand Freud and they thought I was a *whore* because I read Freud's books on sex.

During World War I, I became a very sexy person—a beauty! I was very pretty and I had beautiful breasts. In the summer in Bavaria, I wore dirndls, and I would nicely fill up the little white blouses underneath and every man looked at me. As I grew older, I went on to have many affairs.

●

Throughout my life I had very ambivalent feelings about my breasts. When I was younger, almost all the men in my life liked me *because* of my heavy breasts. But I never wanted to take my brassiere *off!* It was always a battle. I would protest, "Oh, they're too *big*, you know." And they would plead, "Oh, but that's beautiful!" "Oh, no," I'd say, "that's *not* beautiful!" "But I assure you that's just what I like." "Oh, never mind, I wish I didn't have so *much!*" And on it went, back and forth.

If I'd had the ideal Venus de Milo breasts—not the pears, but the apples (*laughs*)—I think my whole outlook on sex would have been normalized. I would have liked to be nude—I would not always have tried to cover up. My heavy breasts made me inhibited and shy and physically restrained. You see, it carried over into other parts of my life that weren't directly related to my breasts. And so I put a lot of emphasis on intellectuality and spirituality and philosophy and other interests which weren't so physical.

There's another reason why I always hated my breasts. They mark me as a woman when I don't want to be a woman. I always wanted to be a man because a man has more sexual freedom, more opportunities, can travel alone. A man could have a profession which, in my time, was impossible for a woman. He could study medicine. All my life I wanted to have the freedom that a man has, and all my life I've tried to be as free as a man. Women were condemned to get babies. Oh, I hated the thought of having babies! I never had one and I'm not sorry.

In the twenties in Berlin, I earned my living as a journalist. I went alone to the choicest bar where you could have oysters and champagne for lunch. I smoked long cigarettes in holders and drank cognac and espresso Turkish coffee. After such a lunch I went back to my editorial office. I lived the carefree life of a man, so I resented having large breasts because they were a mark *against* me. With smaller breasts my career would have been much easier.

I would come to work wearing a monocle on a black strap, and with a suit that hid my breasts. I played the twenties' version of the boyish woman—the flapper. The breastless flapper was the fashion in Germany then, just as it was in America and in Paris. I tried to follow the fashion but it made me think I had *too much* breast! It gave me an inferiority complex.

In order to follow what was chic, I had to be artificially flattened out. There were bras on the market that were especially made to flatten women . . . and you *had* to wear them or be out of fashion. I never could really breathe! I was young then, and it only came to me much later that breasts are something to be proud of. Yet, I could never *really* be proud of them—not after what I went through in my youth.

I often fantasized about surgery of some kind, but I never did anything about it because there were no such operations then. So my experience with my breasts was unhappy.

The image of the female body emphasized in nineteenth-century art was different from that of the flapper ideal when I was a young woman. In the nineteenth century, women wore corsets, had small waists, big behinds, and large, often sagging breasts. As a bohemian I disliked this art and its values. So I was heartbroken that my body was like this nineteenth-century voluptuous woman which the bourgeoisie so idealized. More than anything, I wanted to be a very modern, sleek, twentieth-century woman.

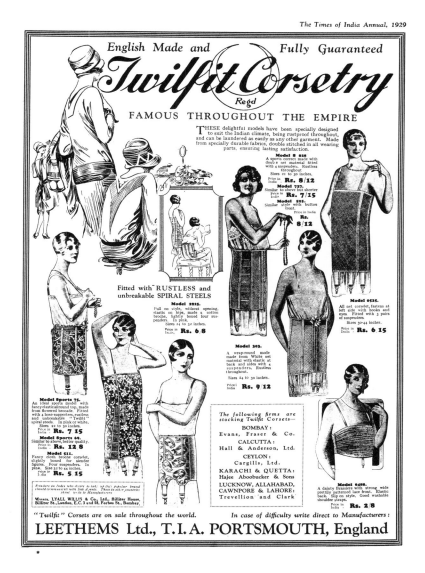

The Times of India Annual, 1929

Even though I had old-fashioned parents, I was more liberated than the American women I met when I came to the United States in the mid-thirties. We Europeans had a less puritan outlook.

After the war, big breasts came back into fashion with the returning soldiers. Away from women, they got hungry! (*Laughs.*) My friends nicknamed me "Bit Tit Sybil," and of course I felt *terrible* about it, but I was very successful. I had big tits but I was slender and, particularly for Americans, that was very good. American men are a little crazy about breasts. They like them too much!

During my young rebellious years back in Berlin, I modeled for artists when I needed extra money. They always compared me to a Maillol sculpture. I had pretty good breasts then so I must have spoiled them by binding and flattening them, because those pretty Maillol breasts got heavier and larger and finally fell down.

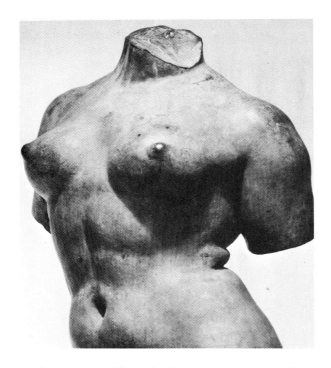

When I was fifty I had a hysterectomy which gave me a hormone imbalance and I had to get hormone injections. My breasts got even *bigger* because of that. That was also the time I went through "the change." Since then, every month I get male hormones mixed with female, and if I don't I go insane!

There were times during my menopause when I got very hot—I was oversexed because of the hormone imbalance. On hot summer days, a few times I walked out on the street wearing just a thin blouse without a brassiere to show myself. *Everybody* looked, and although they didn't approach, we experienced the erotic sensation. For them it was like voyeuristic masturbation and for me . . . well, I was walking through the street like an exhibitionist! (*Laughs.*)

Until ten years ago my breasts were still reasonably acceptable. I could finagle them by lying down and stretching with arms behind my head. So in the sex poses I could cheat a little bit on my breasts. (*Laughs.*) But now I can't. My breasts have gotten softer and raising my arms doesn't help anymore.

When I still had good breasts, I had a bra fetish. I enjoyed wearing elegant, sexy, black lace bras—not anymore. What was underneath counted then. Now, unfortunately, I don't have to undress. One good thing about my breasts is that I get very easily aroused through them. They've been that way ever since I can remember. Being bitten and sucked was always very stimulating in my sexy years, which have slowly passed away.

But I haven't abandoned my sexuality at all. Sometimes I like to stimulate my own breasts. God has given human beings a marvelous thing—masturbation. I take care of myself . . . that really *saves* me! My God, I have to exist *alone!* There's no help! It's been ten years since I've made love.

When I go to sleep at night, I lie on my side and lift my breast over my arm. Somehow this makes me feel better. I comfort myself—I cuddle myself. I have to because there's nobody else to do it! That is a terrible thing. It's a very important thing for people to be touched and held. I recently had a woman here doing massage therapy with me and when she touched me, I started to *cry.* I wasn't sad or anything—it was a completely involuntary release. This was the first time a human being had touched me since my husband died a year ago.

I went completely without tenderness or physical contact with anybody for such a long time. When my husband was alive at least there was human contact just through the presence of another. I gave him my hand—I stroked him—he stroked me—he said a kind word. The last few years he was much too sick to make love or anything, but there was always a physical nearness. Now the world has become so icy cold . . . so cruel.

Nobody looks at me anymore. I'm too old to be attractive to men. I tell you, I used to be looked at by *every* man on the street. But one day I saw a man looking in my direction, but he wasn't looking at me. When I turned around, there was a young woman behind me and then I knew my fun in life was over. That was a sad moment for me. I suddenly felt lonely.

In Europe when I was young, I always walked outside in a tide of admiration. It was a good day when I went out in the morning and some guy said in German, "Hey, *Puppe!*—hey, doll!" Now, nobody cares. I can go anonymously through the world . . . but that doesn't give me a sense of freedom. No, on the contrary, I feel old and insecure.

●

I always had trouble finding bathing suits which made me look decent. Ach! . . . I look so terrible! I look so bad that I don't go to the beach anymore. Now nobody even wears bathing suits anymore—they wear *bras* and *panties!* When you're seventy-nine you can't go around in a bikini! I've seen women my age wearing bikinis on the beach. The *nerve!* How could they? To me it's disgusting to be seen in public in such a condition. I've even seen photographs of old, wrinkled women running around in the *nude* on special beaches. Oh, I think it's terrible! Don't you have any feelings about that?

D: I think it's a good thing.

Why is it a good thing?

D: I think people should see how old people look. There's a whole mystique about the body and aging. The fact that we can't see what the different generations look like cuts off generation from generation and hides the fact that aging is a process that we will all undergo. When we see an old body, we are actually looking at ourselves in the future.

You don't see ugliness between a small breast, a middle-sized breast, heavy breasts, old breasts, hanging breasts, wrinkled breasts, leather-looking breasts? You think *all* breasts are good?

D: No, not exactly, but . . . I don't necessarily equate beauty with size or age. Of course, I've had to confront my own conditioning. But now I can see very large hanging breasts and still find them beautiful. I've seen the breasts of the hundreds of women I've interviewed and most of them are really okay. So I've come to realize that the negative feelings so many women have about their breasts are mostly in their heads, you know. That's the truth.

Maybe my breasts aren't *that* ugly. (*Laughs.*) Probably a lot of it *is* in my head! They're really not *ugly*—they're heavy, but they don't hang that much. My problem is that Venus de Milo is my ideal . . . and they hang compared to *any* Venus! (*Laughs.*) You've interviewed so many women and seen so many breasts by now. How should one be? How should one feel about one's breasts?

"Exactly the proportions of Venus"

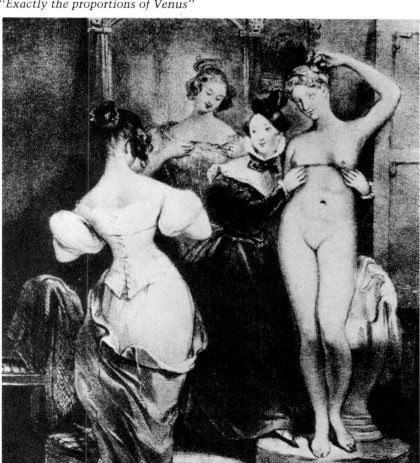

Diana

"Very old," age undetermined • Native American • Mother of two; great-grandmother

I was born long before Native Americans registered births, long before. So I've lost track of how old I am. When it came time to register births, I had to get someone to sign that they knew when I was born to satisfy the government, but no one really knew. So I have been here a long time!

As a child I studied to be a priestess. I spent a great deal of my preparation studying in the mental fields, the spiritual fields, the energy fields, and in the chemical fields of the earth. I was always made conscious of the fact that I was "Woman," the future of the race, the forward march of the race, and the "Woman" who was to carry the light. So that was the way my education came.

I love getting older. I didn't believe in menopause as the modern world thinks of it. I believe in the body takin' its natural state. Now, of course, I no longer menstruate, but I never had the distressing symptoms like nervousness. I didn't have time for them. I never had hot flashes. Nothing happened to my breasts—they didn't get bigger or smaller. I never had any of those things. I think most all of that is culturally learned, I really do, and is a result of poor living.

A lot of things can be psychologically induced. Don't forget that I started studying at a very early age and much of my first studies were about learning to handle the chemical worlds, which include your body, too. We are taught that the mind can produce any condition in the body that can be produced with any alien drugs. So training our minds to produce a beneficial condition in the body is a serious thing with us. For we believe that all people are potential masters, gods and goddesses, if they stay on the "path."

I was born under the star and constellation of "The Priestess," or perhaps Diana in your culture. I was only six months old when my mother passed over, and since we lean with the ancient ways of the world, I was wet-nursed. Then when whooping cough broke out and I took to it, I was put on mare's milk.

I grew up physically active. I worked on the farm, I loved the forests, I rambled, I climbed hills and trees. I was like a Lady Tarzan! I did a lot of deep breathing exercises as part of my physical culture, because we know that we must train the body and the brain in order to develop our mind.

I was raised right on the frontier and in the forest where I could watch all the animals reproduce and feed their little ones, so childbirth and breast-feeding were never any mystery to me. I can't remember asking the questions children ask today because I knew the answers beforehand. I saw it all around me from the time I could crawl.

Among the native people, women don't hide their breasts when they are feeding a baby. Part of the pleasure of childhood is to watch mothers feed their babies. I have noticed that a lot of little girls, if they have lived with nature, will put their dolls to their breasts, trying to get to the mother in them.

When my breasts first began to appear, I knew what was happening—I knew I was growing up. When you're young you think you are *never* going to grow up. You look forward to it and you wait and wait and wait. So when the signs begin to appear, you think, "Wow! Here I am. I have arrived!"

If you haven't lived with nature, getting breasts

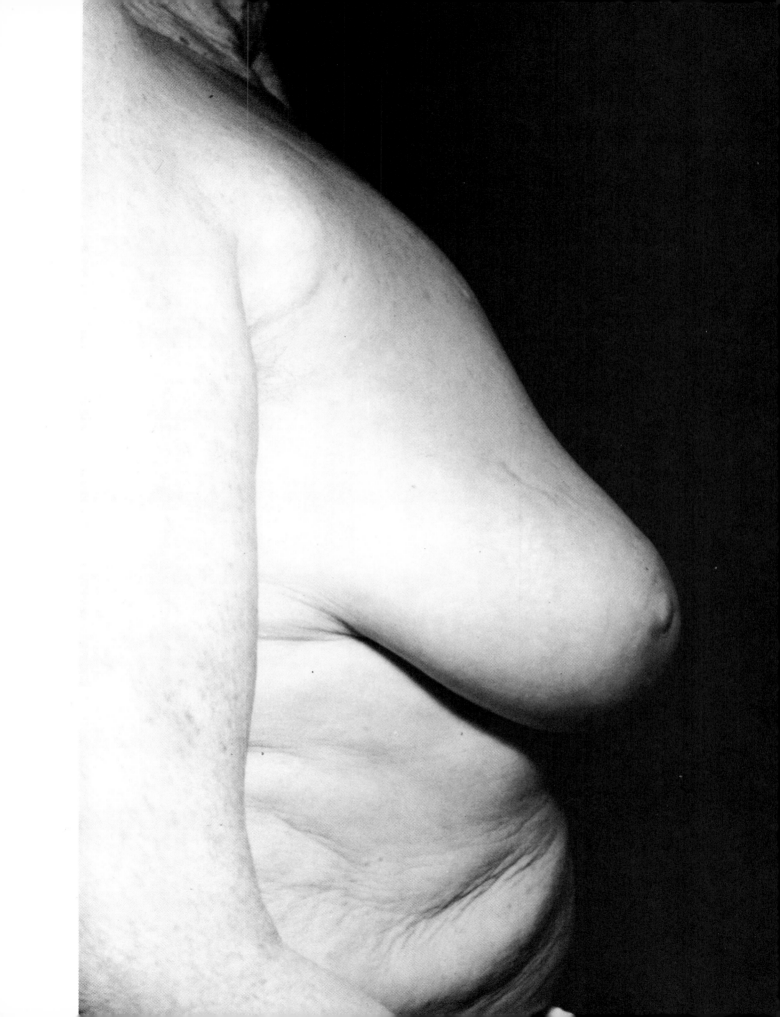

can be traumatic. At first your breasts are sore, and you begin to wonder why. You spend a lot of time thinking about and looking at your breasts. And then pretty soon you start having the feelings in the rest of your body, and so on. But, if you're raised with nature, you more or less know what's happening. Puberty is not anything we were taught; we knew it was just the "Woman" in us awakening.

With us, puberty wasn't hidden the way it is today. We shared it with *all* the people. We have a puberty ritual and it doesn't particularly have anything to do with the breast. That isn't necessary because when we think of "Woman," it involves all of her.

At the first sign of puberty, the first menstruation, that is the ritual day. The ritual is even more important than weddings are in the Western world. Everyone gathers to celebrate all night with their campfires and their food. Then at sunrise the next morning, the whole Nation gathers together to watch her race into the light of a new day and to glory in the fact that she is now "Woman."

●

Children were born in the home when I grew up, so I saw birth long before I was old enough to think about getting pregnant myself. It was all an old story to me. I didn't pay much attention to my body while I was pregnant.

Some women, you know, they are so careful. They stay in the house and cry, "Woe is me—I am pregnant." I didn't make any changes in the way I lived. I was very active during my pregnancies. I have always been an outdoor person and pregnancy was nothing for me. The day before my son was born I climbed the mountains in Michigan in the snow, and I was surprised the next morning when I woke up with "action." I gave birth in three hours!

My first time breast-feeding was amazing. There was this little mouth taking hold and, of course, they are *very* eager. The baby's lips are warm and they're working at the nipple, their hands are manipulating your breast, and then the rest of your body responds. Suddenly you realize that you are feeding the body of another person from your own body. You've known of this— you've seen it and heard it over and over and over again—but you never know it so much as when it's *your* breast and *your* baby.

Among the Native Americans, there is a belief in nonverbal communication. The colleges think it is new, but it's thousands of years old. We practice preconception and prenatal influence, which means we are consciously, directly, and knowingly creating our future race. Long before we conceive, we set our body and our mind and all of our energies to prepare ourselves accordingly. There is no guesswork in our furthering of the race in its forward march, so it is real important that we bring forth someone who is stronger, wiser, and greater than we are.

When a mother is nursing her young, she can transmit *anything* that she wants—it's up to her. She can make her child a "superchild" or she can

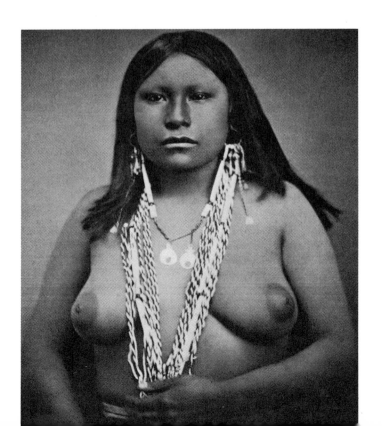

make it a failure. And I don't mean just by failing to love it. I mean that if she doesn't nurse it, that child will not love *itself!* If you do not feed your child in your arms, surrounded with your aura and your love and the energy and the good from your body, then that child will feel unwanted, unworthy, and unloved—a nothingness! That is what is the matter with a lot of the world today!

Native Americans believe that we should each love ourself above anything else in the world. Each one of us is the most perfect one, the most beautiful one, the most desirable one, the brightest light in our world. It's something we are very strong on because we believe that only if we learn to love ourselves, can we begin to love anybody or anything else.

When we sit together in our circle, using energy and building energy and talking energy, the babies must sit in the circle, too. Most of the time they are nursing at the breast so they pick up whatever we are doing or talking about. We are very conscious of the fact that we not only feed our babies with our milk and with our body, but that we feed them also with all our other energies while we are breast-feeding.

To us, with our training in the chemical body, the breast is a part of the gland system and it produces, if we allow it to, on and on and on. In what Western people would consider my menopause there were times when I had milk in my breasts. I have known that to happen to other women, too.

It is even known that there is a tribe on some other continent where by taking an herb the men can make milk flow and feed the babies! There are many miraculous herbs in the earth. So you see, it isn't all that mysterious.

Among us, breast milk has many uses. Each morning in preparation for the baby's daily bath, its eyes are washed out with mother's milk. Milk not only cleanses, but it also has chemicals that feed the tissue of the baby's eyes. And breast milk has been used to save many adult lives. I have known a few times in the past when someone was so low or sick that they could not be fed or there was no other food and they were kept alive with breast milk.

●

The world thinks that among the Native American people, women are looked down on, but they are not. Women are very important in the tribes, especially old wise women—great-grandmothers.

Among the Native Americans, when I say "Woman," I don't mean that she is a woman. English just doesn't express it. I mean she is "Woman," that brings forth the races. She feeds the races with her breast, and with the energy that is She. We have no word for babies—there is no such thing as a "baby" lying at her breast. She feeds the "little man" or "little woman" of the races.

We see a lot of failure in everyday life, and I have to admit that this applies to a lot of Native American women, too. Many have even *stopped* breast-feeding—not because they want to, but because of many pressures on them which have created much fear in their minds. Don't forget, fear in the mind does more damage than anything else. Women in the Western world have been taught fear of many things, especially for their beauty.

Many women believe that their breasts can no longer be beautiful if they breast-feed their babies. I'm no authority, but if women have breast marks, it tells me that they aren't eating and living right. You don't have to have stretch marks and veins—they are unnatural. *My* breasts don't have 'em!

Lack of knowledge of our own bodies, now that is *really* a tragedy! You don't have to go to gyms to stretch and make a muscle woman of yourself. When you're breast-feeding your baby, you also put all the rest of your body into perfect condition again. If you live your life right, you will have the muscles you need and the brain you need and the years you need to do the work that you have to do.

Nature is the most perfect teacher you can have. If you go along with it you can't fail. I really think that the way we have lived in the last generation or two is why a lot of women develop so many of their health problems. It's simply because women don't allow their bodies to have the natural rhythms they need to reproduce, to be happy in the reproduction, and to feel fulfilled in what they are doing.

Regardless of how you try to get away from it, the body responds to the old Laws. There is a saying among the ancient peoples that if you don't go along with the Law, the Law will not go along with you, speaking of the Divine Law of Nature. And if you don't live by that Law, you will lose by that Law.

When women return to the old ideas, when they brainwash this system of sickness and fear out of their bodies and minds, they will come back to being natural, healthy women. It's going to be a long road back.

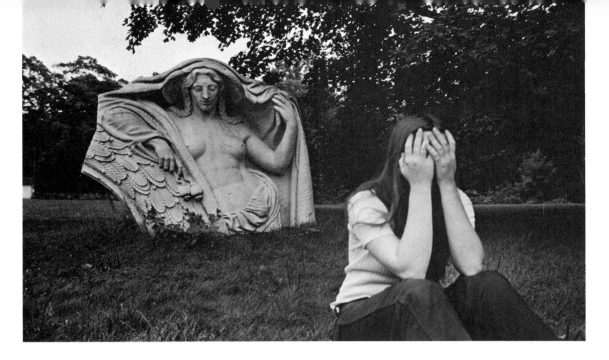

How would you describe your breasts?

Well, my goodness . . . *(undoes blouse and looks at her breasts)* . . . natural, I guess!

Most women today are ashamed and have a tendency to droop their shoulders as if they were trying to hide something, instead of standing straight and proud like "Woman." For ages, hiding the body has been called the "fig leaf" position in the Western world. So I notice that women do the "fig leaf" position up here, too. *(Indicates her breasts.)* They do this *(slouches and crosses arms over breasts)*, instead of doing this *(sits erect)*.

"Woman" is *never* ashamed of her body! There may be places that she won't expose her body because of something around her—some idea, some convention, some disagreeable male approach. But if she has her way, "Woman" won't hide her body very much. You see, if the mind affects the body, then the body affects the mind. So if women hide too much, too often, they become ashamed. And "Woman," as I said, is *never* ashamed of her body!

I recently had a friend who is a medicine man ask me, "Do you know a beach around here where we could go bathing? My woman likes to bathe in the nude, but the beaches along here are so crowded and such a problem with the way people interfere, that I'd like to find a private beach somewhere."

Before the invasion of the people from Europe, our women didn't wear all those clothes and neither did men. But they yielded to a lot of the cultural polish, which they are finding today has only depleted and weakened their bodies and minds. Now they are slowly on the road back.

It seems to me that the modern Western man is very preoccupied with women's breasts. I think it's because they didn't get it when they were babies, or maybe because they were never allowed to fondle women's breasts when they were children. It is nothing for a Native American who is nursing her baby to have a child two or three or four years old walk up and pat the breast and feel it while the little one is nursing. How many men in the Western world could do that as children? So when they get older, you know, they hunt themselves a breast to play with! *(Laughs.)*

When I see these magazines with pictures of

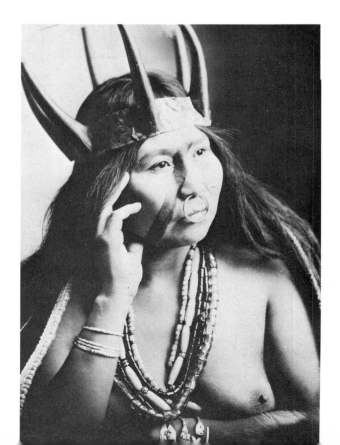

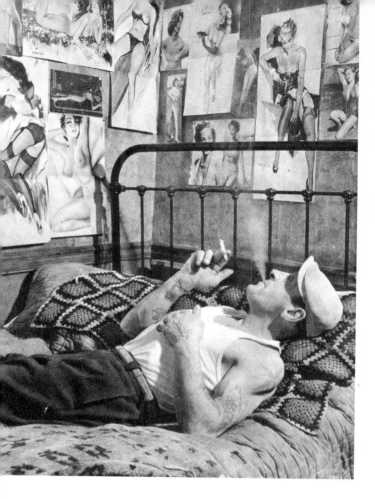

stimulates the buried energy that is "Woman." Women are just now beginning to realize who they are—what "Woman" really is—She who brings forth the races.

I'm happy to see women going back to the natural way. They are trying to move forward into the future by turning the pages back in time, and that's the strange way it works. A lot of them are refusing to have their babies in hospitals and wouldn't even *think* of artificially feeding a baby. They say they are on a "nature trip." Among the ancient peoples, returning to the Divine Law of Nature was prophesied long ago—it was called the "Return to the Circle."

Diana of Ephesus, Rome, 2nd century A.D.

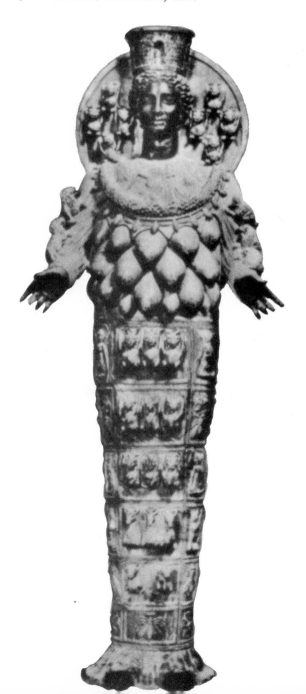

naked women, it is not the women I think about. I'm not at all prudish myself, but I think that the magazines must cater to little boys who have to prove themselves. See, if men need to look at this type of thing it shows me where they are going today, and that's why the women are getting as strong as they are. The men are getting weaker because they are willing to live their lives in their bedrooms and dens with *paper* women! It's a good sign for women and a very sad sign for men.

●

My breasts have meant a great deal in teaching me to be "Woman." Their sensitivity tells me I am "Woman," because women are *sensitive* beings. So breasts are a constant reminder that you are "Woman." And when the breasts remain well-developed through later life as they should, and are not hanging and flabby and full of scar tissue, then there is still that sensitivity in them, and in you to them. As old as I am my breasts are still a constant reminder that I am "Woman."

There is a magic evolving and revolving in *all* women, and knowledge of this has gradually been forgotten over the past few thousand years. Now the time has come when "Woman" becomes more and more conscious of herself, and that

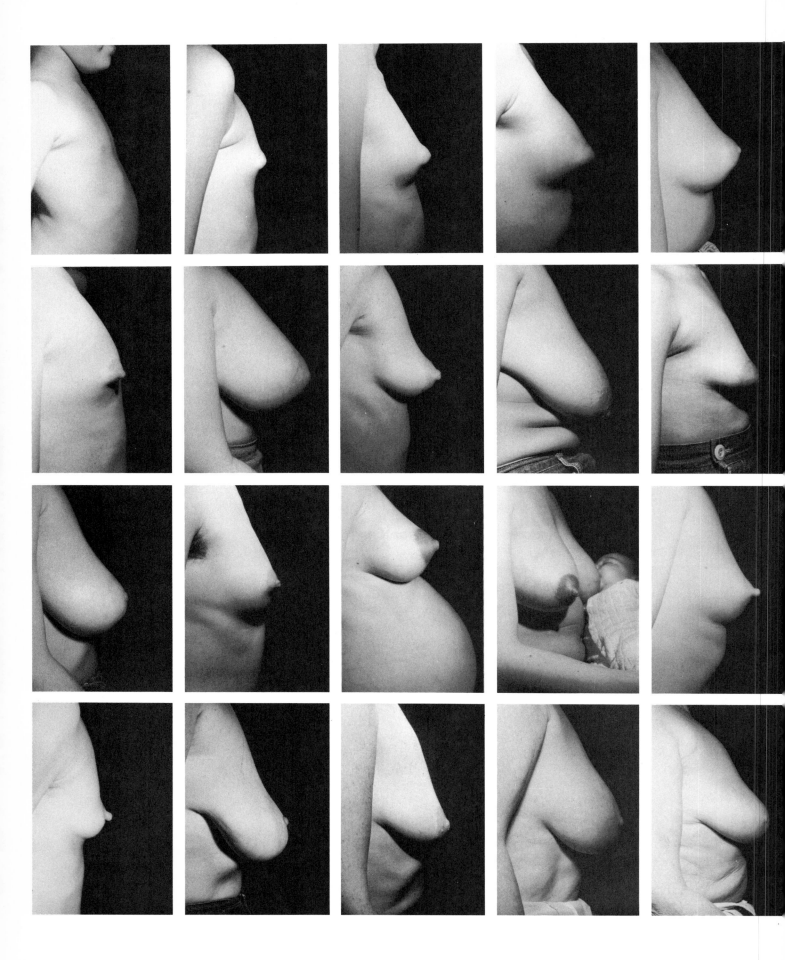

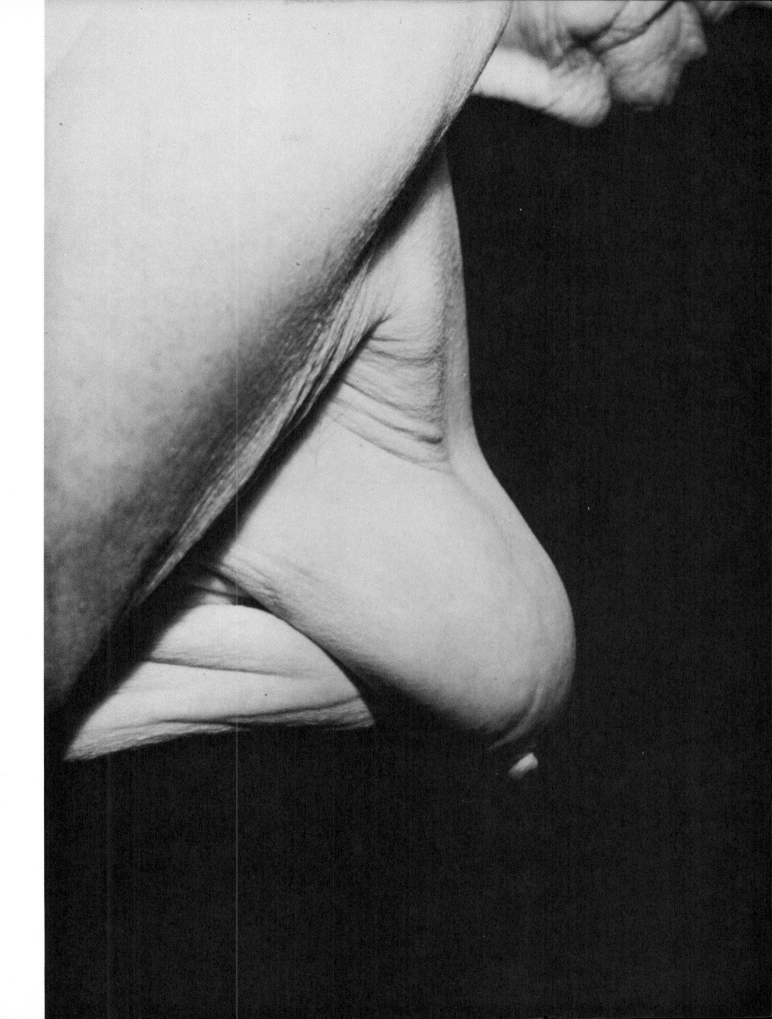

Epilogue

Looking back over the unfolding of the book, we marvel that it was all contained, as within a seed, in our original idea for a photographic catalog. But, it is because women believed in the seed and gave it life that it finally blossomed into the book you have just read.

The women who revealed themselves in the book have opened the doors to a serious dialogue on the issues that surround women's experience with their breasts. Their collective voices have initiated and legitimized an area of consciousness raising that we hope will benefit all women. Though the book's publication marks the end of one phase, it is really the beginning of a larger ongoing process.

●

Time and time again, after being interviewed, women expressed very positive feelings about the provocative experience they had just been through. These reactions demonstrated to us that the questionnaire used to guide their interviews, which they helped to create, was indeed a resource for women's greater self-awareness and understanding.

 • *I'm really intrigued by the questionnaire. It brought up things from the past that I've left behind. It has rekindled my memory and I have a lot to think about now.*

 • *It brought me face to face with something I've dealt with all my life and helped me come to a new understanding of myself. There's always room to learn more about yourself. Who knows herself inside and out? Who covers every angle in her self-analysis?*

 • *While I was talking, I heard myself saying so many negative things about my breasts that I resolved to try not to hate them anymore. And you know, somehow I do feel less negative about them. . . . So the interview has been cathartic and therapeutic for me.*

 • *I never had a conversation like this with anyone and I haven't ever thought about my breasts in a systematic and detailed chronological way before. I feel as though I've gotten to know how I* really *feel about my breasts.*

 • *Watching my reactions to some of the questions has really raised my consciousness. It's made me think about a lot of things besides my breasts, so I actually discovered some things about myself that I didn't know before! I think every woman should go through this.*

These overwhelmingly positive reactions prompted us to make the questionnaire available to all women by including it in the book.

. . . People don't learn very much when they are just passive recipients of information. . . . The information [does] not become our own until we [begin] to pull [it] up from inside ourselves and share what we [have] never before expressed. . . .

—Our Bodies, Ourselves

Though reading about other women is a learning experience and stimulates one's own memories and feelings, even greater self-awareness can be gained by answering the questionnaire yourself. Perhaps you will discover patterns in your own development that influence you today, and even gain new personal insights that extend beyond your feelings about your breasts.

●

We've learned that the process of consciousness raising has two phases. The first involves sharing and learning from each other's personal experiences, thus breaking down the barriers of myth and stereotype. The second involves studying and analyzing what has been learned — its historical background and contemporary implications.

Beyond the many facets of a woman's experience of having breasts, it is obvious from the sampling presented in the book that all too many women have been oppressed by our cultural attitudes toward breasts, and are often damaged psychologically and even physically. Because of this unhealthy circumstance, clearly there is a need to study the subject in greater depth and provide some analysis which can help women by furthering the consciousness-raising process which this book hopefully has begun.

We are already formulating ideas about the many issues surrounding women's breasts, but we recognize that no valid analysis can be made from the relatively small sampling of women who were interviewed to date. Therefore, we invite you to share with us your own experiences with your breasts. Your responses, whether to all of the questions or only to those that relate to you, are most welcome. Every woman's story is valid, whether it duplicates one which appears in the book or not, for it is crucial to determine how common or uncommon particular experiences are.

Contributions of personal testimony from as many women as possible will create an information bank from which a truer picture can be gained and a more comprehensive analysis can be made.

_____

. . . Body education is core education. Our bodies are the physical bases from which we move out into the world; ignorance, uncertainty — even, at worst, shame — about our physical selves create in us an alienation from ourselves that keeps us from being the whole people that we could be.

— *Our Bodies, Ourselves*

_____

●

In addition to the questionnaire which is provided in this book, we have also formulated three seperate questionnaires to explore further the areas of: (1) *puberty and adolescence;* (2) *breast cancer and mastectomy;* (3) *men's feelings about women's breasts.* These are available upon request.

(1) We are currently preparing a book, intended specifically for girls going through puberty and adolescence, which will present a spectrum of breast-related experiences to help demystify what is frequently an anxiety-filled stage of life.

Girls' written responses to the questionnaire will be an important contribution. We urge readers of this book to obtain the questionnaire and make it available to their daughters, sisters, and friends. We also invite school nurses, sex-education teachers, and other educators to have their female students respond anonymously to the questionnaire (perhaps as a class exercise) and subsequently make the responses available to us.

(2) There is a staggering incidence of breast cancer in this country and most women live in dread of the physical, psychological, and social consequences of losing a breast. Beyond this, too many women who have had mastectomies share Helen's trauma of self-revulsion and isolation (page 212).

Though several celebrities have courageously made public their experiences with breast cancer, their individual accounts do not represent the diversity of circumstances — age, marital status, ethnic background, economic class — women find themselves in, or the multiplicity of ways they've dealt with breast cancer.

If you have had breast cancer, whether or not you've had a mastectomy, sharing what you've been through will be very helpful to all women by continuing to get this experience "out of the closet."

(3) Often a woman's experience of her breasts is directly influenced by her experience with men and by men's attitudes and feelings about women's breasts. A detailed exploration of how men feel is essential to the comprehensive analysis we plan. Men of all ages and backgrounds are invited to contribute to the information bank by sending us their written responses to the men's questionnaire.

●

On several occasions women who had been interviewed corresponded with us. One wrote, "I told my family about your book when I was home for Christmas and I wish I'd had a tape recorder to pick up the conversation that resulted. The whole day turned into a boob consciousness-raising happening that we couldn't shake!"

In addition to the wonderful letters of encouragement, we also received magazine and newspaper clippings on a variety of related subjects (bras, plastic surgery on breasts, topless beaches, the prevention and treatment of breast cancer, breast-feeding, and others); examples of exploitive advertising (such as the claim that certain chickens are best because they have the biggest breasts); jokes or comments about breasts heard on TV or in films; and snapshots of women with their breasts exposed in a variety of situations. One woman even went so far as to lift up her shirt in a twenty-five-cent photo booth and send us the results!

We affectionately refer to this self-initiated clipping service as a "breast watch"! We welcome your contribution to it. Pictures of your own breasts with or without your faces showing, of the breasts of aging women and pubescent or adolescent girls (these have been the most difficult to obtain), and of public breast exposure (breast-feeding, beaches, etc.) will be a welcome addition to our ongoing photographic collection.

All correspondence and requests for the above questionnaires should be sent to:
Daphna Ayalah & Isaac J. Weinstock
P.O. Box 1635
Grand Central Station
New York, N.Y. 10017

(For the interest of photographers, the information on the breast pictures in the book is: camera: 35 mm with 55 mm f/1.8 lens; exposure: 1/15 second at f 8-11 (with tripod); film: Kodachrome II, Type A (reset at 32 ASA); lighting: 500-watt 3400 K Photolamp; camera distance from subject: 2 ½–3 feet.)

INTERVIEW QUESTIONNAIRE

Childhood

1. Were you breast-fed? If so, what do you know about it?
2. How and when did you first become aware that women have breasts?
3. How did your mother relate to her breasts? Did she let you see or touch them? How did you feel about her breasts?
4. Why did you think women had breasts (for nursing, sex, other)?
5. Were you taught anything about breasts? What? From whom?
6. Did you ever go around without a shirt on? When did you stop? Why? How did you feel about it?

Puberty / Adolescence

7. Were you prepared for the development of your breasts in any way (by mother / sister / friend / school nurse, etc.)? What were you told? What was your reaction?
8. When and how did you first become aware that your breasts were developing?
9. How did you feel emotionally about your developing breasts?
10. Did they affect you physically (your movement, posture, sense of space, etc.)? Explain.
11. Did you look at or touch your breasts much? Explain.
12. Were you curious about your friends' breasts or adult women's breasts? What did you do about it?
13. Did you share the experience of developing breasts with anyone? Describe.
14. What was your experience with bras (first bra, dating, etc.)?
15. Did your breasts grow suddenly or gradually? Describe.
16. Did you have any hopes or expectations of how your breasts would turn out (shape, size, etc.)? Describe. Were you pleased with the way they were developing?
17. Did you do anything to change or "improve" them (creams, exercises, binding, etc.)? Describe.
18. Did your breasts attract attention? From whom? Describe. How did you feel about it?
19. Did developing breasts affect your relationship with boys / girls? With parents, teachers, others? How?
20. Did your breasts affect your self-image and/or social status? How?
21. Describe your first sexual experience(s) with your breasts. How did you feel physically and emotionally?
22. What part did your breasts play in your adolescent sexual experiences?
23. Did your breasts play a role in the formation of your adult personality? How?

Present Feelings

24. Do your breasts have a "personality" or "character" different from the rest of your body? Explain.
25. How do you feel about your breasts right now? How do the women you know feel about their breasts?
26. Have you ever considered or done anything to change your breasts (e.g., exercises, surgery, hypnosis, etc.)? Describe.
27. Is there an "ideal" breast? If so, describe.
28. How would you describe your breasts (shape, bra size, etc.)?
29. Are your breasts uneven in size or shape? If so, how do you feel about it?
30. Do you have supernumerary or inverted nipples, or hair on your breasts? If so, how do you feel about it? Have you ever done anything to change it? Describe.
31. How have men or lovers reacted to your breasts?

Sex

32. Are your breasts sexually arousing? Describe. If so, when did you first become aware of it?
33. Are your breasts important during sex? Explain. If not, how do you feel about it? How do lovers feel about it?
34. What do or don't you like done to your breasts during sex?
35. Do you pay attention to your breasts while masturbating? Describe.
36. If you have made love to another woman, how did you relate to her breasts? Did it affect the way you feel about your own breasts? Explain.

Men

37. How have men related to your breasts during sex? How do you think men feel about women's breasts? Why? Is it cultural or biological? Do men's feelings affect women? How?
38. How do you feel about the way women's bodies, particularly breasts, are portrayed in men's magazines (*Playboy, Penthouse,* etc.)?
39. What effect, if any, do these magazine images have on women / men? Have you been affected? How? Have women or men you know? Explain.
40. Do you enjoy looking at other women's breasts (in the street, in magazines, at the gym, or elsewhere? Are you ever aroused?) Explain.
41. Are you ever complimented or harassed in public by men because of your breasts? What do they say? How does it make you feel? How do you react? Why do you think it happens?

Bras / Bralessness

42. What kind of bras have you worn in the past? How did they make you feel psychologically? Which style was your most / least favorite? Why (comfort, appearance, etc.)?
43. Do you wear different bras for different purposes (athletics, sexual allure, etc.)? Explain.
44. Have you ever had a memorable or unusual experience with a bra? Explain.
45. Do you wear a bra now? If so, why (support, fashion, etc.)? How do you feel about other women going braless?
46. How do you feel when your breasts are unsupported? Have you ever considered not wearing a bra? Explain.
47. If you do not wear a bra, did you ever? Why did you stop? Did you have to get used to going braless? In what ways?
48. Do you feel different physically or psychologically with and without a bra? Explain.
49. How have other men and women reacted to your going braless?
50. Do you think that wearing or not wearing a bra has affected your breasts? How?

Clothing

51. In relation to your breasts, what type of clothing and bathing suits do you most / least prefer? Why?
52. Do you like clothing that draws attention to your breasts (low-cut, tight, see-through, etc.)? Or clothing that hides your breasts? Why?
53. In what situations have you worn breast-revealing clothing (public or private)? Describe. How does it make you feel? What reactions do you get from your partner? Other men? Women?
54. When you are in situations where other women wear clothing which reveals their breasts, how do you feel about it?

Breast Exposure

55. Are your breasts ever exposed in casual situations among friends (changing clothes, etc)? How do you feel? How do they react? How do you feel when friends expose their breasts in front of you?
56. Do you feel different exposing your breasts in the presence of a man than of a woman in a nonsexual situation? Explain. How do you feel about exposing your breasts in a sexual situation? How is it different?
57. Have you ever exposed your breasts in a public situation (swimming, sunning, etc.)? Why? What kinds of reactions did you get? How do you feel when you see women whose breasts are exposed in public situations (breast-feeding, bathing, etc.)?
58. How do you feel about the fact that women cannot generally go bare-breasted in public as men can (in parks on hot summer days, on beaches, etc)? Should women be able to? Would you like to? Is it discriminatory that women can't? Explain.
59. Why do you think public breast exposure is usually considered "indecent," illegal, and a sexual offense? How do you think the taboo on breast exposure originated?
60. If it becomes acceptable and women begin to go bare-breasted as men do, how would you feel about it? Would you? Why or why not?

Pregnancy / Breast-feeding

61. How did your breasts change during pregnancy? How did you feel about the changes?
62. Did you breast-feed or bottle-feed? Why? Will you breast-feed if you have children? Why?
63. How did you anticipate breast-feeding? What had you heard?
64. While pregnant, did you do anything to "prepare" your breasts for breast-feeding? Explain.
65. *If you did not breast-feed:* How did you prevent your breasts from producing milk after you gave birth? Did your breasts change physically from the way they were before pregnancy? If so, how do you feel about the changes? Did you feel differently about your breasts in any way after giving birth? If so, explain.
66. How did you feel the first time you breast-fed? How did it feel when the milk came in, and later when breast-feeding became routine?
67. Did you have any complications or problems while breast-feeding? Explain.
68. How did the hospital staff react to your breast-feeding?
69. Was breast-feeding ever a sensual or sexual experience? Describe.
70. How did you feel about your breasts while you were nursing?
71. What did you think about while breast-feeding?
72. Was breast-feeding ever a "spiritual" or unusual experience? Describe. Did you develop any special practice (breathing, meditation, etc.) while breast-feeding? Explain.
73. Did you ever nurse among friends or relatives or in public? How did you feel at first and then later on? How did other people react?
74. How did your husband react to your breast-feeding? Did your breast-feeding and the change in your breasts (size, milk) affect the way he related sexually to your breasts? Explain.
75. While nursing, was the sexual sensitivity of your breasts affected in any way? How? Did you relate differently to your breasts during sex then? Explain.
76. How long did you breast-feed your child? What made you decide to wean when you did? Describe the weaning process.
77. How did you feel about your breasts after you stopped nursing?
78. Did your breasts change physically from the way they were before you became pregnant? Describe. How did you feel about the changes? How did your husband or lover feel about the changes?
79. Did your experience of breast-feeding affect you (self-image, view of life, etc.) in any way? Explain.

Health

80. Do your breasts change during your monthly cycle? Describe. If so, do the changes affect you psychologically? How?
81. Do you examine your breasts? How often? How do you feel about male or female doctors examining your breasts?
82. Have you ever had any health problems with your breasts? Explain.
83. Do you know any women who have had a mastectomy? How has it affected them? How did it affect you? Have you ever seen their mastectomy? If so, how did you react?
84. In the event of breast cancer, if you were advised to have a mastectomy, would you? Why or why not? If not, what would you do? What would it mean to you to lose a breast?

Aging

85. Have you ever seen the breasts of old women? How did they appear to you? How did you react?
86. Have your breasts changed with age? Describe. How do you feel about it? Have you ever considered doing anything about it (lifts, etc.)? What?
87. Has the sexual sensitivity of your breasts changed with aging? Describe. If so, how do you feel about it?
88. Has the aging of your breasts affected the way your sexual partner(s) relates to them? Describe. If so, how does it make you feel?
89. Has the aging of your breasts affected your self-image in any way? Explain.
90. Were your breasts affected by menopause? How?

Miscellaneous

91. What word(s) do you use to refer to breasts? How do you feel about other words that are used? Have you ever named your breasts? Explain.
92. Are breasts a vulnerable part of the body? If so, explain.
93. Do your breasts or breasts in general have symbolic meaning for you? Explain.
94. Have your breasts taught you anything? Explain.
95. What have you taught / will you teach your children about breasts (by way of example, verbally)?

For those sending in their responses to the questionnaire, information on the following will be helpful: age, "marital status" (single, married, etc.), education, occupation, religion, where raised, number of children, brief description of life-style. ANONYMITY GUARANTEED

Illustration Credits

286